Ophthalmic Dispensing

By

RUSSELL L. STIMSON
Newport Beach, California

(Third Edition)

Springfield · Illinois

Charles C Thomas · Publisher

Published and Distributed Throughout the World by
CHARLES C THOMAS • PUBLISHER
Bannerstone House
301-327 East Lawrence Avenue, Springfield, Illinois, U.S.A.

© *1971, 1979 by* CHARLES C THOMAS • PUBLISHER
ISBN 0-398-03823-6
Library of Congress Catalog Card Number: 78-17194

First Edition, 1951, by C. V. Mosby Co.
Second Edition, 1971
Second Edition, Second Printing, 1974
Second Edition, Third Printing, 1976
Second Edition, Fourth Printing, 1978
Third Edition, 1979

With THOMAS BOOKS *careful attention is given to all details of
manufacturing and design. It is the Publisher's desire to present
books that are satisfactory as to their physical qualities and artistic
possibilities and appropriate for their particular use.* THOMAS
BOOKS *will be true to those laws of quality that assure a good
name and good will.*

Printed in the United States of America
N-1

Library of Congress Cataloging in Publication Data

Stimson, Russell L.
    Ophthalmic dispensing.

    Includes bibliographical references and index.
    1. Opticianry. I. Title. [DNLM: 1. Eyeglasses. 2. Optics.
WW350 S8590]
RE962.S74   1978   617.7'5   78-17194
ISBN 0-398-03823-6

To my
wife.

PREFACE TO THE THIRD EDITION

It is flattering to have been invited by the publishers to write a third edition of this book, first published in 1951. Consistent with my original intentions, I have added material which I hope will make it possible for the reader to grasp a view of the scientific background of ophthalmic dispensing to the point that my many references can be profitably and enjoyably studied. Since a high percentage of dispensers develop from apprenticeship, my effort has also been to provide amplification of the preceptor's effort.

Again I have been most fortunate to have the assistance and counsel of a devoted secretary to put my thoughts on paper. I shall be everlastingly grateful for the help of Mrs. Dawn Daughtry.

RUSSELL L. STIMSON

Newport Beach, California, 1978

PREFACE TO THE SECOND EDITION

My first thoughts are those of gratitude to the professions and trade for the generous acceptance of the first edition of this book. In no book of this general type can it be said that the author is not also to a great degree an editor. In the twenty years since the first edition, all of the contributors whom I mentioned, except Dr. Paul Boeder, are deceased.

Clarence H. Albaugh, M.D., has been of great assistance in translating foreign literature and Warren A. Wilson, M.D., has been more than liberal with his time in counseling.

I am most grateful to again have found a coterie of helpers in opticianry who have made significant contributions to this second effort: James J. Farino, Erie County Technical Institute; Ernest J. Bahnsen, Ferris State College; John E. Archer, Los Angeles City College; Joseph L. Bacotti, New York Community College; and Charles E. Walsh, Worcester Industrial Institute.

Most fortunately, Mrs. Anna Koeppel, who organized and typed the first edition, was available and willing to again accept the wearisome task of changing a handwritten manuscript into something acceptable by a publisher. My sincerest thanks, Ann!

RUSSELL L. STIMSON

Los Angeles, California

PREFACE TO THE FIRST EDITION

The selection and adjustment of the proper lenses and frames for a prospective wearer of spectacles has become a matter of interest that is not confined to the artisans who prepare them. Therefore this book for practicing opticians is not intended for their use exclusively. To the end that it might be more interesting and instructive to students in courses in ophthalmic optics in the technical schools, optometry schools, or graduate courses in ophthalmology, the introductory chapters have been somewhat amplified. It is hoped that by its arrangement it may be helpful to nurses and technical assistants in refractionists' offices. Remarkable advances in the science of refraction and lens technology in the past decade demand more than a superficial knowledge of opticianry to apply lenses and frames to new problems and new needs. Although ophthalmic lenses are first discussed as a separate physical entity, throughout the remainder of the book they are considered as a component of an optical system in which the ametropic eyes and the patient himself are parts. Hitherto the literature does not seem to contain a unified treatment of lens and frame fitting. It is my hope that it is accomplished in this publication.

So far as is possible the subject has been treated in simple language. A glossary is appended for the assistance of those to whom the material is new. Numerous illustrations are spread throughout the text in which an effort has been made to simply portray the subject matter. References to the literature placed at the bottom of the page on which the subject is discussed are for the use of those who wish to pursue specialized phases more intensively.

During the preparation of this book I have had the unsparing assistance from a number of individuals. Those whom I wish especially to mention are Mr. Ralph Barstow, who originally urged me to set down my notions on paper; Dr. Charles Sheard of the Mayo Clinic, for counsel on the arrangement of the subject matter; Dr. William A. Boyce, for his advice on the chapter on cataract lens fitting; Dr. Alfred R. Robbins, for his suggestions on the chapter on lens evaluation; and particularly Dr. Paul Boeder and Mr. Henry B. Carpenter, for their many suggestions and criticisms in the margins of the unfinished manuscript.

RUSSELL L. STIMSON

Los Angeles, California

INTRODUCTION

As steadily as the importance and the value of ophthalmic services have been increasingly recognized, so too, has it been apparent that ophthalmic dispensing will take on a deeper significance.

Rather slow progress was made in the development of improved technique in the ophthalmic dispensing field until the present century was well advanced. It was then appreciated that only by the establishment of educational standards and more advanced processes in training would dispensing keep abreast of the progress of other branches of eye care in its contribution to human welfare.

Independently, in a number of states in this country and in England, schools of higher education were established to afford the student adequate knowledge in scientific and technical subjects applicable to this field and a thorough training in practical procedures.

The dearth of proper textbooks for private and classroom instruction has been a handicap.

The material in this book is a contribution toward visual perfection in that it affords an essential background to those who would render an adequate service in ophthalmic dispensing. Regardless of the knowledge and skill employed in the refraction, the patient can only receive the desired results when the laboratory instructions are accorded detailed consideration, and then only as the completed device is fitted and adapted in accordance with the requirements of the prescription.

There is a need for a coalition of thought and practice that would impart to the refractionist, the student, and the practitioner a more concise appreciation of both the scope and the limitations afforded by a properly compounded and correctly adapted seeing device and the need for a scientific approach to this objective. This was the motivating force that prompted the author to undertake this manuscript. The results are most gratifying. Many subjects pertinent to the student of dispensing are treated in a manner that should prove invaluable in the classroom and for review by all in the ophthalmic field.

Other books have considered separate phases of this subject. None other has been so comprehensive in treatment of so many of the problems essential to adequate knowledge of the many ramifications involved in dispensing services.

The reader will have a genuine appreciation of the magnitude of the author's efforts and will realize that his lifetime of experience and study well qualified him for the undertaking.

HENRY B. CARPENTER

Syracuse, New York

ACKNOWLEDGMENTS

I wish to express my thanks to the following publishers for the courtesy of the use of excerpts from their publications: King City, Distinguished Service Foundation of Optometry; Boeder, Paul: *An Introduction to the Mathematics of Ophthalmic Optics.* Springfield, Charles C Thomas, 1937; Ogle, K.N.: *Optics.* London, U.K. Optical B & L, Ltd., 1968; Emsley, H.H.: *Emsley's Optical Tables and Other Data,* 1968. Rochester, Shuron/Continental Optical Company, *Pedioptic Frames,* 1961.

After one has used a number of terms and concludes by setting down some of them as a glossary, conscience forces him to refer to authority for clarity and accuracy in his definitions. I have found great assistance in *Dorland's Illustrated Medical Dictionary,* Philadelphia, W.B. Saunders Company; Schapero, Max *et al.: Dictionary of Visual Science, Philadelphia,* Chilton, 1960; Hardy, Morris and Flick: *A Dictionary for Opticians and Optometrists,* London, Hatton Press, 1951.

R.L.S.

CONTENTS

Ophthalmic Dispensing

Chapter 1

HISTORY OF OPHTHALMIC DISPENSING

✦◆✦

Compared with some of the other things manufactured to improve the comfort or well-being of humans, optical lenses and the fitting and dispensing of them as spectacles are comparatively recent. It is unbelievable that in very primitive times someone did not learn that a reasonably transparent material which was made convex on the front surface, like that cabochon cut of a semiprecious stone, would increase the apparent size of anything upon which it was laid. Following that event it is reasonable to suspect that a search turned to the finding of transparent hard materials.

Careful research has failed to disclose any very clear references to lenses in early historical writings. The apparent bending of the end of a straight rod immersed in water was carefully investigated by Claudius Ptolemy, 138 AD, and even the regular increase in the apparent deviation at an increased angle was noted.

Two lenses in a conveyance to rest upon the nose were first mentioned about the end of the thirteenth century. This is not surprising when we recognize their sophistication. (1) The material for lenses was first crystal and later glass. (2) It was necessary to grind and polish a magnifying lens in the form of a sphere and later a hemisphere. In 1927, E. J. Fordyke found some crystal magnifiers in a tomb in Crete which were of the period 1200–1600 BC. Thousands of years elapsed before the lens curves were flattened to produce the relatively longer focussed lenses suitable to be held before the eyes to improve visual performance. It was not until late in the thirteenth century (1268) that Roger Bacon described "the segment of a sphere with the convex side toward the eye with which letters are seen far better and they seem larger. For this reason such an instrument is useful to old persons and those with weak eyes." (3) The invention of a means to secure lenses to the head and before the eyes is most frequently, although controversially, ascribed to Salvino d'Armati, who is mentioned in a statement found on a mural tablet dated 1317 under a bust in the Church of St. Maria Maggiore in Florence. However, a letter dated 1299 by Trettato del Governo da Sandra di Pipozzo di Sandro Florentine remarks, "I find myself so oppressed by age that I can neither read nor write without those glasses they call spectacles, lately invented. . . ."*

A sermon delivered in 1305 by Fra Giordano da Rivalto should qualify him as the godfather of all dispensing opticians. He said, "It is not yet twenty years since the art of making glasses was invented. This enables good sight, and *is one of the best as well as most useful of arts that the world possesses.*"

As time went on, spectacle makers made the lenses, made the holder, (sometimes of leather, wood, or metal) , and sold the products from trays at fairs or in the streets. The selection of lens power was made by the customer. Practically all of the spectacles were used as reading glasses because the first lenses were convex. Baptista Porta, in his book *Natural Magic* (1591) , was probably the first to describe the making and polishing of concave lenses. Thus, the correction of near sighted (myopic) eyes was provided. Shastid† reports that concave lenses began to be employed about the beginning of the sixteenth century. Pope Leo X, for example, is known to have worn a pair in 1517.

The German opticians formed a guild that was probably the first optical organization.

In 1629, King Charles I of England granted a charter to the Worshipful Company of Spectacle Makers, which amounted to a guild. The members controlled the quality of spectacles offered for sale and, within the limits of the city of London, were permitted to destroy any spectacles that did not come up to standard. Two comments that might be made are that (1) it was commendable that quality of product was paramount and (2) a sort of cartel was formed which gave reason for the continuance of the organization. The charter remains active to the present time.

---

*Flick, C.S.: *A Gross of Green Spectacles.* London, Hatton Press, 1951.

†Shastid, T.H., M.D.: An outline history of ophthalmology. *Am J Physiol Optics, VII(3):580-581,* 1926.

Since 1897 it has controlled the education and examinations of all British ophthalmic opticians (optometrists).

Combinations of lenses to make microscopes and telescopes were not accomplished until the seventeenth century. James Gregory described his telescope design in 1669, which was followed soon after by Isaac Newton's design (1721). Both of these telescopes used concave mirrors (not convex lenses) as the light gathering (objective) lenses. In 1667, Hooke recorded his method of making lenses for microscopes. He was followed by Leeuwenhoek, the celebrated Dutch microscopist in 1719.

Benjamin Franklin had tired of changing his spectacles each time his attention changed from distance to near. So, in 1784 he asked his optician to split a pair of his distance and his reading glasses, and then to reassemble the spectacles with distance lens power in the top and reading power in the bottom. Thus he could have clear vision at distance or near, according to which portion of his lenses he used. He had invented the first bifocal lenses. His letters to his friends about that time indicated that the lens power of spectacles was still chosen by the wearer.

Although comparatively satisfactory spectacle lenses were chosen by trial and error, little was known about the optical performance of the components of the human eye. The whole science of physiological optics was yet to be developed. About 1800, Thomas Young, whose vision was not well corrected with available lenses, learned that when he immersed his eyes in a pail of water objects at the bottom of the water could be more easily recognized. Thus he had corrected the large amount of astigmatism of his eyes. About twenty-five years elapsed until, in 1827, Airy lead the way to the making of the cylindrical glass lenses which corrected Young's astigmatism.

Further developments in physiological optics were scant until the publication in 1864 of a textbook entitled *Accommodation and Refraction of the Eye* by F.C. Donders, M.D., of Holland. This book aroused the interest of medical doctors everywhere in the examination of eyes and the prescribing of spectacle lenses for them. When the patients started to bring their lens prescriptions to optical stores, some opticians restricted their activity to the filling of doctors' prescriptions. Others availed themselves of the knowledge in Donders' book and others that followed vigorously undertook to acquire knowledge and improve their ability in sight-testing and the preparation of individualized spectacle lenses.

As time went on the two groups of opticians continued to concentrate upon their specialized activities until finally they were advertising themselves as "refracting opticians" and "prescription opticians." It was natural that medical doctors and prescription opticians became more closely related in their common cause to care for patients' eyes. Refracting opticians, many of whom were related to jewelry stores, were self-sufficient because they were doing the sight-testing and also supplying the required spectacles.

Cuignet, 1873, developed and popularized a means of an objective refracting procedure involving light reflected into the patient's eyes. By the use of a cyclopegic, a drug that hinders the action of the ciliary muscle and thereby retards accommodation, doctors were now able to do a large part of a refraction without the patient's verbal response. This technique called retinoscopy aroused greater interest in eye examinations. The drug (usually atropine or homatropine) also dilated the patient's pupils affording the doctors the opportunity to obtain a better view of the retina and to facilitate diagnosis of systemic, or other, diseases which were affecting eye health.

Some refracting opticians seemed to feel they were existing on sufferance of organized medicine and wished to establish their own legal identity. They chose the name "optometry" (a word used by Donders and others) as the name for their profession and undertook to obtain state licensure to refract eyes without the use of drugs. Although by a strict interpretation of the medical practice acts in many states it was contended by some that refraction was really the province of medicine, state medical societies yielded this small corner of their right to treat the entire person of their patients to this group of refracting opticians (now optometrists) when they were assured there was no intention to use licensure as a "back door" approach to the practice of medicine.

Prescription opticians became well established and in some cities the firms operated several stores. In some states the optometry laws had been written so badly that, although prescription opticians were doing no sight-testing and had their entire allegiance to the medical profession, optometrists contended that these opticians were in violation of the Optometry Act. The only defense in this situation was for the prescription opticians to rally the support of their ophthalmologist friends and obtain some kind of state legislation to be able to continue their businesses. In some states where optometry organizations were strong, the laws restricted opticians' advertising, even to the display of eyewear in their show windows. In some states opticians were deprived of the privilege to make duplicate lenses without a prescription. In other states there was no vigorous agitation about this matter by the local optometrists.

In 1926 a group of dispensing opticians in Philadelphia formed a local, then a national, organization of opticians who were committed to the sole business of caring for medical doctors' patients. Like the original Worshipful Company of Spectacle Makers, a code of ethics was established to enforce high quality service using highest quality materials. This organization was named the Guild of Prescription Opticians of America. Its membership approached a thousand member firms. It moved its home office to Washington, D.C., where its staff could more conveniently intercede to thwart legislation that was construed to be inimical to the progress of dispensing opticians in the care of ophthalmologists' patients. In 1971, it was realized that the small number of opticians represented by the organization made a very small impression upon Congressional Committees. This situation caused many members to believe that the terms of membership should be opened to include all dispensing firms. It was decided to give the expanded organization a new name. Opticians Association of America was chosen. The new constitution relegated the Guild to a minor function of the organization. Its activity is largely a continuation of the work of the Guild Standards Committee. This consists of setting appearance, equipment, and performance standards for dispensing optical stores. Without any means of enforcement, this effort is considered idealistic by many dispensers.

In 1947, the American Board of Opticianry was formed to assist in the establishment of collegiate courses in opticianry and to certify the competence of opticians by written examination.

The first requirement was five years of experience or graduation from an accredited two-year course in Ophthalmic Optics. Certified Opticians who acquired additional experience and met certain conditions were entitled to take a second, and more difficult, examination to become Master Opticians. Within a few years, Mr. Robert Duffins, a member of the Board, made a liberal contribution for the establishment of an Educational Foundation in Ophthalmic Optics to provide scholarships and student loans. There still existed a need for an organization of Certified Opticians to provide continuing education. The International Academy of Opticianry was formed to provide this service. The United States Office of Education, which is a function of the Department of Health, Education and Welfare, has a list of accredited providers of medical and paramedical services. Members of this list are eligible for grants for educational purposes. They are considered as the group eligible to participate in or act as members of advisory groups in regulatory matters. When the American Board of Opticianry made inquiries in preparation toward submitting a petition for the recognition of opticianry, the representatives were told the Board was ineligible because it was a self-perpetuating organization that had no membership which was representative of opticianry. There was a suggestion that if the Educational Foundation, International Academy of Opticianry, and American Board of Opticianry were to combine as an autonomous whole, such an organization might be considered. Thereupon, a special meeting was called and out of the three groups the National Academy was formed.

The O.A.A. invited the N.A.O. to affiliate with it in much the same manner as the Guild of Prescription Opticians. However, it was felt that loss of the Academy's autonomy by becoming a part of a trade organization involved in legislative and political affairs would destroy the possibility of recognition by the Office of Education. If this position is correct, the opportunity for the recognition of opticianry would be hopeless, because there is no other organization that could not be defined as a trade organization. Thus far, there has been no accommodation of the matter.

Courses in opticianry have grown until there are now seventeen high school and two-year college courses teaching optical technology and complete courses in ophthalmic dispensing. The Department of Labor is vigorously promoting an Apprenticeship Plan which is being actively supported by established firms across the country.

Thus a vocation that was formerly wholly constituted of apprentices is meeting present-day technological advances by also sponsoring formal education to help fill the ranks of a rapidly expanding occupation.

REVIEW

1. Who was Salvino d'Armati?
2. Describe the Worshipful Company of Spectacle Makers.
3. Discuss Benjamin Franklin's contribution to ophthalmic optics.
4. What was one of Thomas Young's discoveries?
5. Identify F.C. Donders, M.D.
6. When did Cuignet develop the retinoscope?
7. What is the difference between a refracting optician and a prescription optician?
8. What is the name of the national trade organization of dispensing opticians?

ADDITIONAL REFERENCE

1. Sutcliffe, John H.: *British Optical Association Library & Museum Catalogue*. London, Council of the British Optical Association at Clifford's Inn, 1932.

Chapter 2

ANATOMY OF THE EYE

◆◆◆◆◇◆◆◆

L et us begin with a brief discussion of the eye before which an ophthalmic lens may ultimately be placed. With one exception,* treatises on dispensing have regularly started with an exposition upon lenses and frames. It seems reasonable to first give thought to the eye and its adnexa as well as the deviations in form and function which give rise to the need of an ophthalmic lens and/or prism to improve its usefulness.

Standing before the eye globes are the libs (palpebrae). These are actually folds of the external skin which adapt themselves to the curvature of the globe to cover and protect it. The eyebrow is the upper boundary of the upper lid. The lower lid passes to the cheek without a sharp line of partition. Protection of the cornea is the principal function of the lids. Dust particles and other debris in the air are wiped off in the act of blinking. Moisture is provided from the tear glands to sustain a constant tear film on the corneal surface. The epithelium (outer layer) of the cornea thickens and finally opacifies if the surface is allowed to remain dry for a protracted period. Such an event may occur after burns, ulcers, or lid surgery.

The services of a dispensing optician are required at this point to supply and fit a "moisture chamber" for the relief of the patient. This shield fits snugly around the whole orbital area and according to the ophthalmologist's wishes may or may not have a lens in it to permit vision. It may be fitted to the patient's spectacles or secured by an elastic headband. Of greatest importance is that it remains closely fitted around the orbit and thereby retains the moisture which collects.

The lids also protect the retina by squinting when excessive

---

*Fleck, H., Heynig, J., and Mutze, K.: *Die Praxis der Brillenanpassung.* Leipzig, VEB Fachbuchverlag, 1960.

light strikes the eyes. Squinting becomes a habit for nearsighted individuals who find that distance vision is somewhat improved when the lids form a slit.

The lid margins contain lashes (cilia) which grow more thickly on the upper lid. When the eyes are prominent, the lashes long, and the nasal bone between the eyes is narrow and flattened, a dispensing optician has difficulty in fitting eyewear far enough removed from the eyes to prevent the upper lashes from touching the back surfaces of the lenses.

The eye globe rests in the bony cavity of the orbit. Surrounding the eyeball, except in front, is a loose-fitting sac or sheath which is known as Tenon's capsule. Between this envelope and the bony walls of the orbit is a layer of fatty tissue.

The shell of the eye globe is composed of several coats. The outer tunic called sclera is about 1.0 mm ($^1/_{25}$ inch) thick. It is fibrous and provides most of the stability to the shape of the eyeball. In the posterior portion of the eye, this layer is nearly opaque.

Inside the sclera at the back of the eye is a layer of blood vessels which deliver the nutrition to the eye. This coat is called the choroid or uvea. In reality it is a prolongation of the arachnoid sheath of the optic nerve. As it continues up toward the front of the eye it becomes the ciliary body that surrounds and supports the crystalline lens. As this coat of the eye continues forward it becomes the iris. Inside the choroid layer rests the retina. This layer is composed of nerve endings called rods and cones. Images of external objects stimulate the rods and cones to produce the sense of sight.

Although the eye globe deviates from an exact sphere, it is generally the shape of a ball 24 mm (virtually 1.0 inch) in diameter. There is a slight bulge on the temporal (outer) side. On the anterior (front) surface there is a greater bulge, almost 12 mm (0.47 inch) in diameter which unlike the remainder of the sclera is transparent and normally contains no blood vessels. This is called the cornea. It serves as the window through which light enters the eye. The radius of curvature in the central portion is about 7.8 mm (0.3 inch). The curve gradually flattens toward the limbus (margin). The cornea is about 0.8 mm ($^1/_{30}$ inch)

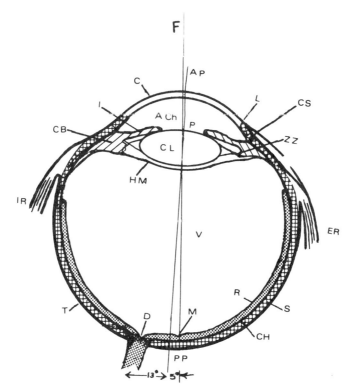

Figure 1. Section of schematic anatomy of the eye. (AP) = anterior pole; (Ach) = anterior chamber; (AP-PP) = optical axis; (C) = cornea; (CB) = ciliary body; (Ch) = choroid; (CL) = crystalline lens; (D) = disc, optic nerve head; (ER) = external rectus muscle; (FM) = fixation axis, visual axis; (HM) = hyaloid membrane; (I) = iris; (IR) = internal rectus, medial rectus muscle; (L) = corneal limbus; (M) = macula; (P) = pupil; (PP) = posterior pole; (R) = retina; (S) = sclera; (T) = Tenon's capsule; (V) = vitreous humor; (ZZ) = zonule of Zinn.

thick. Behind it is a watery substance called the aqueous humor which is constantly being formed. It drains out of the globe through a canal on the under side of the cornea at the limbus. This duct is called the canal of Schlemm.

Directly behind the iris is the crystalline lens which is held in place by a girdle (zonule) that extends from the lens margin to the ciliary muscle. This muscle has both radial and longitudinal muscle fibers. Aqueous humor is formed in the walls of the triangular space behind the iris and the margin of the crystalline lens. The lens is biconvex with more curvature on the posterior (back) surface than on the anterior (front). It is about 4 mm thick in the center.

The lens grows throughout life but has its greatest growth in the first year after birth. The nucleus of the lens has three stages of development. The fetal nucleus is formed between the third and eighth months of fetal life; the infantile nucleus is formed between the ninth month of fetal life and puberty; after puberty it has grown to the adult nucleus. These nuclei grow in layers one upon the other in the form of an onion. As life progresses the nucleus continues to grow and become harder. This loss of elasticity finally interferes with the free functioning of the lens in later adult life. The dimensions of the lens after one year of life are approximately 7.5 mm in diameter and 2.5 mm thick. The lens has grown to 9 mm in diameter and 4 mm thick at twenty years. At age 70 the diameter has increased another 0.5 mm and the thickness by 1.0 mm.

Behind the crystalline lens the remainder of the globe is filled with a gelatinous substance called the vitreous humor. This gel is very unstable, and unusual pressure upon it or a rupture of the membrane that contains it causes the gel to transform into liquid. Fluid then separates out from the remaining gel, leaving it shrunken. The process continues with small threads and fibers becoming interspersed throughout. In some instances the deterioration proceeds until the remaining vitreous becomes congested and finally opaque.

The fourth layer of the eye on the inner side of the back of the eyeball is a thin layer of nerve endings which are the radiations of the optic nerve. This part of the eye is called the retina. The nerve endings are in two forms. The central portion of the retina is populated with about a million neural endings, cylindrically shaped receptors which, because of their shape, are called cones. In the fovea, the center of the macular area, 34,000 cones are compressed in an area less than 0.5 mm ($^1/_{50}$ inch) square. Radiating out from the center of the retina the separation between the cones increases and the interstices are filled with the other form named rods. The function of the cones is to form vision.

In the macular area a very high percentage of these retinal elements have individual pathways to the cortex. Several rods tend to be grouped, hence perception of detail is diminished. Rods are stimulated with much less light than the cones, thus serving importantly in darkness. They are also sensitive to motion.

As the distance from the macula increases, the rods and cones are not so tightly packed. The low percentage of cones compared with rods continues to the margin where there are only rods.

All of these nerve endings leave the retina in the trunk of the optic nerve. This nerve enters the globe through an aperture in the sclera and choroid which is called the lamina cribrosa. This papilla (disc) or nervehead is about 18° nasalward from the macula (central portion of the retina). The nerve fibers of the optic nerve connect directly with the occipital cortex of the brain.

This very brief sketch of the anatomy of the eye has mentioned the essential image-forming parts of the eye. They are used to form an image upon the retina from which neural impulses are transmitted to the visual cortex of the brain.

For comparison purposes a camera is like the eye except that the box of a camera is filled with air instead of fluids. The cornea, aqueous humor, and crystalline lens are duplicated by the lens of the camera. The retina is copied by the photographic film. Like the camera, the image of the objects in front of the eye falls on the back surface.

The muscles outside of the eye globe, the extraocular muscles which turn the eye to a desired position, are the next considera-

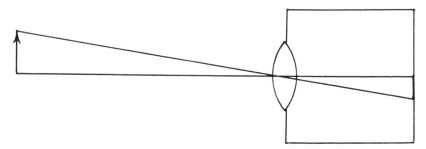

Figure 2. Camera simulates eye.

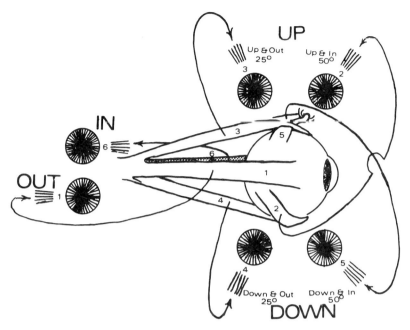

Figure 3. Schematic display of the extraocular muscles and their action. (1) = external rectus; (2) = inferior oblique; (3) = superior rectus; (4) = inferior rectus; (5) = superior oblique; (6) = internal — medial — rectus.

tion. Six muscles are attached externally to the globe of each eye. Four of these muscles form two pairs which are attached on opposite sides of the globe and rotate the globe in opposite directions. The internal (medial) rectus turns the eye in (toward the nose). Opposing it is the external (lateral) rectus which turns the eye out. Above and below are the superior rectus (up) and inferior rectus (down) muscles. Because the muscles converge to the foramen (opening) at the back of the orbit, the action of these muscles is not directly up and down. The convergence of the muscles is about 27°. Therefore, if the superior rectus alone is stimulated it pulls the eye globe up and out and the inferior rectus pulls the eyeball down and out. The two remaining muscles are so attached that they pull almost oppositely at an angle of 51° from the anterior-posterior line of the globe. This oblique action creates an antagonistic action which compensates for torsions caused by the recti muscles in the acts of elevation and depression of the eye.

REVIEW

1. What are the three principal functions of the lids?
2. How is a dispensing optician involved in repairing their malfunction?
3. Name three of the coats (or layers) of the eye globe.
4. What is the approximate curvature of the cornea?
5. What is the function of the ciliary muscle?
6. How do the nerve impulses leave the eye globe?
7. How is a camera different from the eye?
8. How many extraocular muscles surround the eye globe?
9. Name the pairs of muscles which act as opponents.

ADDITIONAL REFERENCES

1. Duke-Elder, W. Stewart: *Text-book of Ophthalmology,* Vol. I. St. Louis, Mosby, 1934.
2. Kestenbaum, Alfred: *Applied Anatomy of the Eye.* New, York, Grune, 1963.
3. Wolff, Eugene: *Anatomy of the Eye and Orbit.* London, Lewis, 1948.

Chapter 3

PHYSIOLOGY OF THE EYE
AND THE OCULOROTARY MUSCLES

◆◆

N ow that the essentials of the components of the optical system have been mentioned, the next step is to examine how they perform to accomplish the acts of vision (perception). This chapter will be a discussion of a small part of physiology, the science of functions, of a few of the parts of the eye.

Discussion of the performance of the eye as an optical instrument presupposes familiarity with some of the fundamental laws of optics. It is necessary to proceed without a discussion of these principles until the following chapter.

Technically, the function of the cornea could be considered a matter of anatomy, but because it performs a very important optical service, further discussion of it will follow. To function ideally as a lens surface, the cornea should be a section of a perfect sphere, at least in the central section where light rays continue through the pupil. Actually the cornea is seldom this perfect shape. The curvature also tends to flatten toward the margin (limbus). Since the average cornea has a radius in the central area of about 7.8 mm, the curvature should be nearly identical with that of a 0.63 inch ball bearing. Such absolute geometrical precision is not found in the constitution of human beings.

The curvature and clarity of the cornea have a significant effect upon the performance of the eye, because about 75 percent of the focal effect is accomplished at this front surface. The commonest deviation, and one which requires an ophthalmic lens to correct it, is when the shape of the cornea is not spherical but ellipsoidal like the center of the side of a football. Under such circumstances light will not come to a point focus. Rays that enter in the long dimension of the ellipse will focus farther away from the corneal surface than the rays which fall on the shorter dimension of the ellipse. This divergence from a spherical shape or lack of concentricity is named for its optical effect. Light through such a surface is termed "astigmatic" (Gr. *á*, primative; *stigma*, spot) because it is not focussed to a single point. This curvature imperfection is not pathological. It is not a disease in this form.

Another distortion of the curve of the cornea is definitely a disease. It is more common among girls than boys and is first noticed about puberty; that is, at ten to fifteen years of age. The tissue of the cornea grows much thinner in the central area and the surface becomes dilated to form a cone shape usually slightly below the center of the pupil. This irregular shape will not focus light truly, hence vision is badly blurred and no spectacle lens is of much benefit to vision. Usually the deformation subsides after a few years and remains relatively arrested. In other instances the thinning of the cornea continues and the deformity increases. This disease was one of the original reasons for the development of contact lenses. With a perfectly shaped glass lens covering the cone and fluid under the lens, the contour of the cornea (now totally immersed) became practically ineffective and usable vision was accomplished. To prevent the back surface of the contact lens from rubbing upon the thinned corneal apex, the contact lens rested upon the sclera (the white surface) of the eye. Present-day corneal contact lenses can be satisfactory for early development of keratoconus and some patients have success for a long period. Ultimately, if the condition progresses to opacification of the visual area, surgical correction by corneal transplant is the only other alternative.*

The clarity of the cornea is diminished and light transmission reduced by many of the inflamations of the cornea known as keratitis. Syphillis and tuberculosis are causes of some of these diseases. Visual acuity is diminished when the lesions are in the central area of the cornea. Ophthalmic lenses have no beneficial effect upon the diffused images produced by these diseases.

Light rays which fall upon the cornea are refracted (bent) to come to a focus about 31 mm from the surface. These focussing rays proceed through the aqueous humor for 3.6 mm until they

---

*Girard, Louis J.: *Corneal Contact Lenses.* St. Louis, Mosby, 1964.

reach the anterior surface of the crystalline lens. The light rays are refracted again as they progress 3.6 mm through the lens. They leave the posterior surface of the crystalline lens to pass through the vitreous humor. The rays are now focussed to meet at the fovea centralis (the center of the macula). The light rays stimulate the cones of this area of the retina which start the neural impulses to the brain. The action of all the components of the eye duplicates the physics experiment of youth—the convex lens which was used as a "burning glass" to bring rays of sunlight to focus in a small spot. Along with the visible light came the heat rays which were used to irritate the back of a hand or scorch the edge of a scrap of tissue paper.

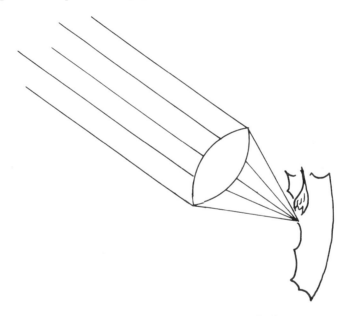

Figure 4.   Heat rays concentrated by lens.

The cornea and crystalline lens have served as two lenses which together provide the proper focal length to produce an image upon the retina. The explanation of what occurs when the retina is stimulated by the light rays is very complex. This is because it not only involves the physiological function at the retinal sur-

face, but it brings into consideration the neural impulses carried
to the brain.

The most sensitive portion of the retina is called the macula. It
is located about 3.5 mm temporalward from the optic disc (the
point where the optic nerve enters the back of the eye). The
radiations of the optic nerve approach the macula from all directions but do not cross it. The macular area is mostly composed of
cones. These nerve endings provide the form sense to vision. At
the center of the macula lies the fovea centralis. It is about 0.3
mm by 0.2 mm in size. Only cones are tightly compacted in this
spot to produce the highest degree of visual acuity. A cone in the
macular area has been found to be about .002 mm in diameter.
For the images of two points (such as two small stars) to be
recognized (resolved) into separate images it would follow that
an unstimulated cone should intervene between the images of the
two points. Referring to the description of the tangent of an angle
in Chapter 4, see Figure 5.

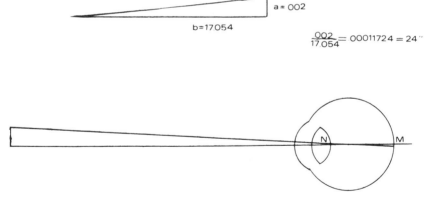

Figure 5.   Minimum angle of resolution.

Thus, under ideal conditions a perfectly functioning eye should
resolve two luminous points at an angle of slightly more than one
minute; that is, two stimulated cones 0.002 mm in diameter, each
of which subtends an angle of 24 seconds are separated by an unstimulated cone 0.002 mm in diameter (subtends an angle of 24
seconds) which covers the diameters of two cones, or 48 seconds.

This is less than what is termed normal acuity (resolution). The diffraction of the pupil margin, the cloudiness of the media of the eye and atmosphere, the recently observed quivering (saccadic) movement of the eye, and the lack of geometrical precision of the cornea all contribute to an end result in that a 5-minute angle, in which each of the legs and spaces of a letter E are one minute, is considered standard (normal) acuity.

Figure 6.   Stimulated and unstimulated retinal cones.

The accepted standard was empirically established. Thorington (1897) reported that many years before when the British Army wished to establish a criterion for perfect vision, a number of expert marksmen were asked to demonstrate the greatest distance at which they could recognize a small letter. The average of the findings was used as a standard for selection of men to be trained as marksmen.

In Utrecht in 1862 Herman Snellen presented a set of test letters based upon a 5-minute angle which he had devised to determine the quality of individual visual acuity. Although there have been many different tests devised since that time, most present-day test charts still use slight modifications of Snellen's letters.

Physiologists and others have contended from time to time that various letter shapes do not measure the *minimum separable* angle but the *minimum legible* angle. To measure the resolving power of photographic lenses and other optical instruments, three bars and two spaces are used.

As a variation of this principle the letter "E" made in various sizes is turned in vertical and horizontal positions to simulate the above test. It is frequently used for preschool children or for

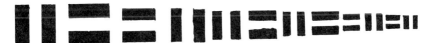

Figure 7.   Resolving power test.

illiterates. Possibly the stigma of it being termed an "illiterate" chart prevents its use for all adults. It does not allow the wide variability in legibility created by some letters such as L V A B. The letter L can be discerned at one-third more distance than a letter B of the same size.

Snellen assigned Roman numerals to the distances at which his test letters were calculated to be identified; thus, LX = 60 meters (200 feet), XXX = 30 meters (100 feet), to VI = 6 meters (20 feet). It was his recommendation that visual acuity be recorded as the testing distance over the letters recognized; such as 6/XXX (20/C feet) to 6/VI (20/XX feet), but his suggestion was disregarded and normal vision is popularly called 20/20. This suggests 20/20 equals 100 percent vision, from which erroneously follows the thought that 20/40 equals 50 percent vision, which is far from the truth. This deterioration of Snellen's notation into a fraction has led to confusion.

Acuteness of vision diminishes very rapidly from the area of the fovea. A simple demonstration of this fact is to hold a well-lighted book page at normal reading distance, then look at a period at the end of a sentence. Holding the book steadily first look intently at the period with one eye closed. Then shift fixation to the last letter of the word before the period. Slowly fix upon each preceding letter. At about the fifth to seventh letter the period will disappear if fixation and attention are carefully held upon the letter. In fact the last letter of the word which is no more than 12 to 14 mm from the letter fixed upon will begin to become blurred. Extensive research has shown that visual acuity declines in the form shown in Figure 8.

The fovea is also the reference point for all images that fall upon the retina. When direct vision is fixed upon an object, all other objects are to the right, left, above, or below that point. The images of these objects fall upon opposite sides of the retina as illustrated, but since the effect of the retinal stimulation is projected back in a straight line in the direction of the stimulation, there is no consciousness of the fact that the sum of these individual points of stimulation produce an inverted image upon the retina.

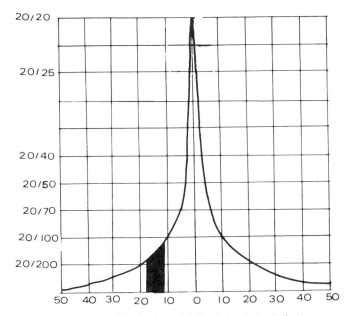

Figure 8. Retinal sensitivity (after Wertheim).

Again, the inverted image on the ground glass of a camera is a simulation of this phenomenon upon the retina. Some writers have dwelt at some length upon the accomplishment of mentally erecting this inverted retinal image. The concept is much simpler

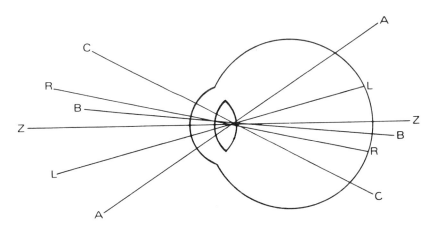

Figure 9. Inverted retinal image.

to understand when it is reduced to only a small object on a blank space before the eye. For instance, four or five small pictures are spread on a large wall, with fixation on the center of the wall. If the pictures at the periphery are moved progressively toward the center and the surrounding pictures finally removed with only the central picture remaining, no violation of the demonstration is made when the elements of this final picture are observed down to the smallest central item. The most minute detail which makes a retinal stimulation *above* the fovea centralis is projected into the space *below* center. This same effect follows for all other directions.

The senses of hearing and seeing are similar in that in both instances the effects of the excitation are returned in the direction of the stimulus. A sound is not sensed in the inner ear within the skull. The sound is mentally projected in the direction of its origin. As experience grows, the precise location can be determined rather accurately. In the same manner the image on the retina is not sensed within the head, the illuminated object is seen (perceived) in space, projected in a straight line retracing the path of the light rays that enter the eye. This combination of physiological and psychological phenomena has been the subject of research for many scientists for a very long time. Prince* states that " 'perception' expresses much more adequately what we are concerned with than does 'vision,' which on its own lacks the cerebral and, what is just as important, the psychological factors involved in our consciousness of our surrounding world." We shall return to these considerations again when binocular vision is discussed.

As previously mentioned, the crystalline lens is the second lens in combination with the cornea which brings light rays from a distant object into focus upon the retina. Quite different from the fixed shape of the cornea, the crystalline lens shape and lens power are altered by the action of the ciliary muscle which surrounds the lens. Few subjects have had so many diverse opinions advanced as the mechanism of the changing of the lens shape and power (accommodation). In 1619 Scheiner proved by an

---

*Prince, J.H.: *Visual Development,* Vol. 1 Edinburgh, E. & S. Livingstone, 1949, p. 4.

optical experiment that an optical system existed within the eye which was alterable and focussable; in other words, the crystalline lens accommodated or changed to meet the requirements of differing distances of objects from the eye. Despite Scheiner's demonstration, eminent authorities presented numerous theories such as (a) two focal planes and the retina between them, (b) the cornea changes shape, (c) the eye globe elongates like a camera, (d) the pupil contracts and creates sufficient depth of focus, and (e) the crystalline lens moves forward and backward.

It was not until more than two hundred years after Scheiner's experiment (1853) that Helmholtz proved undeniably that the lens changed shape when the eye focussed for clear vision of an object close to the eye. In a darkened room, he arranged a square source of illumination to project upon a subject's eye. He noted the relative size and positions of the reflections of the light source upon the cornea, the front surface of the crystalline lens, and the back surface of the crystalline lens when the subject viewed a distant object. Then, without the eye moving, it was focussed upon an object near at hand. The reflection of the cornea did not change in size or position, confirming that the curve of the cornea did not change in the focussing of the eye. However, the large reflection of the slightly curved front surface of the lens became smaller, demonstrating that the convexity of the surface was greatly increased. The change in the size and shape of the reflection from the back surface of the lens was not perceptible. Hence, the front curve of the lens bulged forward, which increased the curvature of the surface and also the power of the lens. Even when these facts were conceded the discussion continued upon how the ciliary body is activated to cause the lens to change its dimensions and curvature. The most recent contributor who has reinforced these conclusions is Fincham.[†]

The currently accepted mechanism of accommodation is that, as the ciliary muscle contracts, the choroid is pulled forward. The anterior (front) capsule of the lens protrudes into the pupillary area of the iris and the shape of the lens is changed. In this process as the lens has increased in thickness the diameter is somewhat lessened.

[†]Fincham, E.F.: *Trans Ophthalmol Soc*, *XXVI*:239, 1925.

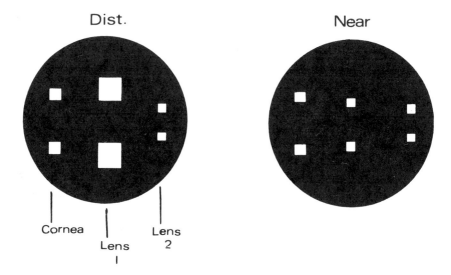

Figure 10.   Lens surface reflections in accommodation (Helmholtz).

Coleman* has added to the knowledge on this subject by the use of ultrasonography from which he emphasizes the importance of vitreous support based upon hydraulic forces.

At birth the lens approaches a spherical shape but rapidly flattens. By the end of the first year the dimensions are diameter 7.5 mm, axis (thickness) 2.6 mm, which at twenty years of age has only changed to 9 mm × 4 mm. The lens continues to grow through all life: at seventy years it measures 9.5 mm × 5 mm. From these data it is seen that accommodation is at its greatest in childhood.   The closest point at which a normal eye can see

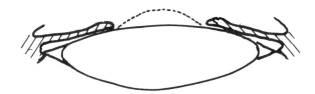

Figure 11.   Schematic presentation of the act of accommodation.

*Coleman, D.J.:   Unified model for accommodative mechanism.   *Am J Ophthalmol,* 69:1063, 1970.

clearly slowly recedes all through life (note the following as measured by Duane) *:

At 10 years $2^7/_8$ inches
12 years   3   inches
16 years $3^1/_2$ inches
20 years $3^3/_4$ inches
24 years   4   inches
28 years $4^1/_2$ inches
32 years   5   inches
36 years $5^3/_4$ inches
40 years $6^1/_2$ inches
44 years   10   inches
48 years   16   inches
52 years   22   inches
56 years   32   inches

An incontrovertible explanation of this reduction in elasticity of the lens has not been made. From the physical aspect, most authorities agree that the friction between the layers of the lens increases for several reasons as life progresses. Many physiologists believe that much of the cause of the reduced lens activity is the gradual weakening of the ciliary body. Possibly it is a combination of both. As shown in Duane's chart, the net result is that the near point of accommodation continues to recede at a reasonably constant rate until about age forty when the decline is increased for about fifteen years.

ERRORS OF REFRACTION

Let us return to the imagery of the eye when the optical components do *not* focus rays of light originating at infinity to a point image. Physiologically, the eye is at its greatest state of rest (no accommodative effort) when viewing an object at great distance. Description of the ideal state follows:

Emmetropia: the eye condition when parallel rays of light incident upon an eye in a state of rest come to a point focus upon the retina.

When one considers that the attainment of such optical perfec-

*Duane, A.: *Am J Ophthalmol,* 5:865, 1922.

tion is dependent upon accuracy to fractions of millimeters in the radius of curvature of the cornea, the curves of the lens, the spacing of the components, and finally the distance to the retina, it is evident that this total combination occurs very infrequently. Like all manifestations of perfection, approximations overwhelmingly outnumber the absolute. Occasionally, emmetropia is referred to as the normal eye, but such a concept has no more foundation in biology than the attainment, for instance, of 165 pounds in weight or 5 feet 8 inches in height.

Hypermetropia: the eye condition when parallel rays of light incident upon the eye in a state of rest have not yet come to a focus when they reach the retina.

Hence the illumination from each very small area of the object presents a small blur instead of point image upon the retina. The sum of all of the luminous points in the object makes an inverted image that is out of focus upon the retina. If the retina is not too far in front of the focus, accommodation will be instantly activated to produce a clear image. If the individual's ability to accommodate is large and the blur is small, it is obvious that this person may not realize he has an error of refraction because his ability to see is satisfactory and the muscular energy required may not be perceptible (manifest). There are a large number of eyes with such condition, latent hyperopia, and a simple sight test with letters (such as is used for an automobile driver's test) would classify these eyes as "normal" or emmetropic.

If this condition were in a greater degree and the retina were farther from the focus, a greater amount of accommodation would be required for clear vision. At some point the extra demand would result in fatigue (asthenopia) and if the accommodation became exhausted then blurred vision would result. This poor eye performance and the other symptoms which would most likely accompany the fatigue (sometimes called eye strain) would cause the individual to seek a refraction (sight-test) and the procurement of appropriate lenses.

Myopia: the eye condition when parallel rays of light incident upon the eye in a state of rest come to focus before they reach the retina.

Only rays of light originating from an object close to the eye will focus upon the retina. Accommodation will give no benefit to this eye for distant vision. Because near vision is clear, this eye simulates an emmetropic eye accommodated for close vision. All distant objects are blurred and no muscular effort will improve vision. In layman's language, this eye is nearsighted.

Myopia, except in high degrees, is not bothersome for activities near at hand. Reading and studying are not difficult, hence nearsightedness and bookishness have long been associated. Until recently, athletics which require good vision for distance was laborious for myopes. Spectacles were a great hindrance. Recently contact lenses have opened the way for many myopic men to become outstanding basketball and football players.

Astigmatism: the eye condition when parallel rays of light incident upon an ellipsoidal cornea are focussed at two different distances and therefore cannot produce a completely clear image upon the retina.

There are five possibilities where these focal distances can fall: (1) neither may have come to a focus at the retina; (2) one may not have come to a focus at the retina; (3) one may not have come to a focus at the retina and the other have already come to focus in front of the retina; (4) one may have come precisely to focus on the retina and the other to have already come to focus before it reached the retina; and (5) both focal distances in front of the retina.

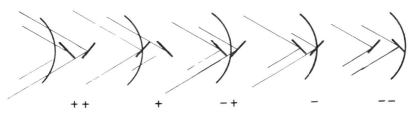

++   +   − +   −   − −

Figure 12. Five kinds of astigmatism.

Although these percentages* may differ somewhat with different races and in different parts of the world, the amount of differ-

*Cavara: *Boll Oculist, i:*301, 1922.

ence is not great.

1.	27%	+ +
2.	13.72%	+
3.	11.3%	± ∓
4.	9.62%	—
5.	38.37%	— —

It would seem that the first project would be to find a means to bring the two focal distances to the same point. The means will be discussed in the next chapter.

Doctor Duane's table of the nearest point that accommodation will focus the crystalline lens shows an approaching problem for later life about age 44. At that time, accommodation will be exerted to 70 percent of its capacity to read at fourteen inches. Since it is a usual experience that the body cannot perform near its total capacity for a very long period of time, it is plain that assistance is going to be needed to allow reading or close work to be comfortably accomplished. The solution is an ophthalmic lens and the service is completed by an ophthalmic dispenser.

Thus far this discussion has made reference to only one eye. Actually the project is much more complicated than it has been presented. Since two eyes are involved and binocular single vision is the desired end result, it is clear that two eyes with images comfortably focussed on the two retinas and with the eyes so directed that the images are simultaneously falling on the foveas of the two retinas is a singular occurrence. Assuming that the retinal images are satisfactory, the performance of the extraocular muscles of the two eyes is almost incredible. With the eyes in a state of rest and fixed upon a distant object such as the moon, the extraocular muscles must converge the eyes microscopically to receive the images of the moon on the foveas. If the eyes (not the head) turn to look at a star, all twelve muscles of the two eyes join in the vergence (turning) of the eyes. As an experiment, note how quickly the eyes can sweep across the sky and stop precisely on such a small object as a star.* Part of this act is innate and part of it is learned. An infant's inaccuracies in reaching for a toy

---

*Campbell, F.W.: The accommodation response of the human eye, *Br J Ophthalmol Opt, 16(4)*:1969.

suspended before him are part of the learning process in the coordination of eyes and hands.

When an object is fixed upon at a near point, the eyes converge while accommodation increases to produce clear vision. This coupling of functions is also a reflex arc similar to the demonstration in the night sky. Proof that at least a part of this association is hereditary is confirmed when lenses are provided for a hypermetropic cross-eyed baby and with relief of accommodation his eyes become straight. The reflex cannot be suspended as is shown when a card is held before one eye while the uncovered eye views an object at near. The covered eye converges approximately the proper amount although it cannot see the object. This unrewarded convergence is known as *accommodative convergence*. It may not be precisely the proper amount, but in interest of single binocular vision it is supplemented with what is called *fusion convergence*. This function is capable of reducing convergence somewhat if the eyes have turned in too far or adding a slight amount of convergence if the eyes do not turn in sufficiently. Thus it is either a positive or negative function.

Since the second nodal point is only 17 mm from the retina, a normal 20/20 letter at 20 feet is only 0.025 mm tall at the retina. This emphasizes the precision with which the extraocular muscles must perform in order to retain this small image precisely upon the fovea. As remarkable as this achievement may be, it is superceded by the act of simultaneously fixing the two eyes upon the same object. Inaccuracy in fixation causes the images to fall upon disparate areas of the retinas and thereby two objects are projected in space (diplopia). The almost micrometric adjustment from the nerve supply to the extraocular muscles for this accomplishment is rarely duplicated elsewhere in the body. As we have noted, even the simple act of elevating or lowering the eye requires action to some degree of all six extraocular muscles. To raise the eye straight up requires the superior rectus; to prevent the eye from rotating (torsion), the inferior oblique must also contract. The lateral (externus) is also stimulated to prevent the eye from converging. The remaining muscles must simultaneously relax. Even this simple eye movement into a secondary position is a very complicated movement.

Double vision is not tolerable and is generally avoided by the phenomenon of fusion. Although each eye receives a retinal image, this faculty causes the eyes to turn to such a position that the images fall upon identical areas of the retinas and thus a single object is projected in space. The unification of the images precedes the conscious awareness of the images. A great deal of discussion and controversy exists among outstanding physiologists, psychologists, and others with reference to how this act is accomplished. Such divergences include whether there is a simultaneous superimposition of the images or a psychic alternation of image replacement of corresponding parts of the image. However it may be, whether it is known as unification or fusion, the phenomenon still makes a significant contribution to our well-being.

The motor reflex that reestablishes a single image after an obstacle interrupts fusion is known as *fusion compulsion*. If a $4^\triangle$ or $5^\triangle$ prism is held in either hand in position to be placed with the base (the thick edge) away from the nose before either eye and, after attention is fixed upon an object across the room, the prism is quickly placed before the eye, momentarily two objects will be seen but swiftly they will merge into one. Repeat the experiment several times. Now turn the prism to the position of base toward the nose. Again introduce it before one eye while looking at the distant object. The same result should be obtained; that is, temporary diplopia followed by single binocular vision. In either or both of these positions, the prism may cause a feeling of "drawing" or effort to sustain single vision. If the prism were to be worn for a period of time, headache or nausea may ensue. Reference to this experiment will be made when the positioning of correcting lenses is discussed.

Continue with the prism experiment by holding the prism Base Up or Base Down. This time two images will be seen one above the other. No reflex or voluntary effort will bring them together and there will be no sense of straining to fuse the images, only the displeasure of double vision. There is a very small fusion amplitude in the vertical meridian.

Years ago a lecturer impressed the function of fusion convergence upon his students with an anecdote. He told how if, in prehistoric times, Og did not have good fusion convergence and saw two wild animals instead of one and struck at the wrong one, he was the victim and therefore brought no meat home to his cave. Thus nature assured there would be no offspring with inherited defective fusion urge.

Ophthalmic dispensers are intensely concerned about this eye function. A cardinal misdeed is to cause unusual stress upon it. The first physiological measurement made before the fitting of lenses is directly related with it. There will be a return to this subject for fuller discussion in later chapters.

REVIEW

1. Why must the cornea function well as an optical surface?

2. What is the name of the condition when the surface of the cornea is ellipsoidal?

3. What is the crystalline lens?

4. What is the angular size of the accepted minimal retinal image?

5. When did Snellen devise the first test letters based upon this image size?

6. How is so-called normal vision rated 20/20?

7. Is vision equally acute over most of the retina? Discuss.

8. How did Helmholtz prove the crystalline lens changes shape?

9. Describe the usefulness of accommodation.

10. Using Duane's findings, when does loss of accommodation restrict comfortable near vision?

11. How does this involve ophthalmic dispensing?

12. Name the three errors of refraction.

13. In the world population is there a great difference in the percentages of hyperopia and myopia?

14. Identify accommodative convergence.

15. What are the alternates if it does not adequately match the requirements of accommodation?

16. Review the compensations made by fusion convergence when a prism was placed before the eyes in different positions.

ADDITIONAL REFERENCES

1. Scobee, Richard G.: *The Oculorotary Muscles.* St. Louis, Mosby, 1947.
2. Adler, Francis Heed: *Physiology of the Eye Clinical Application.* St. Louis, Mosby, 1950.
3. Sheard, Charles: *Visual and Ophthalmic Optics.* Philadelphia, Chilton, 1957.

Chapter 4

OPTICS AND LENSES

◆◆

Formulas to express relationships and physical actions of different optical forms of mirrors, prisms, and lenses are expressed by letters. Letters are used in the same way they were introduced in algebra. However, as far as possible, each letter will continue to represent only one concept. It is sensible to use letters because formulas would become senselessly involved to use phrases of two or more words when a single letter can express the idea.

Capital letters will be used for points as **O** for object, **I** for image, **F** for focal point, **N** for nodal point.

Since points are on lines, **OA** will describe the line from object to the apex of a surface. If, however, the length of a line or distance is the special consideration lower case letters will be used, u for object distance, v for image distance, f for focal distance. To distinguish angles from distances, Greek letters will be used, β, γ, δ, θ, et cetera. Rays will be identified by numerals in parenthesis (1), (2), et cetera. Secondary points which may be found in either the object side or the image side of a surface will be identified with a prime such as F′ for the secondary focal point.

These conventions are intended to reduce the feeling of "mathematical gibberish" which is sometimes associated with the use of letters instead of words.

To shorten the number of formulas required for the purposes of ophthalmic lens dispensing, the directed lines used in plotting quadratic equations in algebra will be used. These are called Cartesian coordinates after René Descarte (1596–1650), who proposed them for analytic geometry. High school students now learn their use in plotting quadratic equations in algebra.

An area is divided into four spaces by two intersecting lines. The horizontal line *(x-axis)* divides the area into upper and lower sections. The vertical line *(y-axis)* divides the area into left and

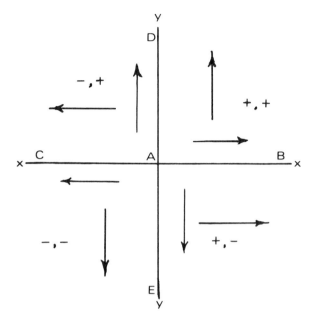

Figure 13. Cartesian coordinates.

right sections. Movement to the right of **A** is positive (+), movement to the left is negative (—), movement up is positive (+), movement down is negative (—). Hence the line segment **AB** is plus, but if the direction is reversed and the movement is to the left, the line **BA** is negative. It follows that with lines having the same terminals it can be stated that **AB** = — **BA**.

Line **AD** is measured *up*. Because the first letter is the starting point, **AD** is plus. **AE** is measured down, so it is negative (—). If **D** and **E** are the same distance from **A**, **AD** = — **AE**.

Light will be shown to originally move to the right in all illustrations.

AXIOMS AND THEOREMS

1. Two magnitudes equal to another magnitude are equal to other: **A** = **C**, **B** = **C**, ∴ **A** = **B**.
2. The sum of the angles of a triangle is 180°.
3. If the arms of an angle extend in one straight line, the angle is called a *straight* angle (180°).

4. If two straight lines intersect, the vertical (opposite) angles are equal.

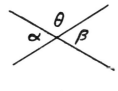

A

Figure 14. Angle relationships.
Figure 14*a*.

Proof: $\angle \alpha + \angle \theta =$ straight angle
$\angle \beta + \angle \theta =$ straight angle
$\angle \alpha$ and $\angle \beta$ are supplements of $\angle \theta$
$\therefore \angle \alpha = \angle \beta$

5. The alternate interior angles of two parallel lines cut by a transversal are equal.

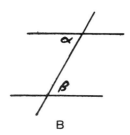

B

Figure 14*b*.

6. The corresponding angles of two parallel lines are equal.

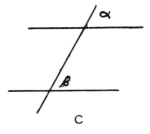

C

Figure 14*c*.

7. In Figure 15, $\angle \alpha = \angle \beta + \angle \lambda$

The sum of the angles of a triangle is 180° (a straight angle).

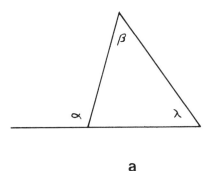

a

Figure 15*a*. External angle of a triangle equals the sum of alternate internal angles.

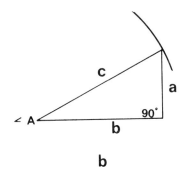

b

Figure 15*b*. Sides of triangle for ratios of functions of angle A.

Proof: $\angle \beta + \angle \lambda +$ the unidentified angle $=$ a straight angle

$\angle \alpha +$ the unidentified angle $=$ a straight angle

$\angle \alpha = \angle \beta + \angle \lambda$

Restated: An external angle of a triangle is equal to the sum of the two opposite interior angles.

The ratio between the hypotenuse, side *c*, and the altitude of the triangle, side *a*, would be expressed as "*a* is to *c*, or *a/c*." If the length of side *c* is chosen to be 1, the ratio becomes *a/*1 or *a*. For all angles less than 90°, side *a* is less than the hypotenuse *c*, hence the ratio is always a fraction.

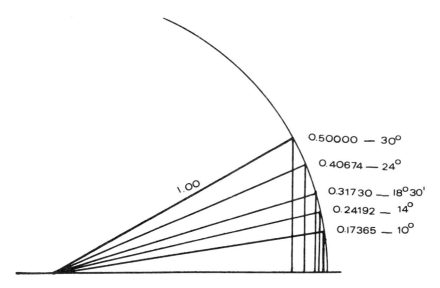

Figure 16. Sines of increasing angles.

At 90° the side *a* increases to the length of side *c*. At this point, the ratio is 1 (1/1 = 1). When the angle passes 90°, the length of side *a* shortens and a series of fractions is reproduced in descending order. Thus, this undulatory group of fractions has described a curve. In Latin, the word for a bend or a curve is *sinus*. From this word the name for the ratio *(a/c)* has been derived. This ratio of sides of the angle (function) is called *sine*, which is abbreviated to *sin*.

Other ways that ratios of the sides of angle **A** can be expressed are *c/a, a/b, b/a, b/c, c/b*. Of these, the next most useful for our purposes is *a/b*. In this ratio, *b* is taken as the base, or *b* = 1. This function is called tangent (tan) of angle **A** and the altitude is outside the arc. Hence, the tangent of a small angle approaches zero. As angle **A** increases to angle 45°, sides *a* and *b* are equal so the ratio equals 1.0000. When the angle increases past 45° and side *a* exceeds the length of *b*, the ratio exceeds 1 and increases very rapidly.

55° = 1.4281
65° = 2.1445

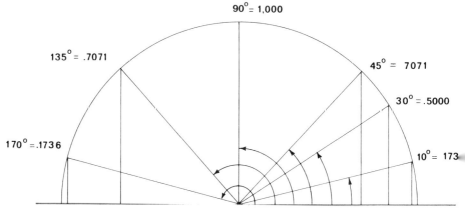

Figure 17. Sines in a 180° angle.

$75° = 3.7321$
$85° = 11.4301$
$90° = \infty$, because c and a are now parallel and the original triangle has disappeared.

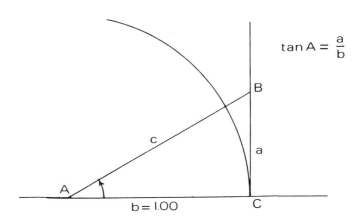

Figure 18. Description of tangent of angle A.

There is still another means by which angles are measured. This means of measurement is very useful in astronomy. The unit of this method of angle measurement is the *radian*. It is that angle in which the arc opposing the angle is the same length as the radius.

An entire turn around point **A** (360°) describes the circumference of the circle. It is remembered that diameter (2 radius) times π (3.1416) is the length of the circumference of the circle. Circumference $=$ D $\times$ π or 2r $\times$ π. It follows that 180° or half way around the circle can be stated as

180° $=$ radius times π, (π r), or
180° $=$ 3.1416 $\times$ radius (or 3.1416 radians)
$\therefore$ 1 radian $=$ 180° /3.1416 $=$ 57.296°

A radian was used by Doctor Dennett as his base for the development of a unit to measure the deviation of prisms (see "Unit of Measurement" later in this chapter).

Now, we have measured the angle at **A** in three ways:

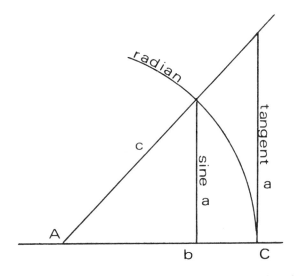

Figure 19. Illustration of sine, tangent, and radian of angle A.

For very small angles, the base line *(b)* approaches the length of the radius **AC** for all three of these means of measuring the angle; that is, sine, tangent, and radian are approximately equal and are therefore considered as equal for many calculations.

At 1°, sin = 0.0175; 0.0175 radians; tan = 0.0175
At 5°, sin = 0.0872; 0.0873 radians; tan = 0.0875
At 10°, sin = 0.1736; 0.1745 radians; tan = 0.1763

OPTICS

Optics in its entirety is the science of the study of light, and light, like other basic forces, is better understood for what it does than for what it is. Philosophers and scientists have propounded theories of its identity; each of these theories explained part of the phenomena of light but is inadequate in other parts. At the present time, the most widely accepted theory is that light consists of fluctuations in the strengths of electric and magnetic fields. These fluctuations are regularly named *waves*. The range of the lengths of these waves is extremely large. It extends all the way from radio waves which are 300 to 30,000 meters or more to gamma rays of radioactive substances 560 quadrillionths of a meter. Of all these wavelengths, only those between four ten-millionths and seven ten-millionths of a meter—or, as is usually written, 400 millicrons (mμ) for violet to 700 millimicrons (mμ) for red—are recognizable as visible light. Radiant energy in short-er wavelengths than violet—from ultraviolet to x-rays and the (γ) gamma rays of radium—are all injurious and finally destructive to the eye and human body.

A characteristic that substantiates the present definition of light is that it moves at the same rate of speed as electricity—namely 186,000 miles per second. From the first crude measurement in 1849 to the present day, there has been a variation of only about 5 percent of this distance. At the rate given, the reflected light from the moon arrives at the earth in less than two seconds. The television pictures from the astronauts required the same transmission time.

Optics is divided into several subjects. Physical optics and geometrical optics will first receive attention. Physical optics is the study of the stimulus called light and the investigation of its laws and properties. Ophthalmic dispensing is directly concerned with only a few of the segments of physical optics, but it is ad-visable that a dispenser, along with gaining technical information, supplement his knowledge of the subject with some collateral reading of physical optics. A high school physics text may serve as an introduction, to be followed by the reading of other texts such as *Optics, An Introduction for Ophthalmologists* by K. N. Ogle (Springfield, Thomas, 1968) and *Physical Optics* by Robert W. Wood (New York, Macmillan, 1934). Those facets of physical optics needed for our purposes will be stated with little discussion.

The portion of optics which is concerned with the movement of rays of light by optical systems is known as geometrical optics. Discussion of ophthalmic optics is by means of geometrical optics although, as is quite plain, basic concepts such as reflection and refraction are in the domain of physical optics.

Propagation of light by a wave theory provides the easiest explanation of some of the basic theories of optics. Since light moves simultaneously in all directions from a source, the wave motion is three-dimensional and difficult to imagine. Reduced to a two-dimensional concept it is much easier to visualize. Most authors use the analogue of waves on the surface of water. A stone dropped into a placid water becomes the center of circles of radiating waves. An object on the water surface undulates in the waves but does not disperse with them. In fact its motion is vertical and at a right angle to the radiation of the waves.

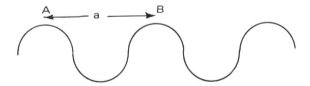

Figure 20. Cross section of light wave.

Figure 20 shows a cross section of the displacement of the smooth surface by waves. The length of a wave is the distance between corresponding points, such as from point **A** to point **B**, which mark the points where the waves rise from the former flat or calm surface. As the wave fronts radiate from the center and the radius increases with distance, the curvature of each wave front becomes flatter. When the waves radiate a great distance, the fronts of the waves lose their curvature and finally become straight. Thus, it is said that rays of light coming from an infinite distance are parallel.

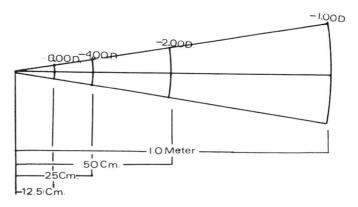

Figure 21. Radiation of wave front.

REFLECTION

Reflected light has some uses in ophthalmic optics. The refractionist often uses a mirror to increase the apparent distance to test letters. A reflected image on the cornea is used as the object for the measurement of the curvature of the cornea (keratometry). Originally this measurement was the *sine qua non* to find the astigmatic error in sight-testing. Now it is a basic measurement in contact lens fitting. Corneal reflections are used as objects for the measurement of interocular distance. Reflected light is used for the inspection of lens surfaces in lens-making. The aerial images of reflections from lens surfaces may be unpleasant for spectacle wearers. Both ophthalmoscopes and retinoscopes use mirrors to reflect light into eyes for the purpose of examination.

In 1678 Huygens proved that the angle of incidence and angle of reflection were equal in his treatise presented to the Royal Academy of Science. No one has presented a simpler description of this phenomenon.

Wave front **AC** from an infinite distance with a flat wave front is incident upon reflecting surface **AB** at point **A**. In the interval while point **C** is arriving at the surface, the ray that fell upon

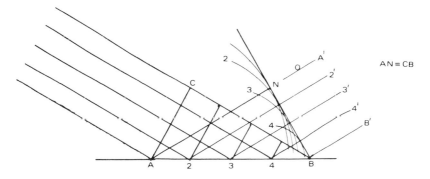

Figure 22. Schematic demonstration of the reflection of a ray.

point **A** is reflected and it will have moved an equal distance to some point upon an arc with radius **AN** = **CB**. **BN** represents the wave front reflected from the surface. Rays (2), (3), and (4) are parallel to **CB** and are reflected similarly. Finally, the tangent to all of these reflections is a straight line **NB**. This line is at the same angle to **AB** as **AC**. Thus, the law of reflection has been demonstrated by construction.

An example of a totally reflecting surface is the polished metal surfaced mirror used in an eye examining room.

The full definition of the law of reflection is that a ray of light falling upon a reflecting surface is reflected at the same angle of reflection as measured from the normal (perpendicular) to the surface as the angle of the incident ray and in the same plane.

Rays of light falling upon a regularly curved surface such as a spherical surface return to or seem to come from a focus. At each point of incidence a tangent plane could be drawn and the reflection could be treated in the way described for a flat surface, but there are methods by which such a tedious method can be avoided. Figure 23 illustrates the tracing of a *paraxial* ray striking a curved surface.

As **D** approaches **A**
DM → **AM**
DM' → **AM'**

From this instance a general formula for all reflected rays from a curved surface can be demonstrated. First, the specific lengths

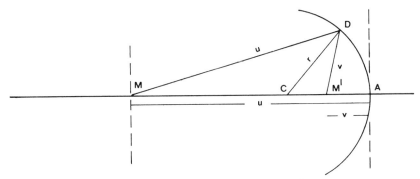

Figure 23. Reflection from a concave surface.

such as **M, AM, AM', DM',** and **AC** are expressed in small letters for lengths, such as u, v, and r. Remember that all lengths are measured from **A** and are directed lines. Hence **AC** $= r$ and **CA** $= -r$. The image distance v will be solved by using the other lengths in simple algebraic equations. The special instance when the object rays are parallel (that is, coming from infinity) will be considered.

In order to show all the angles and lines clearly, Figure 23 is expanded vertically. Hence **DM'** and **M'A** in the figure are obviously not the same length. Since this formula is being derived by geometrical optics with paraxial rays, the angle at **M** is *very* small. This in turn makes the arc **AD** *very* short. When **D** is very close to **A**, the length **DM'** → **AM**. The image distance v is measured **AM'**, therefore **M'A** $= -v$.

Let **AM** $= u$, **AM'** $= v$, and **AC** $= r$.

Since the $\angle$ **CDM** $= \angle$ **M'DC** ($\angle$ $i = \angle$ r) and the normal **CD** is the bisector ($\angle$ $i = \angle$ r) of the angle **D** in the Δ **MDM'**, the following proportion is true:

$$\frac{CM}{DM} = \frac{M'C}{DM'}$$

If the ray **MD** is paraxial, then **A** may be substituted for **D** and the above proportion becomes

$$\frac{CM}{AM} = \frac{M'C}{AM'} \text{ or } \frac{CM}{u} = \frac{M'G}{v}$$

It follows that

$$CM = CA + AM = -r + u = u - r$$
$$M'C = M'A + AC = -v + r$$

Substituting,

$$\frac{u - r}{u} = \frac{-v + r}{v}$$

Simplifying by cross-multiplication of the denominators,

$$uv - rv = -uv + ur$$

Changing signs,

$$-uv + rv = uv - ur$$

Rearranging,

$$rv + ur = 2\,uv$$

Dividing by urv,

$$\frac{1}{u} + \frac{1}{v} = \frac{2}{r}$$

When

$$u = \infty, \text{ so that } 1/u = 0$$

Then

$$\frac{1}{v} = \frac{2}{r}, \text{ or } v = \frac{r}{2}$$

Thus it is shown that rays very close to the axis are reflected by a concave spherical surface to a point that is half the length of the radius of the curve.

Figure 24 demonstrates that, when the incident rays fall on the surface at some distance from the axis and the angle of incidence increases, with each increase in distance from the axis the angles of reflection will correspondingly increase. Hence, these rays will not intersect the xx' axis at **F** but will fall increasingly closer to point **A**. This deviation from the formula for *paraxial* rays is an aberration which is known as spherical aberration.

Such approximations as have been used to develop this formula for the focussing of rays reflected by a curved surface are frequently used in geometrical optics. The use of approximations is not peculiar to optics. For instance, the relationship of the circumference to the radius of a circle, π, is an irrational number. The commonly used 3.1416 is considered sufficiently accurate for ordinary usage, and for quick mental calculations $3^1/_7$ is used, but when great lengths are involved in astronomy the fraction is often carried out further, 3.141592653589793+. The customary limit of the distance of rays from the axis to form a point focus is within 1° at the point of reflection. This will be discussed again with refraction formulas.

Further investigation shows that if the curvature were not

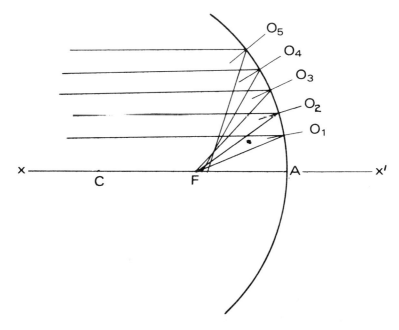

Figure 24. Astigmatic focus by reflection.

spherical and if the radius of curvature were longer (the curve flatter) toward the margin, all the rays could be brought more nearly to the same focal point. This is our first introduction to the use of an aspherical (parabolic) surface. This is the form of the concave mirror used for astronomical telescopes. In order to gather as much light from the stars as possible, the mirrors must be very large. Thus the blurred image from a spherical surface is greatly improved by parabolizing (figuring) the surface. In Chapter 12 this type of surface for ophthalmic lenses will be discussed again.

REFRACTION

At a transparent surface some of the incident rays are reflected as in the case of an opaque mirror, but more than 90 percent of the rays enter the lens material. Although the lens material may seem and also be called transparent, the physical constituents in even the clearest medium absorb a small part of the light that passes through the lens. This light loss is a function of the type of material and its thickness. Some lens materials are designed to absorb a portion of the light transmitted through them. This is accomplished by adding some chemical form of a metal or metals to the material. Such materials are used for sunglasses.

When a ray of light falls on any optical surface normal to that surface, the ray continues in the same direction without deviation. When rays of light fall (are incident) upon a surface at any angle to the normal, the rays are refracted (deviated) from their former direction. The amount of deviation is dependent upon the angle with the normal and the composition (optical index) of the medium (material).

A variation of Huygens construction demonstrating the direction of a refracted ray will be used.

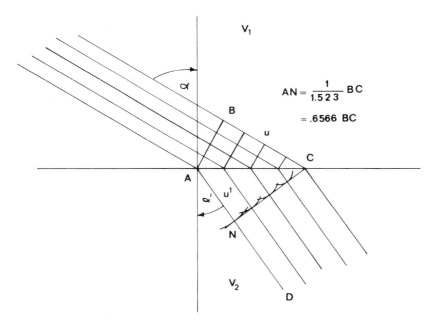

$$AN = \frac{1}{1.523} BC$$
$$= .6566 \ BC$$

Figure 25. Huygens' construction of refracted ray.

Where t = time
 V_1 = velocity of light in the first medium
 V_2 = velocity of light in the second medium
 u_1 = incident ray
 u_2 = refracted ray

Then $t = u_1/V_1$
 $1/u = V$
 $u_2 = V_2 t$
 $u_1 = V_1 t$
 $u_1/u_2 = V_1 t/V_2 t = V_1/V_2$

When the ray from infinite distance falls upon the surface at **A**, point **B** on the same wave front must still travel the distance of u_1 to reach the surface. The time required is the distance divided by the velocity, $t = u_1/V_1$.

While the ray at point **B** approaches the surface, the ray at **A** has entered the second medium. By the time the ray has travelled the distance of u_1, the ray from point **A** will now be the distance u_2 from **A** which would be $u_2 = V_2 t$. The points **N** and **B** must describe lines perpendicular to the direction of the ray because the wave front is flat, since its origin is infinity. With radius V_{1BC}/V_2, a short arc is struck at **A** to demonstrate the points at which this ray may have arrived. If a line is drawn from **C**, where the ray has now arrived tangent to this arc at point **N**, it will describe the new wave front because the tangent is perpendicular to the radius at the point of tangency. The radius is continued through point **D** to show the direction of the ray from point **A** through the new medium. The ray from point **C** is constructed parallel to the line **AD**.

It is observed that the angle of refraction is *less* than the angle of incidence. The law is that when light passes into a denser medium, e.g. from air into glass, the ray is bent *toward* the normal.

REVERSIBILITY OF LIGHT RAYS

The path of light rays is reversible. Therefore, without describing the construction it is manifest that when light rays move from a dense to a rarer medium, such as from glass into air, the angle of refraction is *larger* than the angle of incidence and the ray is bent *away* from the normal.

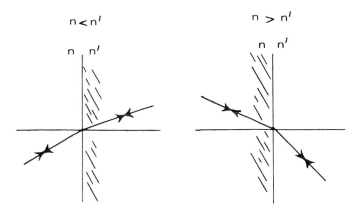

Figure 26. Reversability of light rays.

Although Huygens' demonstration of refraction bears upon the velocity of light in the two media, it shows the relationship of the sines of the two angles as was first described by Willibrord Snell in 1621. This ratio is

$$\frac{\text{sine of the angle of incidence}}{\text{sine of the angle of refraction}} = \frac{V_1}{V_2} \qquad \text{Law (1)}$$

This relationship is a constant for all angles and is named the index of refraction with the symbol n or sometimes μ (mu). Thus

$$n_1 = \frac{\text{sine of the incident angle } \textit{in vacuo}}{\text{sine of the refraction angle in first medium}}$$

$$= \frac{\text{velocity of light } \textit{in vacuo}}{\text{velocity of light in first medium}}$$

For a second medium which has an index of refraction of n_2

$$n_2 = \frac{\text{velocity of light } \textit{in vacuo}}{\text{velocity of light in second medium}}$$

The relationship of n_2 to n_1 is found by dividing

$$\frac{n_2}{n_1} = \frac{\dfrac{\text{velocity of light } \textit{in vacuo}}{\text{velocity of light in second medium}}}{\dfrac{\text{velocity of light } \textit{in vacuo}}{\text{velocity of light in first medium}}}$$

Simplifying the compound fraction

$$\frac{n_2}{n_1} = \frac{\text{velocity } in \ vacuo}{\text{velocity in second medium}} \times \frac{\text{velocity in first medium}}{\text{velocity } in \ vacuo}$$

$$\frac{n_2}{n_1} = \frac{\text{velocity in first medium}}{\text{velocity in second medium}}$$

By substituting from Law (1)

$$\frac{n_2}{n_1} = \frac{\sin i}{\sin r}$$

Which is usually written

$$\frac{n'}{n} = \frac{\sin i}{\sin i'}$$

From which follows

$$n' \sin i' = n \sin i$$

This is named Snell's Law or sometimes Snell's Law of Sines. It is the basic law of refraction and it, or forms derived from it, are involved in all lens problems.

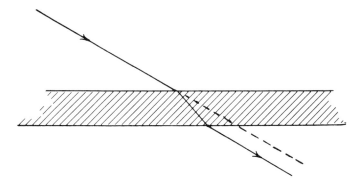

Figure 27. Displacement of oblique ray.

When a ray strikes the surface of a piece of glass with plane parallel surfaces at an oblique angle, the ray continues in its original direction but is displaced. This effect is not noticeable unless the object is near (0.5 meter or less) to the eye. Another phenomenon is that when an object is viewed through a plane parallel piece of glass it seems to be slightly closer (therefore magnified) to the eye. Again this effect is not noticed when the object is at some distance from the eye. The displacement then becomes a very small percentage of the total distance. The percentage angular magnification (which is dependent upon the thickness of the glass, the distance of the object, and index of glass shown by Ogle*) is as follows.

Where t = thickness of glass in meters
u = object distance in meters (object is in or adjacent to the glass)
n = index of refraction

Then $t\left(\dfrac{n-1}{n}\right)$ = % angular magnification

REDUCED DISTANCE

The amount that the object seems to be elevated in the glass was named *reduced distance* by Gauss. It is defined as the actual thickness of the medium (usually glass) divided by the index of refraction of the medium. This gives the apparent position of the magnified image of an object seen through the medium.

A simple demonstration of *reduced distance* is made with a low-power microscope. A mark is made on the top side of a microscope slide and the microscope is focussed upon the mark. Place a piece of plate glass about 0.5 inch thick on top of the slide. The mark will now be slightly out of focus. Refocus the microscope to clear up the image. The distance that the microscope is raised is the apparent elevation of the mark in the glass. This amount subtracted from the total thickness gives the *reduced distance.*

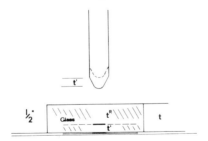

Figure 28. Reduced distance.

Where t = the total thickness of the glass
t' = the distance the image is apparently raised in the glass
t^R = the Reduced Distance

Reduced distance (t' in Fig. 28) is simply the real distance

---

*Ogle, K.N.: *Optics*. Springfield, Thomas, 1968.

divided by the index of the medium (substance) in which the object lays. It is expressed as t/n. The formulas relating to the vertex power of lenses require consideration of *reduced distance*.

The iris of the eye is situated behind the anterior chamber which is filled with aqueous humor $(n = 1.336)$. Hence the pupil of the eye appears to be about three-fourths its real depth because of *reduced distance*.

Small dimensional differences (0.5%) are discernible by a person with normal acuity. Reference is made to this magnification in the discussion of magnification by prescription lenses and also in the discussion of dissimilar ocular images (aniseikonia).

PRISMS

A prism was used in an experiment in Chapter 2 to demonstrate the urge to fusion. When the prism was held with the thick edge (base) up or down, it produced diplopia by displacing one object above or below the other. Occasionally prisms are prescribed for the correction or stimulation of the extraocular muscles. The definition of a prism is a refracting element bounded by two non-parallel surfaces.* The edge or thinnest part of the principal section of a prism is the apex. The thickest part of a principal section is the base.

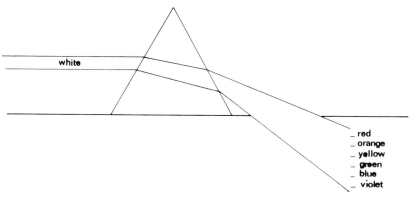

Figure 29. Dispersion of light ray.

*BS. 3521: *Glossary of Terms Relating to Ophthalmic Lenses*. London, British Standards Institution, 1962.

Isaac Newton (1640) demonstrated that white light could be spread (dispersed) with a prism to create a spectrum. Equally important, he showed that the spectrum could be recombined into white light with an identical prism. The fact that glass has an increasing index of refraction for the colors from red to violet caused the light to spread out into the colors of a rainbow.

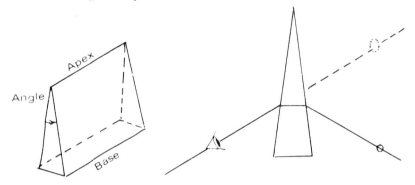

Figure 30. Deviation of light ray.

Although light rays are deviated toward the base of a prism, the eye projects the deviated rays in the direction from which they were received, thereby seeing the object displaced toward the apex.

If a prism is positioned to have the first surface perpendicular to the direction of a light ray, the light falling on the first surface will not be deviated. When the ray strikes the second surface, it will have an incidence angle equal to the angle at the apex of the prism; because the ray is moving from a higher index of refraction into a lower index (air), the ray is deviated from the normal. By Snell's law of refraction, $n_2 \sin \alpha^1 = n_1 \sin \alpha$ (**A**). Since $n_2 =$ air $= 1$ and because the angles are very small,

$$n_2 \sin \alpha^1 = \alpha^1 - \alpha = \alpha^1 - A$$
$$= nA - A$$
$$\text{Prism deviation} = A (n - 1)$$

Since the index of refraction of crown glass used for ophthalmic lenses is usually $n = 1.523$, $(1.523 - 1 = 0.523)$ prism deviation $= \delta = 0.523$. Hence the deviation of the prism is about one-half the angle of the apex.

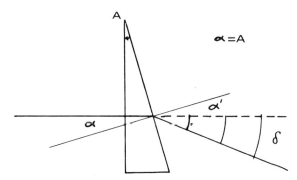

Figure 31.   Geometry of prism deviation.

UNIT OF MEASUREMENT

The first term to denote prism power was the angle in degrees at the apex. Because it was difficult to identify without special equipment and varied with the index of the glass used, it was discontinued before 1900 but the erroneous term "degree" is occasionally heard though "prism diopter" is intended.

Prentice,* in 1890, proposed that the optical effect of a prism be used for the unit and that the displacement be measured on a plane (or wall) perpendicular to the line of vision. Such a unit is not additive, because as the angle of deviation increases the tangent plane of the wall is farther from the eye than in the original measurement.

Ophthalmologist Dennett took exception to this disparity and undertook to provide a unit which was measured on the arc instead of the tangent. He divided a radian (57.3 arc degrees) by 100 and called the unit *centrad*.† Since this amount of deviation (0.57°) is very similar to Prentice's Prism Diopter in small amounts and since the wall of the refracting room was a convenient tangent plane while there was no simple means to set up an arcuate surface, the mathematically precise unit did not survive Doctor Dennett's circle of friends. Practically, the difference in units is almost academic because the vast majority of prisms pre-

---

*Prentice, C.F.: *Ophthalmic Lenses and Other Optical Papers*. Philadelphia, Keystone Press, 1907.

†BS. 3521: *Glossary of Terms Relating to Ophthalmic Lenses*. London, British Standards Institution, 1962.

scribed are less than 10 Prism Diopters (within 5° of the primary line).

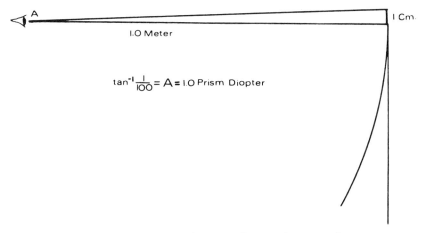

Figure 32. Prism Diopter and centrad compared.

Prentice's proposal was to name the unit "Prism Diopter" and that it be the deviation of 1 centimeter at 1 meter.

$$\tan \frac{1}{100} (.01) = \Delta$$

It can be shown that the effect of a prism is somewhat less than its marked amount if the object is at a near point. In clinical practice this is of no importance because the measuring prism was used at near point and the prescribed prism will be made to the power of the measuring prism.

Since the deviation is in the base-apex meridian, a prism varies in its vertical and horizontal prism effects if it is placed at an oblique angle. Resolving the resultant vertical and horizontal prism power of oblique prisms was an arduous chore for a dispensing optician in days gone by, but improved refracting procedures and equipment tend to produce lens prescriptions uniformly resolved into prism bases horizontal and vertical. Present-day lens surface generating machinery and lens-analyzing instruments (lensometers) are designed to produce and inspect compound prisms as the prescription is written.

Lest it be charged that this item has been overlooked, to find the single prism power that is the equivalent of two prisms with bases at right angles or the reverse problem of resolving a prism with a diagonal base-apex line is vector analysis.

(a) Combine 1.5$^\Delta$ Base Down with 2.0$^\Delta$ Base In.

Draw lines to represent the powers of the prisms on polar co-ordinate paper. The length of the diagonal (hypotenuse) is the prism power of the combination. It can be easily determined by the circles on the paper.

Using two units for 1 Prism Diopter (for accuracy), the Base In prism is marked at 4 spaces while the Base Down prism is located at 3 spaces. When the rectangle is completed, it is seen that the diagonal is 5 spaces (2.5$^\Delta$) long. The axis of the prism is tan α = 1.5/2 = 3/4 = 0.7500 = tan 36° 52'. Hence, the combination is resolved as 2.5$^\Delta$ axis 37° Base In and Down.

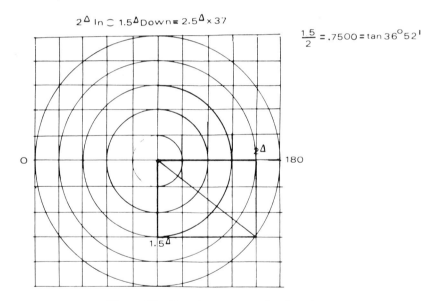

Figure 33. Prentice compound prism chart.

(b) Combine 2$^\Delta$ Base Out 2.5$^\Delta$ Base Up.

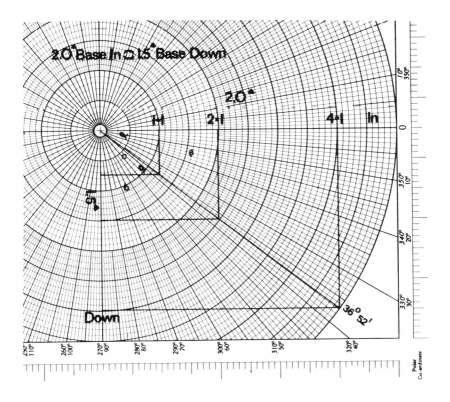

Figure 34.

When plotted, we find the diagonal to measure 6.4^Δ and the axis of the prism $= 2.5/2 = 1.2500 = \tan 51° 20'$ above the 180 line or axis 129 Base Up and Out for the right eye or axis 51 Base Up and Out for the left eye.

(c) Resolve 5^Δ at axis 145 Up and In for the Left Eye into its Base In and Base Up components.

Draw a line from center to the fifth circle at axis 145. Since this axis is more than 90°, it will be measured as the distance from 180° or 35°.

When the tangent table is consulted, $\tan 35 = 0.7002$. For this problem, the tangent is equal to 0.7 which identifies the relationship of the lengths of the sides of the rectangle, i.e. as 7 is to 10.

Referring to the drawing, the horizontal (base) line is only slightly more than 4 units, the vertical side by the calculation should be 0.7 as long or 2.8. From this we can conclude that the single prism is generated by 4ᐃ Base In and 2.75ᐃ Base Up.

THEORY OF LENSES

Consistent with the notion of a wave theory, since light radiates simultaneously in all directions from a point source and since it moves at the same velocity in all directions in the same medium (for example, air), the wave fronts describe spheres of increasing radius. This progress of light radiating from a source is referred to as *vergence*.

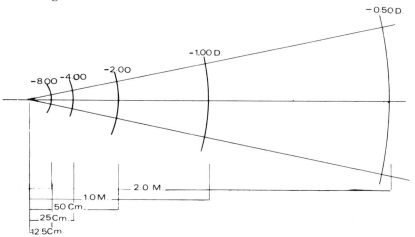

Figure 35.   Divergence of a light ray.

Close to the source when the radius is very short there is great curvature to the wave front, but as the distance from the source increases, the curvature of the surface diminishes until finally at an infinite distance the wave front is flat and perpendicular to the direction of the light. It follows that the curvature of the wave front is the reciprocal of the distance. If the distance of the wave front from the source is measured in meters the vergence is known as Diopters. The vergence at one meter is 1 Diopter which is written 1.00D. When the wave front has expanded to 2 meters with half the former vergence = 0.50D.

Light diverging from a point is called negative (—) vergence. Conversely light which converges toward a point is known as positive (+) vergence. It follows that lenses which cause parallel light to diverge are named minus (—) lenses and those lenses that direct parallel rays toward a point focus are termed plus (+) lenses. Lenses and their effects can be diagrammed as in Figure 36.

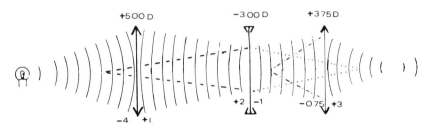

Figure 36. Wave-front lens calculations.

Using the notion of vergences, the light path through a series of lenses can be diagrammed. By this tedious process an artillery range finder was redesigned for the Air Corps during World War I because no optical engineer was available at this particular lens shop who could use the conventional ray tracing (not wave front) method.

These calculations and all similar lens work involve a great deal of multiplication and division of numbers with five or more digits. Long ago, a means to simplify this work was the project of mathematicians. The solution to the problem follows.

LOGARITHMS

In 1590, Lord Napier, a Scotsman, observed that when the exponents of a number were increased in an arithmetic sequence the powers of the number increased geometrically. For instance, look at the numeral 2. Its first power is itself, 1×2 or $2^1 = 2$, but the square of 2 is 2×2 or $2^2 = 4$. It follows that

$$2 \times 2 \times 2 = 2^3 = 8$$
$$2 \times 2 \times 2 \times 2 = 2^4 = 16$$
$$2 \times 2 \times 2 \times 2 \times 2 = 2^5 = 32$$

It would seem logical that all of the numbers falling in the intervening spaces between these powers of 2 would have fractional exponents. For example, the number 6 is more than 2^2 (4) and less than 2^3 (8). By this reasoning $6 = 2^{2.xxxx}$. Napier's invention was to discover the mathematical formula which would find these fractional exponents and then list the individual solutions. The value of this reasoning was that it could be applicable to any other number (base), as well as 2. Further, when these fractional exponents were *added*, the sum would give the *product* of the numbers. Research proved the hypothesis to be true, so Napier proceeded with the laborious task of producing such a list. He published his first results in 1614 (twenty-five years later). Because Napier chose an incomensurable number *e* as the base for his calculations, his natural or hyperbolic system is confined to theoretical mathematics.

He named this table A Table of Logarithms. This new word was formed from the Greek words *logos* (proportion) and *arithmos* (number).

He was assisted in this work by his intimate friend, Briggs. After Napier died (1617), Briggs concluded the development of the work by using the number 10 as the base number. This selection as the base number is very important because it fits our decimal system of notation. For example:

$$10 \times 10 = 10^1 + 10^1 = 10^2 = 100$$
$$10 \times 100 = 10^1 + 10^2 = 10^3 = 1,000$$
$$100 \times 100 = 10^2 + 10^2 = 10^4 = 10,000$$

The logarithms of numbers between the given powers may be estimated such as $8523 = 2.93059$. For purposes of identification, the whole number (2) of the logarithm is called the *characteristic* and the decimal fraction is called the *mantissa*. These words are seldom used.

Although these pages of numerals (see Fig. 37) may seem formidable, they are not as mysterious as they look. The sequence

FIVE-PLACE LOGARITHMS (Continued)

N.	0	1	2	3	4	5	6	7	8	9
300	47 712	727	741	756	(770)	784	799	813	828	842
301	857	871	885	900	914	929	943	958	972	986
302	48 001	015	029	044	058	073	087	101	116	130
303	144	159	173	187	202	216	230	244	259	273
304	287	302	316	330	344	359	373	387	401	416
305	430	444	458	473	487	501	515	530	544	558
306	572	586	601	615	629	643	657	671	686	700
307	714	728	742	756	770	785	799	813	827	841
308	855	869	883	897	911	926	940	954	968	982
309	996	*010	*024	*038	*052	*066	*080	*094	*108	*122
310	49 136	150	164	178	192	206	220	234	248	262
311	276	290	304	318	332	346	360	374	388	402
312	415	429	443	457	471	485	499	513	527	541
313	554	568	582	596	610	624	638	651	665	679
314	693	707	721	734	748	762	776	790	803	817
315	831	845	859	872	886	900	914	927	941	955
316	969	982	996	*010	*024	*037	*051	*065	*079	*092
317	50 106	120	133	147	161	174	188	202	215	229
318	243	256	270	284	297	311	325	338	352	365
319	379	393	406	420	433	447	461	474	488	501
320	515	529	542	556	569	583	596	610	623	637
321	651	664	678	691	705	718	732	745	759	772
322	786	799	813	826	840	853	866	880	893	907
323	920	934	947	961	974	987	*001	*014	*028	*041
324	51 055	068	081	095	108	121	135	148	162	175
325	188	202	215	228	242	255	268	282	295	308
326	322	335	348	362	375	388	402	415	428	441
327	455	468	481	495	508	521	534	548	561	⁻'
328	587	601	614	627	640	654	667	680	693	
329	720	733	746	759	772	786	799	ᵒ¹ᶜ	⁻⁻⁻	
330	851	865	878	891	904	91⁻	930			
331	983	996	*009	*022	*035	*0⸍	¹			
332	52 114	127	140	153	166					
333	244	257	270	284	297					
334	375	388	401	'4	ᐟ7					
335	504	517	530							
336	6⸍	647	�ᶿ0							
337	⸴	⸳								
338										
339	53									
340										

Figure 37. Sample page of logarithm table.

of numbers down the left side can be used for 3, 30, or 300 or any power of 10 × 3. The identification of the power of 3 is indicated by the *characteristic* before the fraction (logarithm). For 3, which is between 10° and 10¹, the characteristic is 0 with the fraction added, hence,

$$3 = 0.47712$$
$$30 = 1.47712$$
$$300 = 2.47712$$

Across the top of the page are decimal fractions of the numerals on the side. For example: 3004 = 3.47770. Thus, the complete table identifies all the numerals from 1 to 10,000.

To Multiply

EXAMPLE: 31 × 2

$$\log 31 = 1.49136$$
$$+ \log \ 2 = 0.30103$$
$$\overline{1.79239}$$

Turn the pages of the table until .79239 is found. In the table, it is at 620. However, the product must be more than 10 and less than 100, so the answer is 62, which had already been done mentally. But now a more difficult multiplication can be done just as easily.

EXAMPLE: 477 × 69

$$\log 447 = 2.67852$$
$$+ \log \ 69 = 1.83885$$
$$\overline{4.51737}$$

Between 10⁴ = 10,000 and 10⁵ = 100,000, 3291 = .51733 and 3292 = .51746, so the product is between 32910 and 32920. The last digits of the numbers to be multiplied are (47) 7 and (6) 9, so 7 × 9 = 63. Hence the precise product is 32913.

EXAMPLE: 4063 × 403

$$\log 4063 = 3.60885$$
$$+ \log \ 403 = 2.60531$$
$$\overline{6.21416}$$

When the table is searched for .21416, it gives the number 1637, which must be expressed in a quantity greater than 10⁶ (1,000,000) and less than 10^7 (10,000,000). Therefore, 1,637,000 is the product.

It is obvious that this is not the precise product. However, the error is not more than 1/10,000 or 0.1 percent. An error of this size is permissible for most calculations. However, if the product must be more precisely known, a seven-place (not five place) table would be consulted.

To Find nth Root

EXAMPLES $\sqrt[5]{3125}$

$$\log 3125 = 3.49485$$
$$\div \quad 5 = 0.69897$$

Using the table, we see that the fifth root of 3125 is 5.
Proof: $5 \times 5 \times 5 \times 5 \times 5 = 3125$

Numbers Less Than Zero

Numbers less than zero have minus characteristics, such as

$$.2 = -1.30103$$
$$.07 = -2.84510$$
$$.0035 = -3.54707$$

However, it is easy to make mistakes when $+$ and $-$ numbers are added, so it has become a custom to show the characteristic with 10 subtracted from it, such as

$$-1.30103 = \overline{9}.30103 - 10$$

In practice the -10 is seldom written, so the list above becomes

$$.2 = \overline{9}.30103$$
$$.07 = \overline{8}.84510$$
$$.0035 = \overline{7}.54707$$

These large characteristics are immediate signals that the number is a decimal fraction. Let us apply this to a typical optical problem, where n is the index of refraction of the medium, in this instance optical glass.

To Multiply

EXAMPLE: $(n - 1) \times 0.975$

$$n - 1 = 1.53 - 1.00 = .53$$
$$\log \quad .53 = \overline{9}.72428$$
$$+ \log \quad .975 = \overline{9}.98900$$
$$\overline{\overline{9}.71328}$$

This falls between 71332 and 71341 in the log table, thus the number is between .5167 and .5168. However, (5) 3 $\times$ (97) 5 = 15. Hence the last digit is 5 and 0.51675 is the precise product.

To Divide

EXAMPLE: 18264 $\div$ 71

$$
\begin{array}{r}
\log 18260 = 4.26150 \\
-\log \quad 71 = 0.85126 \\
\hline
3.41034
\end{array}
$$

This is between 41027 and 41044, so the number is between 2572 and 2573. On the right hand side of the pages of Logarithm Tables are groups of numerals. These are used for extrapolation in those instances when the sum or differences of logarithms falls between numerals in the tables. In this instance the difference of the two numbers in the table between which 41034 falls is a difference of 17 (41027 and 41044). The number 41034 is 7 more than 41027. In the set of numbers for 17, 6.8 = 4. Since it is the closest to 7, its value of 4 is added to the antilog 2572 which makes the quotient 2572.4.

In most calculations, this extension arrived at by extrapolation is unnecessary. The error is less than one ten-thousandth of the quotient.

Continue with some more exercises of your own invention in multiplication and division. The practice in the use of the table will prove beneficial in future use of the special Table of Trigonometric Logarithm Functions for problems involving angles.

SPHERICAL ABERRATION

As previously demonstrated with a curved reflecting surface (Fig. 24), the rays that strike the surface close to the axis of the reflector have the longest focal distance; rays that strike the surface at the margin reflect to cross the axis nearer the reflecting surface. By Snell's Law, refracted rays are a ratio of the sines of the incident and refracted rays. Reference to a sine table shows a constant decrease in difference between the sines as angles increase in size. Hence, marginal refracted rays, like reflected rays, focus closer to the surface.

sin 5 = .08716
sin 10 = .17365, a .08649 increase
sin 15 = .25882, a .08517 increase
sin 20 = .34202, a .08320 increase
sin 25 = .42262, a .08060 increase
sin 30 = .50000, a .07738 increase

From this information it becomes obvious that refraction formulas must have limitations to be workable. First, the formula must refer to rays very close to the lens axis, and second, the formula must be in terms of geometry (lines) and not trigonometry (angles).

Rays very close to the axis at a curved surface are called *paraxial* rays. Emsley, in his *Aberration of Thin Lenses* (1956), provides an excellent discussion of paraxial rays. "These rays are those which are incident upon a lens surface so close to the axis of the surface that the trigonometric functions (sines and tangents) are identical." If you refer to your Natural Function Table, you will note that a four-place table shows sines and tangents for less than 1° are the same. At 1° they are each .0175. It is obvious that this is again an approximation. A five-place table would show that they begin to differ slightly below 1°, and a seven-place (Vega) would show a difference still closer to zero. However, for all practical purposes, 1° is satisfactory because an error of less than one ten-thousandth is inconsiderable in terrestrial calculations.

It is now apparent that Snell's Law must be expressed in geometrical units (lines) and a formula must be derived.

With the use of logarithms to help simplify the work, let us apply Snell's Law to calculate the paths of several parallel rays through a convex surface at different distances from the axis of the curve. Four rays are chosen at 0.5, 1.0, 2.5, and 5.0 cm from the axis. The radius of the curve is chosen as 10 cm. The index of refraction of the second medium n' (glass) is 1.523.

The distance in the second medium (n') from the surface to where the refracted ray crosses the axis is the focal length. As expected, this length reduces as the incident ray strikes the surface at each increased distance from the axis.

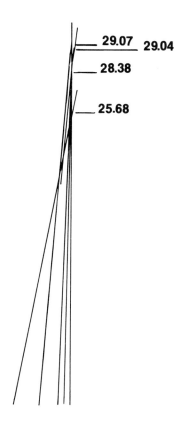

Figure 38. Spherical aberration of a curved surface calculated.

The calculations will be done either by arithmetic or logarithms. As an exercise, recalculate each focal length by the other method. Retain these notes for future reference.

Snell's Law (n' sin 1' = n sin 1) has been reexpressed using the data in Figure 38 to read: $n_1 \sin \theta_1 = n_2 \sin \theta_2$

The 0.5 Cm RAY

sin $\angle \; \theta_1$ = h/r = 0.5/radius = 0.5/10 = 0.0500
0.0500 = 2° 52′ = angle of incidence
sin $\angle \; \theta_2$ = (sin θ_1)/n′ = .0500/1.523 = .03283 = 1° 53′ = angle of refraction $\angle$ of deviation = $\angle \; \delta'$ = $\angle \; \theta_1$ − $\angle \; \theta_2$ = 2° 52′ − 1° 53′ = 0° 59′

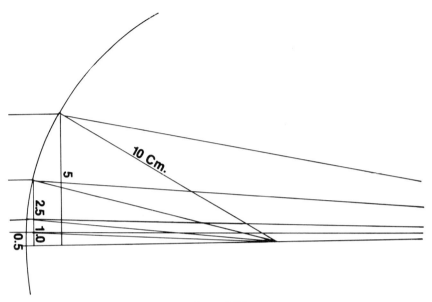

Figure 38R.

$\tan \angle \ \delta' = a/b$; $b_1 = a/\tan \delta = 0.5/.0172 = 29.07$ cm, the distance from the surface to the point where the ray crosses the axis. This is the focal length of the 0.5 ray.

The 1.0 Cm Ray

$\log \sin \angle \ \theta_1 = 1.0/10 = \overline{9}.00000 = 5° \ 44.3'$

$\log \sin \angle \ \theta_2 = \quad \log .10000 = \overline{9}.00000$
$\qquad \qquad \qquad - \log \ 1.523 = 0.18270$
$\qquad \qquad \qquad \qquad \overline{\qquad \qquad}$
$\qquad \qquad \qquad \qquad 9.81730 = 3° \ 46'$

$\delta_2 = 5° \ 44.3' - 3° \ 46' = 1° \ 58.3'$, $\log \tan \ \delta_2 = \overline{8}.53700$
$b_2 = \quad \log 1.0 \quad = 0.00000$
$\qquad - \log \tan \ \delta_2 = \overline{8}.53700$
$\qquad \qquad \qquad \overline{\qquad \qquad}$
$\qquad \qquad 1.46300 = 29.04$ cm, the focal length.

The 2.5 Cm Ray

$\sin \angle \theta_1 = h/\text{radius} = 2.5/10 = 0.2500 = 14° \ 29'$

$\sin \angle \theta_2 = 0.2500/1.523 = 0.1642 = 9° \ 27'$

$\delta_3 = 14° \ 29' - 9° \ 27' = 5° \ 2'$

$b_3 = 2.5/\tan \delta_3 = 2.5/.0881 = 28.38$ cm, the focal length.

The 5.0 Cm Ray

$\log \sin \angle \theta_1 = 5/10 = \overline{9}.69897 = 30°$

$\log \sin \angle \theta_2 = \quad \log \angle \theta_1 = 9.69897$

$\qquad\qquad\qquad - \log 1.523 = 0.18270$

$\qquad\qquad\qquad\qquad\qquad \overline{9.51227} = 18° \ 59'$

$\delta_4 = 30° - 18° \ 59' = 11° \ 1'$; $\log \tan \delta_4 = 9.289633$

$b_4 = \qquad \log 5 \qquad = 0.69897$

$\qquad - \log \tan \delta_4 = \overline{9}.28933$

$\qquad\qquad\qquad\qquad 0.40964 = 25.68$ cm, the focal length.

This demonstrates why the parallel rays of light which strike a refracting surface do *not* produce the textbook point image. This violation of the ideal point image is termed an aberration, specifically, spherical aberration. These calculations show that if the effects of a refracting surface are to be compared, it would be necessary to know the distance the rays striking the surface were separated from the axis.

It is noted that the difference in the focal length of the 0.5 and 1.0 rays is very small. If these distances were reduced to 0.1 and 0.2 they would be almost identical. This observation promoted research to find a new refracting formula in which the functions of angles were not used. In such a formula the rays would have to have such small angles of incidence that their sines and tangents would have to be identical.

BASIC GEOMETRICAL OPTICS REFRACTION FORMULA

Boeder (1937) prepared a simplified derivation of the formula now needed. To comply with the limitations described, $\angle \beta$ in Figure 39 must not be more than 1°. If it is made that small, then *h* will actually be much shorter than shown.

If $\angle \beta = 1°$, its sin $(h/r) = .0175$

The actual length of DC = r in Figure 39 is 43 mm.

Hence, $h = 43 \times .0175 = 0.7525$ mm

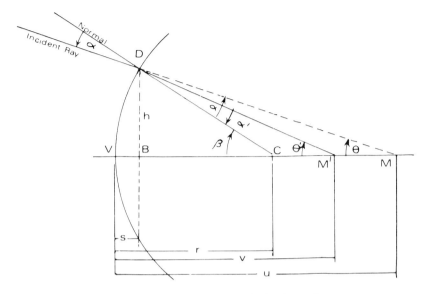

Figure 39. Abscissa formula derived (Boeder).

Thus, Figure 39 is enormously exaggerated in the vertical meridian in order to display the angles.

In $\triangle$ DBC, tan $\angle \beta =$ BD/BC $= h/(r - s)$

In $\triangle$ DBM, tan $\angle \theta =$ BD/BM $= h/(u - s)$

since $\angle \beta =$ the external $\angle$ of $\triangle$ CDM, $\angle \beta = \angle \alpha + \angle \theta$

To express $\angle \alpha$ in terms of the other angles, $\angle \alpha$ must be transferred to the left side of the equal sign:

$- \angle \alpha - \angle \beta + \angle \theta$

Changing signs, $\angle \alpha = \angle \beta - \angle \theta$

Since all angles are small and the ray which is directed toward M is paraxial, h is also very small (0.0007 meters) and its square ($h^2 = 0.00000049$ meters) is negligible. It follows that, in like manner, the distance **VB** $= s =$ sagitta and is measured by the lens measure formula ($s = h^2/2r$) which in this instance becomes negligible because of h^2.

It follows that $(r - s) \rightarrow r$ as $\angle \beta \rightarrow 0$

and $(u - s) \rightarrow u$ as $\angle \theta \rightarrow 0$.

Then $\angle \beta$ becomes h/r and

$\angle \theta$ becomes h/u

$$\angle\ \alpha = \angle\ \beta - \angle\ \theta = \frac{h}{r} - \frac{h}{u} = h\left(\frac{1}{r} - \frac{1}{u}\right)$$

And, in like manner

$$\angle\ \alpha' = \angle\ \beta - \angle\ \theta' = \frac{h}{r} - \frac{h}{v} = h\left(\frac{1}{r} - \frac{1}{v}\right)$$

For paraxial rays Snell's law

n sin α = n' sin α'

Reduces to

n α = n' α'

Substituting to clear the angles from the equation

$$n\ h\left(\frac{1}{r} - \frac{1}{u}\right) = n'\ h\left(\frac{1}{r} - \frac{1}{v}\right)$$

Removing parentheses after dividing by h

$$\frac{n}{r} - \frac{n}{u} = \frac{n'}{r} - \frac{n'}{v}$$

Rearranging

$$\frac{n'}{v} - \frac{n}{u} = \frac{n'}{r} - \frac{n}{r}$$

and

$$\frac{n'}{v} - \frac{n}{u} = \frac{n' - n}{r}$$

This formula has accomplished our purpose, the angles and all of the terms, with the exceptions of the indices of refraction, are linear measurements very close to the x-axis (abscissa) of the construction.

u = object distance
v = image distance
r = radius of curvature of surface
n' = index of refraction of second medium
n = index of refraction of first medium

Acknowledging redundancy to obtain emphasis, we will review the subject of scale.   In the illustrations this formula has been derived by using paraxial rays which in turn reduce the angle of incidence to 1° or less, which causes all vertical dimensions to become negligible. These conditions make all drawings, constructions, and illustrations impossible if they are held to scale. The tangent of 1° with a base the width of an average book page is about 4 inches × .01745 = .06980 inches or about 1.5 mm. The lines would be almost superimposed if drawn to scale. Another violation of scale is found in the presentation of an object or image at infinity. If the object were actually at infinity, it would be infinitely small and have no vertical dimension.

Even the sun at 93 million miles from the earth and a diameter of 865 thousand miles produces an angle of 31 minutes. This small angle produces an image of the sun, not a point focus. Thus we have returned to approximations in which the possible errors are regularly small enough to be neglected. To describe the action of rays of light, a convenient height is chosen for the illustration and infinity is reduced to part of the width of a book page.

The substance of the previous paragraph is obvious if the situation is thought through, but I must confess that books on geometrical optics without amplification of these notions were most difficult without the assistance of a teacher. One eminent author delayed his definition of paraxial rays until page 152 of his text. Yet, as is plain, the subject is based upon the notion of light rays that scarcely deviate from the lens axis.

The formula for paraxial rays last derived is sometimes called the *conjugate foci formula*. In 1910 Southall referred to it as the *abscissa-equation* and justifiably so. The entire consideration is in the direction of the x-axis with scant heed of the vertical ordinate (y-axis). It is also named the *lens makers'* formula.

Although this formula is fundamental to geometrical optics, it is seldom applied in the form derived because there are very few instances where the image is formed in the second medium after refraction at a single surface. The human retina does receive the image of the refraction of light by the cornea, but these rays are refracted again by the two surfaces of the crystalline lens about 5 mm behind the cornea. A camera uses the image formed at the back of the box, but the index of the medium inside the box is (air), the same as the medium outside the camera.

Returning to the human eye, it is not adapted to immersion in water. The formula has the term $n' - n$ which determines the difference in the angles of incidence and refraction. If our eyes are opened under water, almost all of the refraction at the corneal surface is obliterated because the refractive index of water and fluids (aqueous and vitreous) within the eye are almost identical. The crystalline lens (approximately + 15.00D.) is the only effective optical element as compared with the nearly + 60.00D. of a normal eye. The only relief is a swimming goggle with a lens which has flat surfaces and air behind it to allow the cornea to function normally.

Hence the formula must be expanded to include the refraction at the second surface of a lens. In actual experience, the surfaces of a lens are separated by the thickness of the lens. Hence, to be very precise, the ray must be traced from its refraction at the surface of the denser medium (usually glass), then through the glass in which the velocity of the light is reduced according to the particular index of refraction, then refracted again at the second surface into a third medium, usually the same as the first (air). These steps are time consuming and unless the lens is very thick the reduced velocity of the ray in the glass has a small effect on the focal length of the lens.

A common practice is to approach the calculation as if the lens had no thickness. With this approach, the lens formula reduces to only two surface refractions. This approximation is referred to as a *thin lens* formula.

Some optical instruments are first drafted with *thin* lenses. When production is contemplated, the lenses are refigured as *thick* lenses in which the lens profiles and media (glass formulas) are considered to nullify or materially reduce aberrations (both monochromatic and chromatic).

It is now appropriate that some attention be given to the relationship between the sizes of the object and image, that is, the magnification generated by the refraction.

m = magnification
0 = object
I = image
The definition is $m = I/0$

This magnification refers to an image size either smaller or larger than the object.

The extension of the incident ray to Q, a very small distance from the x-axis, forms the very small angle α. MQ shows the object 0.

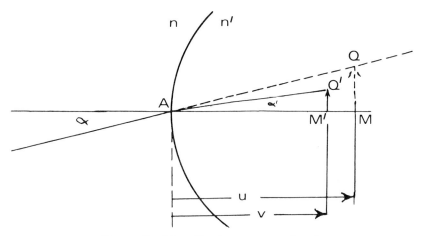

Figure 40. Magnification at a curved surface.

Because α is small, tan $\alpha = \alpha$

$\alpha = MQ/u$ so $MQ = \alpha u$

and

$\alpha' = I/v$ so $I = \alpha'v$

Therefore

$m = I/0 = \alpha'v/\alpha u$

But the angles must satisfy Snell's law restated for paraxial rays

$n\alpha = n'\alpha'$

from which

$n/n' = \alpha'/\alpha$

Substituting n/n' for α'/α in the expression for m, we finally have

$m = nv/n'u$

It should be noted that these formulas have all been limited to a single refracting surface and not to a lens. It is essential to have a clear comprehension of the formation of an image in the second medium. Light that strikes the cornea is imaged upon the retina within the eye and without returning to the first medium (air) as it does in the case of a spectacle lens.

EXERCISE

Find the image distance (v) which is the length of a simplified or *schematic* eye; find the height of the retinal image of a 20/20 letter (.0087 m) in the eye.

When u $= 6.0$

r $= .006$

n $= 1$

n′ $= 1.336$

And $\dfrac{n'}{v} - \dfrac{n}{u} = \dfrac{n' - n}{r}$

$$\dfrac{n'}{v} = \dfrac{n' - n}{r} + \dfrac{n}{u}$$

Then $\dfrac{1.336}{v} = \dfrac{.336}{.006} + \dfrac{1}{6} = 56.16$

$$\dfrac{1}{v} = \dfrac{56.16}{1.336} = 42.04$$

$$v = \dfrac{1}{42.04}$$

$v = .024$ meter

$$m = \dfrac{nv}{n' u} = \dfrac{.024}{1.336 \times 6} = \dfrac{.024}{8.016} = .003$$

$0 = .0087$

$I = .0087 \times .003 = .000026$ meter

Thus, if a 20/20 letter which is 8.7 mm high is placed 6 meters from a schematic eye which has all of the lens power on the front surface and which has a radius of curvature of 6 mm and an index of refraction of 1.336, the image will be formed at 24 mm from the surface and will be .026 mm high.

When the refracted ray has emerged from the second medium and has changed direction again, the optical performance of a lens has been described.

THIN LENS

The foundation for the discussion of lenses is a *thin lens*. It is another mental concept and not a reality. It has no center thickness and its power is the sum of the powers of the two surfaces. It is represented by a straight line with caps at top and bottom to identify whether it is convex or concave. It is very convenient to use in first approximations of designs for optical instruments.

The Gauss system of calculation for lens systems reduces any series of lenses to a *thin lens* called the *equivalent lens*.

Our discussion of lenses will emphasize single lenses surrounded

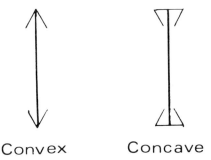

Convex   Concave

Figure 41. Thin lens representation.

by air. In ophthalmic dispensing the consideration is the *secondary focal point* (**F'**).

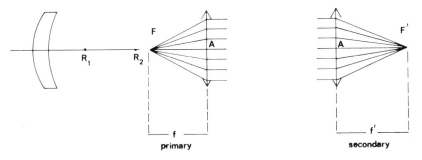

primary   secondary

Figure 42. Focussing of rays by a thin lens.

The distance of a focal point (**AF**) from the lens is known as the *focal length (f)*. For example, $AF' = f' \ AF = - f$.

The formula to find the total refracting effect of the two surfaces of a lens is found to be the sum of the *abscissa formula* which was derived for a single surface, applied to the two surfaces:

$$\frac{n'}{v_1'} - \frac{n}{u} = \frac{n' - n}{r_1} \text{ and } \frac{n}{v_2'} - \frac{n'}{v_1'} = \frac{n' - n}{r_2}$$

When v_1' (the image of the first surface used as the object of the second) is eliminated by adding the two equations and dividing through by n (the refractive index of the first and last mediums), we have the basic formula for the refraction of *paraxial* rays through a *thin* lens:

$$\frac{1}{v} - \frac{1}{u} = \frac{n' - n}{n} \left(\frac{1}{r_1} - \frac{1}{r_2} \right)$$

When $u = \infty$, $1/u = 1/\infty = 0$ and disappears from the formula. From this, if we assign $1/f = 1/v$ which is a constant because it is derived from the constants of the lens $(r_1, r_2, n', \text{and } n)$,

$$\frac{1}{f} = \frac{n' - n}{n}\left(\frac{1}{r_1} - \frac{1}{r_2}\right)$$

From Axiom #1, since $\left(\frac{1}{v} - \frac{1}{u}\right)$ and $\frac{1}{f}$ are each equal to the right side of the equation, they are equal to each other:

$$\frac{1}{v} - \frac{1}{u} = \frac{1}{f}$$

When the focal length is measured in meters, the unit of ophthalmic lenses is easily found:

$1/f =$ Diopter

If $f = 1.0$ meter, then $1/f = 1/1 = 1.00$ Diopter

$f = 0.5$ meter, then $1/f = 1/0.5 = 2.00$ Diopters

$f = 0.25$ meter, then $1/f = 1/0.25 = 4.00$ Diopters

This use of the reciprocal of focal length is a godsend in combining lenses and relieves the labor of manipulating fractions in such cases as adding focal lengths of two surfaces or two lenses:

$$\frac{1}{f_1} + \frac{1}{f_2} = \frac{1}{f}$$

THICK LENS

Since ophthalmic lenses have thickness, the formulas developed for infinitely thin lenses are not applicable. To construct a formula in which thickness is recognized, we return to the formula for a single lens surface

$$D_1 = \frac{n_1 - n}{r_1} = \frac{1}{f_1}$$

and for the second surface

$$D_2 = \frac{n - n_1}{r_2} = \frac{1}{f_2} \tag{A}$$

As we have found, paraxial refraction at a single surface is stated:

$$\frac{1}{u_1} + \frac{1}{v_1} = \frac{1}{f_1} \tag{B}$$

The image distance of the first surface (v_1) is taken as the object distance (u_2) of the second surface. Since this distance is on the right hand side of the surface (image) space, it receives a minus

(−) sign when it is considered in the object space of the second surface, because the lens thickness separates the two surfaces,

$$u_2 = d - v_1, \text{ where } d = \frac{t}{n} = \frac{\text{lens thickness}}{\text{refractive index}}, \text{ the reduced distance} \quad (C)$$

Thus the formula for the second surface is

$$\frac{1}{u_2} + \frac{1}{v_2} = \frac{1}{f_2} \tag{D}$$

It is plain that v_2, the image distance from the vertex (pole) of the second surface, is the back focal length of the lens, and by definition, $1/v_2 = D_v$, the vertex power of the lens. Now let us rearrange these separate formulas, replacing focal lengths with diopters to simplify the formula to find D_v.

If u_1 is very large

$$1/u_1 = 1/\infty = 0$$

which reduces formula (B) to

$$1/v_1 = 1/f_1 = D_1 \text{ and } v_1 = 1/D_1$$

Then from (C)

$$u_2 = d - \frac{1}{D_1}$$

Substituting these expressions in formula (D)

$$\frac{1}{d - \dfrac{1}{D_1}} + D_v = D_2$$

When this is restated with only D_v on the left

$$D_v = D_2 - \frac{1}{d - \dfrac{1}{D_1}}$$

changing signs

$$D_v = D_2 + \frac{1}{\dfrac{1}{D_1} - d}$$

By multiplying the second term on the right side by D_1/D_1, the denominator is simplified to read:

$$D_v = D_2 + \frac{D_1}{1 - dD_1} = D_2 + D_1 \left(\frac{1}{1 - dD_1} \right)$$

Now, if the expression in the parentheses is simplified by dividing 1 by $(1 - dD_1)$, the quotient becomes a continuing fraction $(1 + dD_1 + d^2 D_1{}^2 \ldots)$. Since d is a small fraction (.005 or less), its square (.000025) is inconsiderable and the terms past the first one are ignored.

The formula now reads

$$D^v = D_2 + D_1 (1 + dD_1) \ldots$$

Removing the parentheses, it becomes

$$D^v = D_2 + D_1 + dD_1^2 \ldots$$

This approximation is accurate to within 0.02D. for a + 10.00D. lens 5 mm thick.

When D_2 and the lens thickness are known, and the front lens curve is needed to produce a strong lens such as a lens for aphakia, the formula is then rearranged to find D_1

$$D_1 = \frac{D_v - D_2}{1 + d(D^v - D_2)}$$

Returning to the formula for magnification for a single refracting surface

$$m = \frac{nv}{n'u}$$

is now further simplified because the medium is air on both sides of a *thin* lens. The formula would now read:

$$m = \frac{v}{u}$$

The lens becomes a fulcrum like the pivot of a pair of shears.

$$m = \frac{v}{u} = \frac{30}{80} = \frac{3}{8} = 37.5\%$$

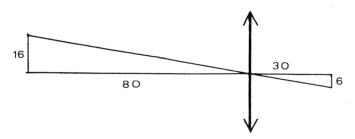

Figure 43. Magnification of a thin lens shown.

REVIEW

1. Identify the use of
   a. Capital letters—such as **A, M, N, F.**
   b. Small letters—such as u, v, h, f.
   c. Greek letters—such as $\alpha, \beta, \gamma, \delta$.

d. Numerals—such as (1), (2), (3).

2. Describe Cartesian coordinates. In what direction from the origin (A) would a point be positive in both meridians (directions)?

3. What is the sum of the angles of a triangle?

4. The sine of an angle is the ratio of the lengths of which two sides?

5. About how many arc degrees are there in one radian?

6. Does visible light represent a very large portion of the radiant energy spectrum?

7. What is the relationship of wavelength to frequency?

8. Name two uses of reflected light in ophthalmic optics.

9. What is the relationship of an incident ray and its reflection?

10. Why do parallel rays at the margin of a large concave mirror not fall upon the same point as those very close to the axis? What is this phenomenon called?

11. When light moves into a denser medium (say, air to glass) in which direction is a ray bent (refracted) ?

12. What happens when an object adjacent to a surface of a plane parallel slab of glass is viewed through the glass from a short distance?

13. When a ray strikes (is incident upon) a glass prism, in which direction is the ray refracted?

14. If the ray is viewed after it leaves the prism, in which direction is the object on the other side of the prism displaced?

15. What is the angle of deviation?

16. Describe the prism unit proposed by Prentice.

17. Describe a paraxial ray.

ADDITIONAL REFERENCES

1. Percival, A.S.: *Optics, a Manual for Students.* London, Macmillan, 1899.
2. Boeder, Paul: *An Introduction to the Mathematics of Ophthalmic Optics.* Fall River, Distinguished Service Foundation for Optometry, 1937.
3. Southall, James P.C.: *Mirrors, Prisms and Lenses.* New York, Macmillan, 1939.
4. Linksz, Arthur: *Physiology of the Eye,* Vol. I. Optics. New York, Grune, 1950.
5. Robertson, John K.: *Introduction to Optics Geometrical and Physical.* Princeton, Van Nostrand, 1961.

6. Huygens, Christiaan: *Treatise on Light.* New York, Dover, 1962.
7. Jolie, M.: *The Principles of Ophthalmic Lenses,* 3 Vols. London, Association of Dispensing Opticians, 1967.
8. Emsley, H.H.: *Emsley's Optical Tables and Other Data.* London, Optical Bausch & Lomb, 1968.
9. Ogle, Kenneth N.: *Optics. An Introduction for Ophthalmologists.* Springfield, Thomas, 1968.
10. Morgan, M. and Peters, H.: *The Optics of Ophthalmic Lenses.* Berkeley, U of Cal Pr, 1948.
11. Fry, Glenn A.: *Geometrical Optics.* Philadelphia, Chilton, 1969.
12. Bennett, A.G.: *Ophthalmic Lenses.* London, Hatton Press, 1968.
13. Levene, J.R.: *Clinical Refraction and Visual Science.* London, Butterworth, 1977.
14. Michaels, D.D.: Visual Optics and Refraction. St. Louis, C. V. Mosby, 1975.

Chapter 5

OPHTHALMIC LENSES

◆◆◆

LENS MATERIALS

Reference was made in Chapter 1 to the assumption that the first lenses were made from transparent natural stones before glass was manufactured. Brazilian quartz crystal, called pebbles, was made into ophthalmic lenses for a mystical benefit until the early part of this century. I have laboriously edge ground these lenses on a plano lap with #60 grain carborundum. The lenses were made by lapidarists. Little was done toward altering the early glass formulas until long after Newton had done his experiments with dispersion (separation of colors) through glass prisms. He was of the opinion that the chromatic aberration of glass prisms and lenses was inherent and uncorrectable. It was more than a century later that Dolland, an English optician, combined convex lenses made of regular glass with concave flint (lead) glass lenses, which disperse light more widely, to reduce the common color fringes surrounding images of common glass lenses. Few improvements in glass formulas or lens design were made until the development of photography in the middle of the nineteenth century.

A little later in the century, the War Department in Germany championed the thought that the army which can see the farthest and the clearest has an important advantage over its opponent. To accomplish this purpose, the optical factory of Carl Zeiss at Jena was heavily subsidized. In association with Schott, the glass maker, (guided by Dr. Ernst Abbe) they brought forth new glasses in which new chemical elements were used to produce new refractive indices and constringence. At the same time, optical instruments and lens systems were redesigned and invented. By the end of the century, Jena was the optical instrument center of the world.

In due course, these new developments radiated to ophthalmic lenses. About 1920, barium glass was used in fused bifocals to produce color-free reading portions. Recently, Schott has produced a high index glass, Hilite, in which titanium is used instead of lead, thus making a very low density glass. Since ophthalmic lenses are now uniformly toughened by air or chemical tempering, a special glass was presented in which more nitrate and other chemicals make it ultra-strong when it is chemically tempered.

In the early 1940s, a competitor for glass was developed by Pittsburgh Plate Glass Company's subsidiary, the Columbia-Southern Chemical Corporation. It is a thermosetting polyester resin, CR39. It is about half the weight of glass and much more impact resistant. It has made possible the use of very large lenses because of its light weight. It can be ground and polished in much the same way as glass. It accepts dye to give the effect of tinted glass. Since this is a surface treatment, the tint is of even density for all lens powers.

After a brief discussion of the principles of lenses, let us turn to the specific lenses used in ophthalmic dispensing. Most of the curved surfaces are spherical, and when both surfaces are sections of spheres, the lens is called a spherical lens. When the curves of a spherical lens are so chosen that the center of the lens is thicker than the edge, the lens is called a convex or *plus* lens. The power of the lens is largely determined by the amount of convexity (difference between center and edge thickness), so it follows that lenses of the same power can have markedly different profiles (cross sections) as in Figure 44. Sometimes it is said that lens *a* is *bent* to make shapes *b* and *c*. In Figure 44 all three convex lenses have the same power. In practice, one sees the flat lenses (*a* and *b*) in trial lens sets and ophthalmic instruments. Spectacle lenses are usually deep curved (meniscus) like *c*.

A convex lens converges light rays. If the rays are parallel when they strike the lens, they will be brought to a point focus (Fig. 45*a*). If they are already converging, the angle of convergence will be increased. Even if the light is diverging, the effect of convergence will be applied so that the light will diverge less, in some instances even converge after passing through the lens.

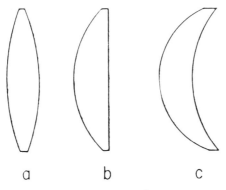

Figure 44. Lens forms.

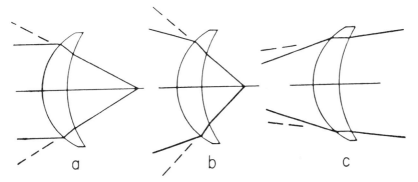

Figure 45. Refraction of different incident rays with convex lenses.

An object seen through a convex lens is magnified. If the lens is moved slightly while attention is paid to the magnified image, the image will seem to move. The movement of the image will be in the direction *opposite* to the movement of the lens, that is, when the lens is moved down the image glides up, and vice versa. To summarize, four methods to identify a plus spherical lens are given:

1. The lens is thicker in the center than it is at the edge.
2. Parallel rays (sunlight or a light across a room) can be brought to a point focus.
3. Objects viewed through it are increased in size.
4. If the lens is moved while looking through it at a distant

object, the image seems to move "against" the movement of the lens.

An equally important series of spherical lenses are concave or *minus* in form. As might be expected, their attributes are diametrically opposed to those of a convex lens. These lenses are thinner in the center than at the edge and diverge light rays. Parallel rays of light are spread out as if they were coming from a point in front of the lens (Fig. 48). Sunlight or illumination coming from a point at some distance from the lens will not be concentrated

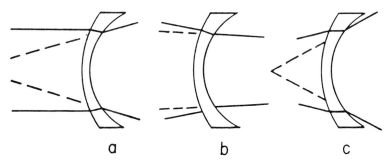

a　　　　　　　b　　　　　　　c

Figure 46. Refraction of different incident rays with concave lenses.

toward a point focus. If the lens is held a short distance from a wall or screen, a halo will be seen around the lens, as the light is diverged. When an object is viewed through the lens, it will be reduced (minified) in size; and when the lens is moved, the reduced image will seem to move in the same direction as the lens, only faster. Thus it is seen that a minus spherical lens has a series of characteristics quite different from a plus lens:

1. It is thinnest in the center.
2. It has a virtual focus, that is, it diverges the light.
3. It is a "reducing glass (objects seen through it are smaller).
4. It shows a "with" movement when the lens is moved while an image is being viewed.

NEUTRALIZATION

An essential concept concerning lenses should be grasped at this time. Its very obviousness could cause its usefulness to be disregarded. The attributes of magnification, minification, shape, and ray deviation of convex and concave lenses have been considered. As might be expected, the algebraic sum of equal power convex and concave lenses in contact nullify one another and the total effect is a plano lens. For example

$$+4 - 4 = 0$$
$$-7 + 7 = 0, \text{ and so on.}$$

Take two trial set spherical lenses of equal power and opposite signs and hold them snugly together. Objects viewed through the combination do not move when the lenses are moved and are not magnified or minified. The lenses perform as a piece of plain plate glass.

Another demonstration should follow. Take such a combination as + 1.00, + 1.50, and −2.50 which equal 0. This group of lenses will perform as before. Take + 1.75, + 0.50, − 1.00, and −1.25 which again total 0, and they will have no lens power if held in contact when grouped in any order.

This characteristic of superimposed lenses of opposite power is known as neutralization. It is the physical optics complement of chemical neutralization such as acid and alkali. In former times it was the only means by which lens powers were found. Convex testing lenses were made to specified focal lengths which were determined by the use of sunlight. These were used to guide lens makers in correcting the curves of concave lenses by neutralization. Thereupon the concave lens could be used as a testing or *standard* lens to make convex lenses. The trial set used by a refractionist is such a group of standard lenses. Until about sixty years ago all spectacle lenses were verified by neutralization.

When meniscus and toric lenses came into use, a problem arose. The curves of the prescription and test lenses did not match. This spacing of the lenses led to some erroneous conclusions.

The only point at which neutralization was dependable was in the axial area where the lenses were in contact. Aberrations and power effects in the margins were averted by some opticians who placed an aperture stop between the lenses to permit light through the axial area only. Judgment as to which was lens power and which was aberration often led to some very heated discussion as

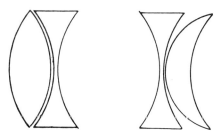

Figure 47.   Lens neutralization.

to whether a particular lens was acceptable.   Usually the opinion of the senior determined the issue.

When ophthalmic lens factories increased in size and physicists and engineers began to be added to their staffs, some of the old precepts about lenses which had been learned by experience were slowly replaced by scientifically sound reasoning.   Among the early presentations was the realization that the neutralized power of a deep-curved lens was the power at the front side of the lens. Many "practical" opticians objected to this thought which was presented to them by "college men" who were not opticians in the first place!   Because the aberration at the margin changes when the lenses are turned over, many of these recalcitrants swore they had met the issue when they put the trial lenses on the side toward their eyes to neutralize.

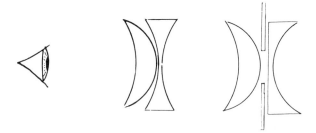

Figure 48.   Means to overcome marginal aberration.

Others who recognized the reasonableness of attempting to measure the power from the back surface had very small (10 mm) flat test lenses made which could be neutralized with trial lenses. These were put in contact (as near as possible) with the back surface. All moderately strong lenses showed a difference in power when neutralized from the front or back side. This demonstration stirred up a "hornets nest" with "'practical" opticians who were reluctant to yield to the new ideas.

In 1908 the Optical Society (London) adopted a report of its Optical Standards Committee in which a table was presented that gave the neutralizing and back surface power of trial case lenses. In 1912 M. von Rohr introduced "scheitel refraction" which translates to *vertex refraction* or back surface (not front surface) refraction or power. A.E. Glancy (1929) produced tables that showed the differences in lens powers between vertex and neutralized measurements.

TABLE I

6.00 Base Meniscus	Vertex	Neutralized
+4.00	+4.17	+4.06
+6.00	+6.32	+6.08
+8.00	+8.53	+8.09
—4.00	—3.98	—3.98
—6.00	—5.98	—5.92
—8.00	—7.98	—7.91

When uncut lenses, which were ground to be correct lens power at the center (or vertex) of the back surface, were first distributed there was a minority who decried what they contended was a breakdown of quality control at the factories.

The whole matter was brought to a head when Bausch and Lomb produced a dioptrometer (later, Vertometer®) and American Optical Company produced a Lensometer® both based upon Abbe's focimeter. This optical instrument, described in Chapter 17, measures the power at the back surface. Again the "fur was flying" because it showed that all strong plus lenses which neutralized well were considerably too strong on the Vertometer or Lensometer. Slowly the lens grinders and refractionists yielded and all of the turmoil is only a memory for "old timers."

Another series of convex and concave lenses is those with a

cylinder-shaped surface on one side. Large numbers of cylinder lenses in trial sets are flat on one side; the cylindrical curve on the opposite side is curved like Figure 49 *a* and *b*. In the same way that a spherical lens can be "bent" so long as it does not change the relationship between center and edge of lens, so can the same cylindrical lens power assume different profiles. When a cylindrical curve is "bent" as in Figure 49*c*, it is called a *toric* curve. This word is derived from *torus*.

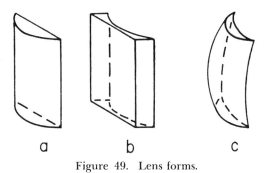

a   b   c

Figure 49. Lens forms.

Optically, these lenses perform quite the same. It is evident that this lens is the same thickness from top to bottom through the center. With no difference in thickness (the same as plate glass) there is no convergence or divergence of light through this meridian. Across the same lens at a right angle, it is quite different. As in a convex sphere, there is a marked difference in thickness between center and edge. One would reason, and correctly, that this lens converges light through one meridian and has no effect at all upon rays in the meridian at a right angle to the first. Parallel light would be converged to a line focus. If an object were viewed through this lens, it would be magnified in one direction and left unchanged across the other, like the reflection in the mirrors at the "Fun House" in an amusement park. The direction through which there is no magnification is called the axis of the cylinder. If the lens is moved slowly up and down when the axis is held in the same position, as Figure 50*a*, there will be no apparent movement of the object viewed, but if the lens is moved crosswise, the object will take on the characteristic "against"

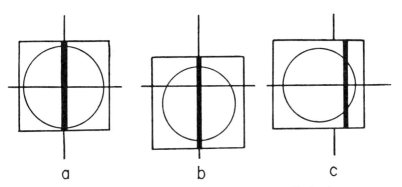

Figure 50. Target displacement of convex cylinder lens.

movement of a plus spherical lens.

Another novel and important test with a cylindrical lens is made by holding the lens in front of a crossline (or a door or window frame) with the cylinder axis vertical so that the intersection of the cross seems to be in the center of the lens. When the axis of the convex cylinder is precisely in the direction of either of the lines, neither of them will be broken (Fig. 51a). If the lens is slowly rotated on its center to the left, the crosslines will take on a "scissors movement." The vertical line will move to the right (Fig. 51b), and the horizontal line of the crossline will follow the direction of rotation of the lens.

This suggests that a cylindrical lens has the effect of both a convex and a concave lens at right angles to one another. This phenomenon should be remembered when transposition is discussed.

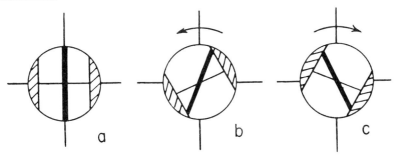

Figure 51. Target displacement of rotation of convex cylinder lens.

When the lens is rotated in the opposite direction, the crosslines will assume the position in *c* after the lens axis has passed the vertical position. If the individual lines of the crossline are noted, the vertical line near the axis of this plus cylinder always moves opposite to the rotation of the lens, while the crossline at right angles has the characteristic of a minus lens, in that it moves "with" the rotation of the lens.

Thus it is seen that a plus cylindrical lens has the same characteristics of a plus spherical lens with these additions:

1. A meridian (the axis) in which there is no focal effect.
2. Maximum curvature in the meridian opposite the axis.
3. Axis identified by rotation test on crosslines.
4. Magnification in the direction of a right angle to the axis.

As in the case of spherical lenses, minus cylindrical lenses are also used to diverge rays of light. In like manner these lenses are identified by their opposite effects:

1. Minification of objects in the meridian at a right angle to the axis.
2. In the rotation test the scissors movement is reversed and the crosslines seem to open rather than close. That is, the line through the axis moves "with" and faster than the rotation of the lens, while the opposite line moves away from the direction of rotation.

The greatest number of ophthalmic lenses in use is lenses that combine the two forms (sphere and cylinder). This is conveniently accomplished by placing the cylindrical surface on one side and a spherical surface on the other. The end result is a spherocylinder that displays a *combination* of the identifying characteristics described.

Since the power of a spherical lens is the same in all directions, the lens is described for prescription purposes when the sign and dioptric power are given, for example:

+0.25D. Sph. (or D.S.)
−5.75D.

Note that the lens powers are designated by at least three digits. Make it a practice to place a cipher before fractional amounts and write ciphers after the decimal point.

Write 0.50, not .50 or .5
Write 5.00, not 5.0 or 5.

The description of a cylinder-shaped lens must also include the position of the axis. Old texts on refraction show several methods of indicating the cylinder axis, which caused considerable confusion. By international agreement*, the horizontal position is known as 0° or 180°. Viewed from the front side of the glasses, meridians are designated counterclockwise beginning with 0° at the patient's left and increasing to the limit of 180° (Fig. 52).

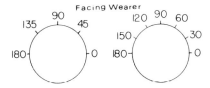

Figure 52. Cylinder axis roation.

After the power of the cylindrical lens, D. Cyl. or D.C. can be written. These abbreviations are not as important, however, as the letters after a spherical lens, because the axis identification shows that the power refers to cylindrical diopters. The word axis is abbreviated to "ax" and frequently to ✕. The degree sign is easily mistaken for a cipher and should not be used. For example 15° is easily read 150. The "combined with" sign ⊃ which was formerly used between sphere and cylinder to prevent confusion in prescription writing has slowly gone into disuse. When all of the rules are observed, lens formulas read

+ 0.12 D. Sph., or
+ 11.50 D.S. + 2.50 D.C. ax 15, or
− 5.00 D. Cyl. ✕ 90

TRANSPOSITION

By its very definition a cylindrical lens has *more* curvature in one meridian than it has on a right angle to it. Or from another point of view it has *less* curvature in one meridian than it has in

---

*Technischer Ausschuss für Brillenoptik (T.A.B.O.), 1917.

the meridian at a right angle. Either view is correct and upon occasion in daily practice the cylinder power must be viewed from one of these views exclusively. If the cylindrical power is on the plus side of the lens, there is only one way to describe it. There is more plus power in one meridian than the other and the difference is a plus cylinder effect.

For example

$$+7.75D.$$
$$-\ +6.50D.$$
$$\overline{+1.25D.\ \text{Cyl.}}$$

If, however, the cylindrical curve is ground on the concave surface, then both of the signs are minus, and the difference between the curves is the power of a minus cylinder:

$$-5.50D.$$
$$-\ -3.00D.$$
$$\overline{-2.50.\ \text{Cyl.}}$$

The lesser curve in each instance is called the *base curve*.

The prescription and/or the style of lens determine which side of the lens is used for the cylindrical surface. For example, the first marginally corrected lenses required a plus cylinder, more recent designs use concave cylinders. Practically all multifocals require minus cylinders.

It becomes apparent that a means of conversion or transposition is necessary. When the "more" or "less" idea is applied to the power of a cylindrical or spherocylindrical lens, the alternate expression can be found by a comparatively simple operation.

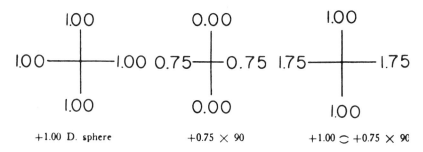

Figure 53. Lens powers "on cross."

For example, if a +0.75D. Cyl. axis vertical (90) is added to a + 1.00D. Sph. (Fig. 53), the total lens effect is +1.00 in the 90° meridian. In the opposite meridian the total power of the cylinder is added to the power of the sphere which makes +1.75D. (or +0.75D. more) in the 180° meridian. If the prescription is written in the regular form it reads

+1.00D. Sph. +0.75D. Cyl. × 90

When the point of view is reversed, it can be said that the total lens effect is +1.75D. in the 180° meridian and that −0.75D. is added in the 90° meridian to produce the power of +1.00D. This is written

+1.75D. Sph. − 0.75D. Cyl. × 180

ADDITIONAL EXAMPLES:

1. −4.00D. −1.50D. × 75

   The power is − 4.00D. at axis 75 and
   1.50D. more or − 5.50D. at the opposite axis 165;
   Or, the power is − 5.50D. at axis 165 and
   1.50D. less or − 4.00D. at the opposite axis 75
   which is written − 5.50D +1.50D. × 165.

2. − 1.75D. × 45

   The power is 0.00D. (plano) at axis 45 and
   1.75D. less or − 1.75D. at the opposite axis 135;
   Or, the power is − 1.75D. at axis 135 and
   1.75D. more or plano at the opposite axis 45
   which is written − 1.75D. +1.75 × 135.

3. − 0.75D. +2.00D. × 110

   The power is − 0.75D. at axis 110 and
   2.00D. more or +1.25D. at the opposite axis 20;
   Or, the power is +1.25D. at axis 20 and
   2.00D. less or −0.75D. at the opposite axis 110
   which is written +1.25D. − 2.00D. × 20.

The expressions in each example are equivalent. Whether the lens is actually ground according to one formula or the other in each case is not determinable on a lensometer or by the optical effect upon an eye behind it. The rule by which this transposition is accomplished is given below. It is applicable to all cylindrical and spherocylindrical lens prescriptions.

1. Add the powers of sphere and cylinder algebraically.
2. Change the sign of the cylinder to the opposite sign.
3. Change the direction of the axis by 90°.

EXAMPLES:

1. Transpose $+1.75D. -2.25D. \times 65$

    1. $-0.50D.$ (Powers added)
    2. $+2.25D.$ (Sign changed)
    3. $\times \ 155$ (Opposite axis)

    $-0.50D. \ +2.25D. \ \times \ 155$

2. Transpose $+0.50D. -0.50D. \times 120$

    1. $0.00D.$ (Powers added)
    2. $+0.50D.$ (Sign changed)
    3. $\times \ 30$ (Opposite axis)

    $+0.50D. \times 30$

A simple method by which to find the opposite axis of the cylinder, when the axis is 100 or more, is to add the first two digits:

    115: $1 + 1 = 2$, opposite axis $= 25$
    160: $1 + 6 = 7$, opposite axis $= 70$
    137: $1 + 3 = 4$, opposite axis $= 47$

When the axis given has only two digits, subtract 1 from the first digits:

    90: $9 - 1 = 8$, opposite axis $= 180$
    73: $7 - 1 = 6$, opposite axis $= 163$
    15: $1 - 1 = 0$, opposite axis $= 105$

Thus the prescription can easily be transposed to provide the formula of the lens, for the cylinder surface is to be ground on either the convex (plus cylinder) side or concave (minus cylinder) side as the case may require.

PRISMS

Occasionally a prescription is written for a prism or wedge-shaped glass. Without curve, this optical form does not focus (converge or diverge) light. It merely deviates (bends) the direction of the light beam. This phenomenon is carefully explained in Chapter 3. When a prism lens is interposed between the eye and any object, the object is not magnified or reduced but it is apparently displaced toward the thin edge (apex) of the prism. In reality light is deviated toward the base of the prism, but since we mentally project objects in the direction from which light enters the eye, another illusion is created. Figure 54 shows how the viewer has the impression of displacement in the opposite direction.

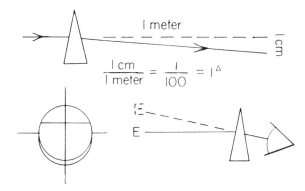

Figure 54. Target displacement by prism.

Prisms have four important uses in ophthalmic optics: (a) by the displacement of images, they can be used to measure the amount an eye or pair of eyes is turned, such as the angle of deviation in a case of strabismus (crossed eyes) or the amount in Prism Diopters that the eyes can be caused to converge; (b) prisms are used to stimulate or inhibit convergence in visual training (orthoptics); (c) binocular vision is dissociated for some visual tests with prisms; and (d) prisms are prescribed to be worn continuously for the relief of double vision in certain cases such as extraocular muscle paralysis or paresis, or extra-axial portions of anisometropic prescriptions (slab-off.)

The unit of measurement of prisms and prism deviation most commonly used is the *Prism Diopter*. Other units have been used by some, but the convenience of the unit suggested by Prentice (1890) * has much in its favor for small measurements. It is indicated by the exponent $^\Delta$ which distinguishes it from the degree sign. One Prism Diopter is the power to deviate a ray of light 1 in 100 that is, 1 cm at one meter (Fig. 54). It may also be expressed

*Prentice, C.F.: *Ophthalmic Lenses*. Philadelphia, Keystone, 1900, pp. 101-124.

$\tan^{-1} = 0.01$. Since the unit is a measurement of the tangent of an angle, only the distance from prism to screen and the amount that the light is deviated are necessary to find the power of the prism. In turn, this unit gives the tangent of the angle of rotation of the eye. For example the displacement of $13^{\triangle} = $ arc tan $0.1300 = 7°24'$. Upon further consideration, visual projection explains why the deviated rays through convex and concave lenses produce the effect of magnification and minification. The increased angle of the converged rays makes them appear as if they come from a greater distance from the center of the lens as shown in Figure 55*a* and the reverse effect of a minus lens is shown in Figure 55*b*.

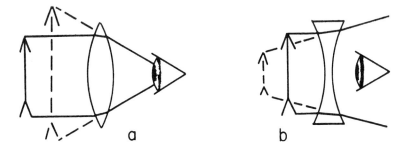

Figure 55. Lens magnification or minification.

Prisms are infrequently prescribed without lens power. Therefore, a lens may have spherical, cylindrical, and prism power, in which case it would demonstrate the characteristics of all of these lenses simultaneously: it would (a) show "with" or "against" movement in all directions (sphere), (b) show more movement in one direction than at right angles (cylinder), (c) show scissors movement on rotation (cylinder), and (d) displace the crosslines (prism).

In common with the other scientific subjects, the vocabulary of optics has changed as the knowledge pertaining to the subject has increased. If the literature of the past hundred years is reviewed, it will be found that the same property or function of a lens may have been given several terms. In other instances, the same word may have been used by different writers to define quite different things. In the past fifty years some standardization has been accomplished. Units and some definitions have been established by international agreement,* and by national organizations such as British Standards Institution and American National Standards Institute.

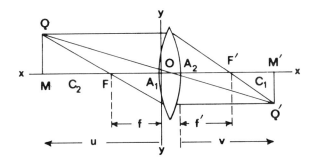

Figure 56. Conjugate foci construction.

Many authors observe the following conventions and terms. The letters to indicate a line **MM'** denote a measurement left to right called positive; the reverse of this direction **M'M** from right to left is called negative. A point (usually the vertex of a surface) is taken as the point of *origin of a system of rectangular coordinates.* The axis of the surface, the horizontal line, is chosen as the *x-axis* and the intersecting line at the point of origin *y-y' is the y-axis.* Measurements made in an upward direction from the *x-axis* are positive and those made downward are negative. Thus, the line-segment **M'Q'** in Figure 56, because it extends below the x-axis, carries a negative sign. All angles measured counterclockwise are positive (**QOM**) and those measured clockwise (**M'OQ'**) are negative. All measurements are made from point of origin (**A₁C₁**, **A₁M**, etc.) except measurements of focal distance, which are measured from the focal point to the lens (**FA₁ F'A₂**). The line connecting the centers of curvature **C₁C₂** in Figure 57 is defined as the *optical axis* of the lens. The point on each lens surface through which this axis passes is a *pole or vertex* of the surface.

Revue D'Optique Theorique et Instrumentale, Paris 1925, Tome 4, pp. 332-339, 390-395.

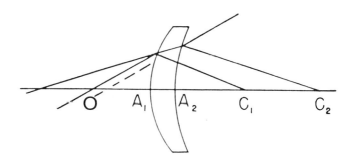

Figure 57. Optical center of meniscus lens.

To Summarize:

A_1M = u = object distance (−)
FA_1 = f = primary focal distance (+)
A_1A_2 = t = lens thickness (+)
A_1C_1 = r_1 = radius of curvature of first surface (+)
A_2C_2 = r_2 = radius of curvature of second surface (−)
$F'A_2$ = f' = secondary focal distance (−)
A_2M' = v = image distance (+)
MQ = y = object height (+)
$M'Q'$ = y' = image height (−)
O = optical center of thin lens

It is convenient to use the cross section of a thin double-convex lens to identify these conventions. In this case the point **O**, through which a ray of light from an extra-axial point crosses the lens axis without deviation, it called the *optical center of the lens.* The following is the formula by which it is located:

$$A_1O = \frac{r_1}{r_1 - r_2}\, t$$

Therefore, in Figure 56 this point is midway between the surfaces because the curves are symmetric $(r_1 = -r_2)$ and $A_1O = t/2$ or one-half the thickness. Double-convex lenses are rarely used for spectacle lenses. The cross section of a plus meniscus lens of the same dioptric power as is commonly seen (Fig. 57) shows that the radii of curvature of both lens surfaces are positive and therefore the distance A_1O is always negative, and the optical center lies outside the lens on the convex side. Thus the so-called center dot put on a spectacle lens when it is held in a plane parallel to a target or crossline chart marks the pole or vertex A_1 or A_2 of the lens. The line connecting with a similar dot on the opposite surface denotes the optical axis of the lens. The position of the optical center of the lens is unknown because it is a function of the curves or form of the lens. The true position of the optical center can be demonstrated if a double-convex lens is tilted on its midpoint while it is held in front of a crossline; there is no displacement of the lines. If a meniscus lens of equal power is rotated in the same way while the concave curve is held toward the eye, the target moves in the same direction as the lens, thus showing that the center is in front of the lens. This test is frequently used in instrument optics to locate nodal planes and principal planes of lenses.*

In ophthalmic terminology, usage defines either pole of the lens surfaces as the *optical center*. Therefore the marking device on a lens-centering device or a lensometer puts a dot on what is regularly called the lens center.† Practically, no significant error is introduced so long as the axes of a pair of lenses are held in the same horizontal plane. It is apparent that, if the plane of one lens of a pair of spectacles were tilted (rotated) on a point other than the optical center, objects would be displaced before one eye. *Center* thickness of a lens refers to the thickness measured by gauge or calipers at this point (A_1A_2). Since the points are poles of the optical axis of the lens, the thickness of a convex lens is greatest here. Contrariwise, a concave lens is thinnest at the *optical center*.

Texts on geometrical optics describe the several points or planes from which the focal lengths can be measured and then derive the formulas for the evaluation of these lengths and their functions. These points, like the optical center of a lens, take new positions inside or outside of the lens with each change in form, power, and thickness. A certain amount of difficulty and confusion surrounds

---

*Jacobs, D.H.: *Fundamentals of Optical Engineering.* New York, McGraw, 1943, pp. 22-24.

†Wagner, A.F.: *Experimental Optics.* New York, Wiley, 1929, pp. 69-71.

Cox, A.: Optics. New York, Pitman, 1949, pp. 24-28.

Fry, G.A.: The major reference point in a single vision lens. *Am J Optom,* 24:1-7, Jan. 1947.

these formulas and concepts. The subject was first clarified by von Rohr in his original work on *corrected lenses*.‡ He developed the convenient concepts of *vertex refraction* and *vertex distance*. He defined the very tangible and invariable distance from the posterior pole or vertex to the secondary focus F^1A_2 as the vertex distance and the reciprocal of that distance $(1/F'A_2)$ as the vertex power.

All modern day trial-lens sets, refracting instruments, lens-measuring instruments, and ophthalmic lenses are calibrated in units of vertex power. This unit of measurement was called the *vertex diopter* (Dv) at the outset but now usage has dropped the adjective and *diopter* refers to vertex power. This unit is the reciprocal of the focal length measured in meters. Thus it follows that a lens with one meter vertex focal length $(F'A_2)$ has a power of one diopter (1.00D.); a lens of 2 meters focal length, $F_1A_2 = 2m$, $1/2 = 0.50D$.; a lens of $\frac{1}{4}$ meter length, $F_1A_2 = 0.25$, $1/.25 = 4.00D$. Paradoxically, the diopter, a delightful application of metric measurement, is not divided in tenths. It is divided in eighths and the decimal fraction is carried to only two places. Therefore a trial lens set or refractive instrument begins 0.12, 0.25, 0.37, 0.50, 0.62, 0.75, 0.87 and 1.00.

CORRECTING LENSES

With this brief introduction to ophthalmic lenses, their effects as correction lenses can be observed. In the case of the so-called ideal or normal eye (emmetropia), objects are clearly seen at distance without any physiological effort of focussing (accommodating) ; hence no correcting lens is required for best visual acuity. The light from distant objects is focussed by the optical system of this eye upon the retina as a sharply defined image. In optical terms, the *far-point* of the eye is at infinity—rays of light from infinity (20 feet or farther) are conjugate with the retina (Fig. 58) .

Such perfect eyes are in the minority, as is revealed by the large number of spectacle wearers. The optical systems of most eyes

‡von Rohr, M.: *Die Brille Als Optische Instrument.* Berlin, Julius Springer, 1921, pp. 27-34.

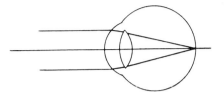

Figure 58. Emmetropic eye.

would focus parallel rays of light from distant objects in front of or behind the retina and therefore vision is blurred to some degree without the assistance of a correcting lens or, in some instances, accommodation. Again in optical terms the far points of these eyes are not at infinity.

When an eye is so constituted that parallel rays come to focus in front of the retina and would produce an image on the retina only when the rays emanated from a point nearer to the eye, this eye has a condition termed nearsightedness (myopia). The point from which the light must come, the far point, is in front of the eye (Fig. 59).

This effect is easily demonstrable with a camera that has a ground glass. Set the lens focus at infinity and view the image upon the glass. Each individual point of the object is focussing upon the glass and the image is very clear. Now rack the lens forward and watch the clarity of the distant objects deteriorate as

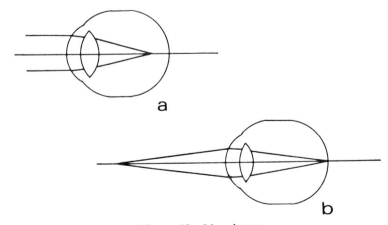

Figure 59. Myopic eye.

shown in Figure 59*a;* the focus of the image has been moved forward from the ground glass. If now an object is placed rather close to the camera, the image of it will be clear as shown in Figure 59*b.* Referring to the formula for paraxial refraction at a single surface

$$\frac{1}{f} - \frac{1}{v} - \frac{1}{u} \quad \text{or} f = v \quad u$$

as the distance of the object, *u,* diminishes, the distance to the image, *v,* increases.

In a more common condition called farsightedness (hyperopia), parallel rays do not come to focus within the distance to the retina. In other words, parallel rays of light would be directed toward a point situated behind the retina. Again distant vision would be blurred because the images do not fall on the retina. In this case, however, since the optical system of the eye is not of sufficient power to focus rays from infinity on the retina, it will only make matters worse to bring the object closer to the eye. It becomes apparent that the only rays that will focus upon the retina of this eye must be somewhat convergent when they strike the eye surface (cornea). That is, they must move toward an imaginary far point situated behind the eye (Fig. 60).

Gullstrand worked out the constants—radii of curvature, indices of refraction, eye length, and so forth (1909)—which succeeding

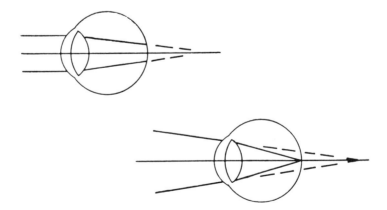

Figure 60. Hyperopic eye.

research has shown is sufficiently accurate to be continued to be used. He gave anterior focal length of the eye as 17.055 mm (or .017055 meters). It follows that $1/.017055 = 58.64D$. If the eye were hyperopic 1.00D., meaning that the focal length of the eye were longer than the physical length of the eye, this dioptric power 58.64D. — 1.00D. would be reduced to 57.64D., producing a new anterior focal length *(f)* of 17.35 mm or an increase of 17.35 — 17.05 = 0.3 mm. But the posterior focal length is measured in the vitreous (refractive index 1.336), hence this increase must be multiplied by 1.336 (1.336 × 0.3) = .4008. Thus we observe that 1.00D. hyperopia refers to the retina being only 0.4 mm in front of the best image. These minute deviations immediately demonstrate that the illustrations of ametropia in all texts are gross exaggerations intended to clarify the reasoning. Let us refer to Figure 60. These eye globes are almost to scale. The far point is shown to stand about 15 mm behind the retina or a focal distance of about (24 + 15) = 39 mm (1/.039) = 25.64D. or an unbelievable hyperopia of (58.64 — 25.64) = 33.00D. Like illustrations and diagrams used in the discussion of the refraction of light rays near the lens axis, the student must be prepared for mental allowances.

These references to the optical power of the refractive system of the eye return to the notion of neutralization. Simply stated, the ophthalmic lens prescribed is the lens that neutralizes the lack or excess of dioptric power of the eye. To refer to the example cited above, the obvious prescription lens would be + 1.00D. sphere to account for the deficiency (57.64 + 1.00) = 58.64 D., the constant given by Gullstrand. The myopic eye is one in which the dioptric power is in excess of 58.64, say 60.14, would require — 1.50D. sphere to lengthen the focal length to produce an image of a distant object upon the retina.

As the diagrammatic illustration is drawn it suggests that the image not having come to focus at the retina will be a blurred upright image. This is not what really happens. As this drawing is made and many others like it in texts on refraction, it refers to only one infinitely small object. In reality all of the points in the object not on the optical axis follow the laws of refraction described in "Reversability of Light Rays" in Chapter 4.

Object points above or below nearly come to a focus and each result in an almost infinitely small blurred area on the retina. The total effect is a blurred image. Return to the camera and focus it for infinity, now place a minus (concave) sphere of 1.00D. to 2.00D. before the camera lens. The image is blurred at once. It is still inverted. There are two ways to clear the image. The obvious one is to remove the minus lens. The other is to rack the lens out to two to four feet. This latter compensation is analogous to the act of accommodation by the crystalline lens. The eye (camera) has made the physiological effort required to account for the lens power deficiency of the eye.

The ideal or emmetropic eye receives parallel rays of light from a distant object as a clearly defined image upon the retina without the physiological effort of accommodation, and normal vision is the result. A refractionist's efforts with the aid of lenses is to produce, where it is possible, the same effect. A simplified rule to accomplish this purpose is to ascertain the position of the far point of the eye and place before the eye that lens whose focal point coincides with the position of the far point of the eye. A quick review of the light paths in the discussion of lenses and ametropia shows the reasonableness of this rule. By way of example, rays of light that were parallel before striking a convex lens emerge as rays that are converging to the focal point beyond the lens. By definition, a hyperopic eye must receive rays converging toward its far point to be in sharp focus upon the retina. Thus, when the lens would focus at the far point of the eye, a distant object is sharply imaged upon the retina. The dioptric power that meets this condition constitutes the ophthalmic prescription (Fig. 61).

At once it is realized that more data may be significant, and in many instances indispensable, if the ophthalmic lens is to duplicate the optical effect of the lens used for examination. By definition, the power of the lens is such that its focal point coincides with the far point of the eye. Therefore, if the posterior vertex of the spectacle lens is not set in precisely the same plane—that is, same distance from the eye as the back surface of the trial lens, the points will not coincide. The dioptric effect of the correcting lens will then be too little or too great as the case may be. The

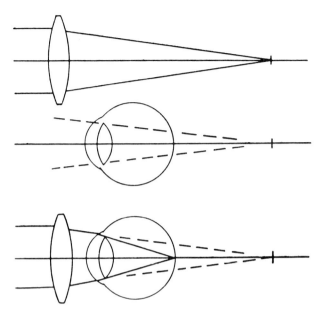

Figure 61. Lens correction of hyperopic eye.

formula by which this alteration in lens power can be evaluated is as follows:

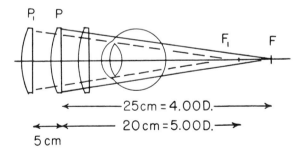

Figure 62. Effect of lens position.

If a convex lens of 25 cm focal length (+4.00D.) is placed in plane **P**, as shown in Figure 62, the focal point is at **F**. If the lens is moved to **P'** (5 cm to the left of the original position), the focal point moves to **F₁**. In the new position, the focal point is only 20 cm (25 — 5 = 20) from the original lens plane and therefore has the dioptric effect of +5.00D. Thus, the dioptric effect of this convex lens at the eye has been materially increased. Quite the opposite takes place when the position of a concave (minus) lens is changed. The primary focus of this lens is in front of the eye. When the lens is moved away from the eye, the effect is that of a weaker lens, that is, one with a greater focal length. The new position of the focal point of the concave lens is —30 cm (—25 — 5 = —30) from P, the first position, and therefore has the effect of only —3.33D. in that plane (Fig. 62).

Therefore
$$Da = \frac{100}{f - d}$$

Where Da = altered dioptric power
        f = focus of lens in cm
        d = displacement of lens in cm

A very useful approximation of this alteration in lens effectivity can be found by the use of the formula:

$$\text{Change per millimeter of displacement} = \frac{D^2}{1000}$$

in which D is the dioptric power of the lens. Applied to the above case, it becomes

$$\frac{4 \times 4}{1000} = .016 \text{ mm}$$
$$.016 \times 50 = 0.80D.$$

Thus it is seen that this estimation of the effect is rather an average. It does not differentiate whether the lens is moved forward or away from its focal point and thereby neglects the difference in effect which has been shown.

The change in the effect of lenses is not marked in low-power lenses and because a large percentage of prescription lenses is rather weak, this alteration in prescription power is sometimes neglected. To be sure, a lens of only 2.00D. would be altered about .004D./mm of change of position and therefore would have to be about 30 mm closer to or farther away from the eye to add the effect of 0.12D. Obviously, the effect of vertex distance in such an instance is negligible. However, the fact that the formula involves the square of the dioptric power of the lens does accelerate the effect. A lens with 5.00D. in any meridian shows a change of about .025D./mm.

Oftentimes more than one trial lens is required to produce the desired lens combination. Obviously several lenses cannot simultaneously stand the same distance from the eye. Present-day refractive instruments and trial sets are so designed that all the lenses have the effect of standing in the plane of the rear lens and therefore the spectacle lens of the indicated total power that is fitted in the same plane as the back lens of the series will have precisely the same effect as the sum of the indicated trial-lens powers. Old style trial sets and instruments were not compensated to be additive and therefore errors were introduced that became quite significant when two or more trial lenses were used. As a matter of precaution, many users of these nonadditive lenses make it a practice to measure combinations of strong lenses with a lensometer while the lenses are still spaced in the trial frame. As could be expected, the optical effect sometimes varies materially from the total of the powers indicated.

In the discussion of lens forms, rays of light were always shown to move toward the lens parallel with the lens axis and finally focus at some point on the extension of that axis. When rays of light strike a lens at an angle to the axis of the lens, the light does not focus at the same distance from the lens as the axial rays. In other words, the dioptric power of a lens changes when it is tilted. If a pencil of light strikes a lens obliquely, the emergent rays are astigmatic and will no longer come to a point focus. Thus a spherical lens acts as a spherocylindrical lens with the axis of the cylinder in the direction of the axis of rotation (Fig. 63).

A precise calculation of this effect is a laborious project but a satisfactory approximation can be found by the application of two simple expressions derived by Martin:*

$$\text{The new sphere} = D \left(1 + \frac{\sin^2\theta}{3} \right)$$

$$\text{Cylinder} = D \ \tan^2\theta$$

Where D = power of sphere

θ = angle of obliquity (tilt)

*Martin, L.C.: *Technical Optics.* New York, Pitman, 1948, vol. 1, pp. 37-38.

Ophthalmic Dispensing

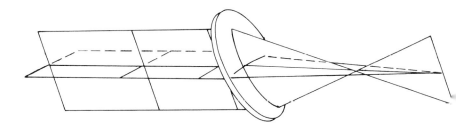

Figure 63.   Astigmatism generated by a tilted lens.

Table II shows the significance of this effect applied to a 1.00D. lens:

TABLE II
1.00D. SPHERICAL LENS TILTED

Degrees	Sphere Power	Induced Cylinder
0	1.000	0.000
5	1.0015	0.010
10	1.0102	0.031
15	1.0223	0.072
20	1.0406	0.138
25	1.0632	0.231
30	1.0833	0.347

The introduction of cylinder power that is induced by the inclination of lenses often creates a greater disparity between the effect of the trial lenses and the spectacle lenses than discrepancies in vertex distances.   The error induced in most prescriptions by alteration of the distance between lens and eye (vertex distance) is mostly spherical.   When the effect of the power is decreased by small amounts, accommodation can frequently compensate.   Excessive plus power would blur vision slightly for distance, but again the overcorrection would be tolerated at near.

A common violation of the optical terms under which the ophthalmic lens prescription was found must be recognized.   Modern refracting instruments hold the trial lenses perpendicular to the visual axes in primary position and the lens centers and axes are on or very near the lines of fixation, thus directing the lens axes through the centers of rotation of the eyes, that is, at the terminals of the Helmholz Base Line. In practice, most ophthalmic lenses are angled 4° to 12° with the face plane; the lens axes are thus directed above the centers of rotation to a position to which the eyes cannot turn, allowing the axes of fixation to follow the lens axis in any field of fixation. The inclination of the spectacle lenses is determined by other factors discussed on pages 327-329, where the power of the lenses and disparity between the planes of the trial lens and spectacle lens are discussed.

If the power of the prescription lens is sufficiently great, the effect of the prescription lens is materially altered.

1. The power of the sphere is slightly increased.
2. A cylindrical element is induced for which accommodation cannot account.
3. Since the spectacle lenses are tilted on the horizontal meridian, the new cylinder axis is 180. When the original prescription is not axis 90 or 180, a crossed-cylinder effect is generated which alters the lens power and resultant cylinder axis.

Again, these modifications of lens effectivity are insignificant in lower powered lenses. For instance:

$+1.00 +0.50 \times 90$ prescribed from trial lenses in vertical position becomes $+1.09 +0.43 \times 90$ if the lens is tilted 15° from vertical. This small increase would scarcely be noted because the axis of the cylinder in the prescription is 90°. With a small change in power and axis, the same change in conditions causes important differences:

A. $+1.00 +0.75 \times 180$ becomes $+1.02 +0.82 \times 180$

B. $+2.00 +1.00 \times 135$ becomes $+2.04 \dfrac{+1.00 \times 135}{+0.14 \times 180}$

These, in turn, combine to $+2.09 +1.04 \times 138$. A further discussion of the effect of tilted lenses is continued in the chapters on prescription analysis and cataract lens fitting.

The primary function of a correcting lens is to focus parallel rays of light upon the far point of the ametropic eye. If the optical center of the prescription lens is placed at the primary focal point of the eye (about 16 mm in front of the cornea), rays from

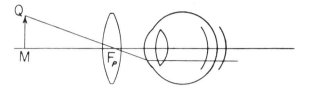

Figure 64. Correcting lens set at anterior focus of eye.

an object **MQ** in Figure 64 produce the same size image for any eye length. Repeated research has shown that most spherical refractive errors are axial—that is, the optical system of the eye agrees closely with the measurements found by Gullstrand—and that the size of the globe is the main contributing factor. It has likewise been shown that astigmatic errors are largely caused by variations in the refractive power of the eyes (curvature of the cornea). Hyperopia due to inadequate refractive power in an eye of normal length produces an image size increase of approximately 1.8 percent per diopter of lens power when corrected. Myopia due to excessive curvature alone shows an equal reduction in image size. A large number of eyes show a combination of axial and curvature ametropia. In any of these latter instances, the position of the primary focal point (**F**) will have moved from the calculated position of 15.7 mm in front of the cornea. When the prescription lens is not placed at the primary focal point of the eye, the retinal image-size is altered. The reduction or increase in image-size is small. Within the limits of $+10.00$ and -25.00D., the effect is contained between $1.06 \times$ (6% magnification) and $.90 \times$ (10% minification).

It seems that when the images in both eyes are increased or reduced by equal amounts, tolerance for the change can be quickly developed in most cases. A very small difference in the image sizes between the two eyes causes distress in some instances. Prolonged research at Dartmouth Eye Institute by Ames and others[*]

[*]Berens, C.: *The Eye and Its Diseases.* Philadelphia, Saunders, 1936, pp. 284-286.

Ames, A., Glidden, G.H., and Ogle, K.N.: Size and shape of ocular images. *Arch Ophthmol*, 7:576, 1932.

Ames, A., Ogle, K.N., and Glidden, G.H.: *J Opt Soc America*, 22:538, 1932.

indicates that differences of 1 percent to 5 percent cause symptoms similar to those of uncorrected errors of refraction. It is obvious that these highly refined physiological measurements and the ophthalmic optics involved immediately become quite complex.

E. D. Tillyer presented a formula in detail in his patent No. 2077134 (1934) in which the correlation and interdependence of magnification, shape, and power are thoroughly explained. Approximations based upon paraxial rays are developed that prove to introduce no serious error. Not only are the effects of image-size described, but each lens function is reduced to a simple workable formula. Morgan and Peters[†] discuss some examples using his formula.

In the magnification formula

$$M = \frac{1}{(1 - cD_1)} \cdot \frac{1}{(1 - zD_v)}$$

the first factor involving dioptric power of the front surface of the lens, D_1, is called the shape factor. In the second part, D_v, the vertex power of the lens is involved and this factor is called the power factor. Thereupon the formula becomes

Magnification $=$ Shape $\times$ Power

They then show that for any fixed distance, the magnification of a lens depends upon

D_v, the vertex power

$c = \dfrac{d}{n}$, the reduced lens thickness

$d =$ the lens thickness

D_1, the front surface power

z, the distance from lens vertex to the center of rotation.

Change in magnification per millimeter of thickness is $(x\ D_1/15)\%$, where $x =$ increase in mm.

EXAMPLE

$D_1 = +9.00$, $x = 2.0$ mm thickness increase

$$\frac{2 \times 9}{15}\% = 1.2\%$$

[†]Morgan, M., and Peters, H.B.: *The Optics of Ophthalmic Lenses.* Berkeley, U of Cal Pr, 1948, pp. 88-91.

Change in front surface power is:

$\frac{xd}{15}\%$ where $x =$ increase in front surface power

EXAMPLE

Front surface power changed from +6.00D. to +10.00D., increase of +4.00, lens is 3.0 mm thick.

$$\frac{4 \times 3}{15}\% = \frac{12}{15} = 0.8\%$$

Change in distance of lens from eye is

$$\frac{zD_v}{10}\%$$

Where Z equals an increase or decrease of distance between lens vertex and center of rotation (z), increase is positive, decrease is negative.

EXAMPLE

a. A +4.00D. spherical lens is moved 3 mm away from eye.

$$\frac{3 \times 4}{10}\% = 1.2\%$$ magnification

b. A +1.50D. spherical lens is moved 6 mm closer to the eye.

$$\frac{-6. \times 1.5}{10}\% = -.9\%$$ decrease or minification

c. A −8.00D. spherical lens is moved 3 mm closer to the eye.

$$\frac{(-8.) \times (-3)}{10}\% = \frac{24}{10}\% = 2.4\%$$ magnification increase

The dioptric power of all lenses produces some magnification, as is shown by the second factor of the magnification formula:

$$P = \frac{1}{1 - zD_v}$$

Since the vertex of the prescription lens is usually placed about 25 mm from the center of the rotation of the eye, each diopter of power generates 2.5 percent change of image size.

$$\frac{1}{1 - 0.25 \times 1.00} = \frac{1}{.975} = 1.025$$

It follows that this change induced by the power of the lens is affected by the profile or shape of the lens. If this were a +1.00D. sphere and made 2.1 mm thick from glass with a refactive index of

1.52 with a series of front surfaces of +1.00D., +4.00D., +7.00D., and +10.00D., the shape magnification would increase with the curvature of the lens by the formula

$$S = \frac{1}{1 - cD_1}$$

as given and the total magnification would be obtained by $M = S \times P$. Therefore the magnification of a +1.00D. sphere in these forms would increase as follows:

TABLE III
MAGNIFICATION OF 1.00D.

Front Curve	Shape × Power		Total
1.00	1.001 × 1.02	=	1.021
4.00	1.006 × 1.02	=	1.026
7.00	1.010 × 1.02	=	1.030
10.00	1.014 × 1.02	=	1.034

To this point, the lens and eye have been considered as a fixed optical unit. The point of greatest retinal sensitivity (macula) has received the image of the distant object. Except for the discussion of tilted lenses, the projected optical axis of the correction lens pierced the macula. This ideal relationship obscures some of the requisites of an adequate prescription lens in real life.

Unlike almost all other optical systems, the eye and lens combination does not move together. When the position of a telescope, camera, or microscope is changed, all the lenses of the system retain their original optical alignment. When the direction of gaze is altered, the eye rotates, but the spectacle lens remains fixed. The center of rotation of the eye is about 13 mm behind the front surface (cornea) of the eye. The imaginary line that connects the center of rotation, C in Figure 65, and the object upon which vision is fixed is called line of fixation, *zz*. When the eye is rotated, and different sectors of the visual field are viewed, the far point of the eye also moves about the center of rotation. As the far point of a myopic eye is moved about, an imaginary spherical surface is generated in *front* of the eye. This surface is called the far-point sphere. The original requirement of a correcting lens was that it have its focal point at the far point of the

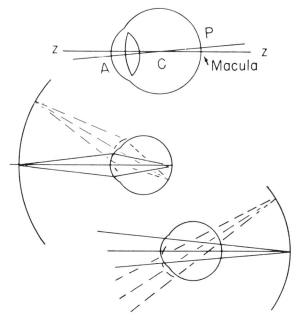

Figure 65.   Far-point spheres of myopic and hyperopic eyes.

eye. It is now apparent that, if the lens meets the new requirements, the marginal (extra-axial) portions of the lens must also
focus parallel rays from a distant object at corresponding points
on the surface of this far-point sphere at all points. The far-point
sphere of the hyperopic eye is traced in the space behind the eye.
Again, the focal points of the marginal areas of the convex correcting lens must fall on the sphere with a constant radius of the distance from the center of rotation to the far point.

   In the discussion of tilted lenses, it was shown that light which
does not strike a lens at a right angle (normal) to a lens in the
axial region does not come to a focus at the same point as in the
case of axial rays. This condition of astigmatism is one of a group
of aberrations encountered in the peripheral portions of all lenses.
It is the most offensive of all, but fortunately is largely correctable
by the simple device of proper choice of lens profile.

   Wollaston (1804) described the meniscus form of lens that
would be necessary in order to provide what he called "periscopic

spectacles." He found the formulas for a series of spherical lenses without astigmatism that focussed on the far-point sphere over a large angle. It was more than a hundred years, however, before the proper calculations were completed and the lenses that fulfilled the formula were produced in quantity. Marginally corrected spectacle lenses were made by Carl Zeiss, Jena, Germany, and called Punktal. This series of lenses was revised and made in this country by Bausch & Lomb Optical Company. Neither of these lenses was extensively used because each prescription required individual base curves and, therefore, they could not be produced outside of a large lens factory. No provision was made for many prescriptions requiring prisms, bifocals, absorption glasses, and so forth.

About 1920 Tillyer with American Optical Company and Rayton with Bausch & Lomb Optical Company separately undertook to simplify marginally corrected lenses so they could be satisfactorily produced in smaller lens laboratories. Their efforts were highly successful. Tillyer® (1926) and Orthogon® (1928) lenses were followed by "best form" (marginally corrected) lenses from all leading lens-makers.

The most recently designed lens series have cylinders ground on the back surfaces of the lenses. This design averts the slight dioptric increase generated when a spherocylindrical lens with the toric curve on the front surface is used at a finite distance. Some lens manufacturers have delayed the huge investment in machinery to convert to this lens form. Strong cylinder lenses with concave cylinders appear and also fit better in frames. Prescription shops find minus cylinders easier to produce from a smaller inventory of semi-finished blanks.

A lens that is designed to maintain its focal point on or as close as possible to the far-point sphere of the eye it corrects must be placed in a certain position to fulfill the requirements of the formula. By common consent the posterior pole (vertex) is placed 27 mm from the center of rotation of the eye. The distance from the cornea to the center is taken as 13.25 mm, so the calculated position of the lens is 13.75 mm from the cornea. However, the Masterpiece® II series (AOCo.) has included parameters of less and more than that amount. The lens axis is coincident with the fixation axis in the primary position. Between the limits of +7.00D. and −20.00D., single vision lenses are regularly available in which the marginal astigmatism has been reduced to negligible amounts when compared with the units of measurement as Tillyer's calculations for Patent No. 1,588,559 indicate in Table XXXIV.

Despite the calculated vertex distance of 13.75 mm, it is common practice to disregard this part of the formula and to examine the eyes and fit the spectacles as close to the eyes as the lashes will permit. It follows that most lenses are set at distances from 9 to 11 mm from the cornea. Thus, convex lenses tend to be fitted slightly stronger and concave lenses weaker than would be required if the lenses were set at a greater distance from the eyes. The magnification of the lenses is also slightly affected in the opposite direction. Neither of these effects is considerable except in very strong lenses.

Another violation of the terms of the original calculation must be considered. Very few spectacle lenses are fitted with the optical axis horizontal, that is, coincident with or parallel with the visual axis in primary position (Fig. 64). Most lenses are tilted in toward the cheeks at an angle of 4° to 12° to the face plane. Correction for this error is described in Chapter 7.

PRISM BY DECENTRATION

It has been shown that when flat surfaces are inclined toward one another, a prism is formed. The optical function of the prism is to deviate rays of light as shown in Figure 54. When curved surfaces incline toward one another, the prism effect is added to the lens effect. By their very form, the surfaces of all convex and concave lenses are inclined toward one another, either toward the lens center or toward the periphery. Thus it is apparent that a lens has the effect of an infinite number of prisms of increasing angles with their bases toward or away from center. This concept of prism effect produced by lenses is a fundamental in ophthalmic dispensing. Figure 66 shows that the prism or deviation increases as the distance from the lens center is increased. It is apparent that if a ray of light which is parallel to the lens axis, but decentered some distance from the axis, strikes a lens it will be deviated toward the thickest part of the lens. The amount of this deviation or prism effect is dependent upon the power of the lens and the distance the ray is decentered from the lens axis.*

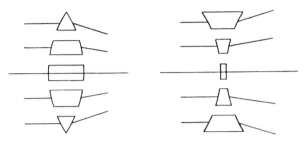

Figure 66. Peripheral ray deviation of lenses.

In Figure 67, all rays parallel to the axis zz' pass through $\mathbf{F'}$ the posterior focus of the lens. Ray $\mathbf{MB}$ at a distance y cm from the axis is refracted toward $\mathbf{F'}$. At the distance f meters, this ray has been deviated the distance y' cm. Then, since a Prism Diopter one-hundredth (as 1 cm is to 1 m) of the distance between the prism and the screen:

$$\text{P.D. } (\Delta) = \frac{y'}{f} = y' \, D$$

Where

$$y' = \text{Amount of decentration in cm}$$

$$D = \frac{1}{f} = \text{Diopters of lens power}$$

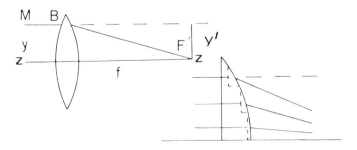

Figure 67. Deviation of refracted rays.

*Bennett, A.G.: *Graphical Methods of Solving Optical Problems.* London, Hatton Press, 1948, pp. 20-25.

As a mnemonic, a 1 Diopter sphere decentered 1 cm (10 mm) makes one Prism Diopter.

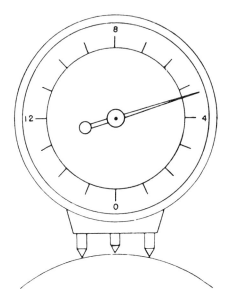

Figure 68. Geneva lens measure showing +4.75D.

OBLIQUE CURVATURE OF CYLINDERS

An optician's lens-measure (Fig. 68) which measures the curves of lens surfaces in diopters can be used to demonstrate this function of a cylindrical surface. When the measure is applied to the surface in the direction of the axis of the cylinder and rotated 5° or 10°, the hand will scarcely move on the dial. The same limited movement will be noted at the opposite meridian. If, however, the instrument is set at an angle of about 45°, the change in curvature will be more rapid with small changes in position. An approximation of the curvature effect in any meridian of a cylinder can be made with a protractor and lens-measure.

For convenience, Table IV has been prepared to show the percentage of the curvature of the cylinder at 5-degree intervals. It is interesting to note that the total of the curvatures at right angles always equals 100 percent of the lens power. Further, the differ-

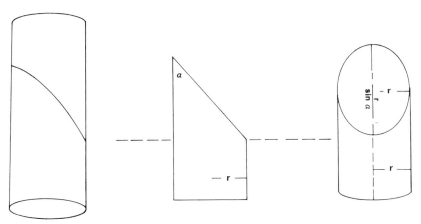

Figure 69.

ences in percentage of curvature follow a progression that can be easily remembered. After the first figure, the difference between 5-degree intervals increases by one each time up to 9 and then reduces one at a time to .97.

TABLE IV
CURVATURE OF CYLINDERS

Degrees From Axis		% of Curvature	Degrees From Axis		% of Curvature
0	180	00	45	135	50
5	175	01	50	130	59
10	170	03	55	125	67
15	165	07	60	120	75
20	160	12	65	115	82
25	155	18	70	110	88
30	150	25	75	105	98
35	145	33	80	100	97
40	140	41	85	95	99

For example, find the curvature in the vertical meridian of 2.50D. Cyl. $\times$ 65.

The cylinder axis is 25° from the vertical meridian. At that point, the curvature of the cylinder is 18 percent of its dioptric power.

$$2.50 \times .18 = 0.45D.$$

Considerable confusion developed in the late nineteenth century in the use of cylindrical lenses for the correction of astigmatism. The use of a nonluminous retinoscope was very difficult for many practitioners, and some refractionists found a certain amount of astigmatism at an axis which did not provide maximum acuity. Additional trial lenses including cylinders were used to arrive at the best visual acuity. Occasionally cylindrical lenses at different axes were combined with the cylinder power found by retinoscopy to the end that prescriptions such as the following were written:

$$+0.75 \times 90 \ \supset + \ 0.50 \times 140$$

As late as 1916, I ground lenses for a refractionist who did not allow these involved prescriptions to be combined into equivalent spherocylinders. This meant that a flat semifinished cylinder had a flat cylinder ground on the other side at 50° away from the cylinder on the first side. There was no way to simplify the work because the doctor used a lens measure to assure himself that there was a cylinder on each side of the lens.

COMBINING OBLIQUELY CROSSED CYLINDERS

Charles F. Prentice* first solved the problem of combining two obliquely crossed cylinders when he applied the vector analysis involved in the parallelogram of forces. The trigonometric method of S. P. Thompson† become the accepted procedure.

$$P = \sqrt{F_1{}^2 + F_2{}^2 + 2F_1F_2 \cos 2\gamma}$$

$$Q = \frac{F_1 + F_2 - P}{2}$$

$$\tan 2\alpha = \frac{F_2 \sin 2\gamma}{F_1 + F_2 \cos 2\ \gamma}$$

Where F_1 = the power of the first cylinder
F_2 = the power of the second cylinder
P = the cylinder of the new spherocylinder

---

*Prentice, C.F.: *Ophthalmic Lenses*. Philadelphia, Keystone Pr, 1900, pp. 53-84.
†Southall, J.P.C.: *Mirrors, Prisms, Lenses*. New York, Macmillan, 1933, pp. 320-326.
Waters, E.H.: *Ophthalmic Mechanics*. Ann Arbor, Edwards Brothers, 1947, p. 49.
Martin, L.C.: *Technical Optics*, Vol. 1. New York, Pitman, 1948, pp. 37-38.

Q = the spherical element
γ = the angle between the axes of the crossed cylinders
α = the value of the angle to be added to the lesser of the original axes to give the axis of the cylinder in the new equivalent.

For all practical purposes in regular ophthalmic procedures this problem can be quite satisfactorily plotted by the vector method on $8\frac{1}{2} \times 11$ inch *polar coordinate* paper:

1. First transpose the lenses to plus cylinders.
2. Represent the power of the cylinder (A) with the axis nearer zero (180°) in the upper right hand quadrant. For the sake of accuracy, choose the largest possible unit.
3. Find the *angle between the cylinder axes* and multiply the amount by 2. Add this amount to the first cylinder (A) axis and plot the second cylinder (B) in this direction, turning anticlockwise.
4. Complete the parallelogram. (Use a compass, if available, for accuracy.) Draw the diagonal. The length of this line is the power of the new plus cylinder (C).
5. Locate the line that bisects the angle (not the side of the parallelogram) between the diagonal and the axis of cylinder (A). This is the axis of the new cylinder (C).
6. The spherical element arising from this combination is found by this formula:

$$\text{New sphere} = \frac{\text{cylinder A} + \text{cylinder B} - \text{cylinder C}}{2}$$

EXAMPLE:

To +8.50 +4.50 × 15, add +2.50 −2.00 × 5.

(This is not a hypothetical case. It is the combined effect of the change in corneal curve and position of spectacle lens as found at a second refraction after cataract surgery.)

1. After transposition to plus cylinders, the combination reads
+8.50 +4.50 × 15 (A)
+0.50 +2.00 × 95 (B)
2. The +4.50 cylinder is the (A) first cylinder because the axis is the closer to the horizontal. The plotting paper is 100 mm in radius, so 20 mm is chosen to represent +1.00D. (The next larger unit would carry 4.50D. off the chart.)
3. When 15° is subtracted from 95°, the angle between the axes is

found to be 80°, and multiplied by 2 equals 160°. When this angle is added to 15°, the axis of cylinder (A), the total equals 175°. Cylinder (B) is plotted in this meridian.
4. The diagonal of the parallelogram is very nearly 55 mm or +2.75D. cylinder.

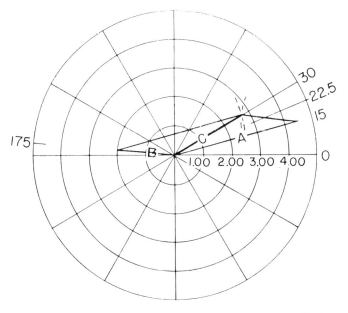

Figure 70. Graphical calculation of obliquely crossed cylinders

5. The diagonal is almost precisely on axis 30°. Therefore the midline between 15° and 30° is 22½° which can be found by several methods.
6. The spherical power generated by the combination of cylinders is

$$
\begin{array}{ll}
+4.50 & (A) \\
+2.00 & (B) \\
\hline
+6.50 & \\
-2.75 & (C) \\
\end{array}
$$

$$
2)\ \overline{+3.75}
$$
$$
+1.87
$$

The total value of the combined spherocylinders becomes

$$
\begin{array}{l}
+8.50 \\
+0.50 \\
+1.87\ +2.75 \times 22\frac{1}{2} \\
\hline
+10.87\ +2.75 \times 22\frac{1}{2}
\end{array}
$$

An easier method of plotting and solving crossed cylinder is described by Emsley in his *Optical Tables and Other Data* (Bausch & Lomb, London, 1968) and requires fewer lines and therefore is subject to fewer errors. It requires a special protractor which is easily constructed on an $8\frac{1}{2} \times 11$ inch sheet of polar coordinate paper. The regular protractor degrees are divided by 2. Thus the whole revolution is numbered from 0 to 180. The circles on the paper are scaled to represent diopters of cylinder.

The routine to use the chart follows:

1. Transpose the cylinders to the same sign.
2. Double the power of the cylinders and plot points on the appropriate axes.

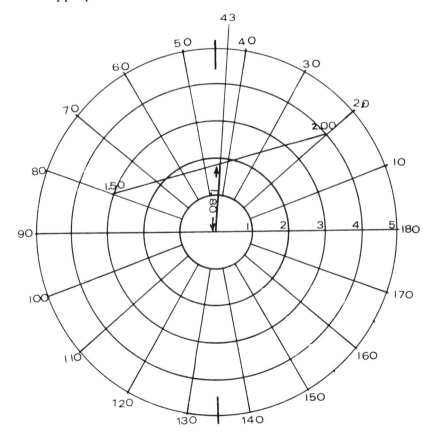

Figure 71.

TABLE V

OBLIQUELY CROSSED CYLINDERS*

Values of $k = F_1/F_2$

α°	8	6	5·33	5	4	3·33	3	2·67	2·5	2	1·67	1·6	1·5	1·33	1·25	1	α°
0	0 / 9·00	0 / 7·00	0 / 6·33	0 / 6·00	0 / 5·00	0 / 4·33	0 / 4·00	0 / 3·67	0 / 3·50	0 / 3·00	0 / 2·67	0 / 2·60	0 / 2·50	0 / 2·33	0 / 2·25	0 / 2·0	180
5	¼ / 8·99	¼ / 6·99	1 / 6·32	1 / 5·99	1 / 4·99	1 / 4·32	1 / 3·99	1¼ / 3·66	1¼ / 3·49	1¼ / 2·99	2 / 2·66	2 / 2·59	2 / 2·49	2 / 2·32	2 / 2·24	2½ / 1·99	175
10	1 / 8·95	1¼ / 6·95	1¼ / 6·28	1¼ / 5·95	2 / 4·95	2¼ / 4·29	2¼ / 3·95	2¼ / 3·62	3 / 3·46	3¼ / 2·96	3½ / 2·63	4 / 2·56	4 / 2·46	4½ / 2·30	4½ / 2·22	5 / 1·97	170
15	1½ / 8·88	2 / 6·89	2¼ / 6·22	2¼ / 5·89	3 / 4·89	3½ / 4·23	3½ / 3·90	4 / 3·57	4 / 3·40	5 / 2·91	5½ / 2·58	5½ / 2·51	6 / 2·42	6½ / 2·26	6½ / 2·17	7½ / 1·93	165
20	2 / 8·79	2¼ / 6·80	2¼ / 6·13	3 / 5·80	4 / 4·81	4½ / 4·15	5 / 3·82	5½ / 3·49	5½ / 3·33	6½ / 2·84	7½ / 2·52	7½ / 2·45	8 / 2·36	8½ / 2·20	9 / 2·12	10 / 1·88	160
25	2½ / 8·68	3 / 6·69	3 / 6·03	4 / 5·69	4½ / 4·71	5½ / 4·05	6 / 3·72	6½ / 3·40	7 / 3·23	8 / 2·75	9 / 2·43	9½ / 2·37	10 / 2·28	10½ / 2·12	11 / 2·04	12½ / 1·81	155
30	3 / 8·54	4 / 6·56	3½ / 5·90	4½ / 5·57	5½ / 4·58	6½ / 3·93	7 / 3·61	7½ / 3·28	8 / 3·12	9½ / 2·65	11 / 2·33	11 / 2·27	11½ / 2·18	12½ / 2·03	13 / 1·95	15 / 1·73	150
35	3 / 8·39	4 / 6·41	4½ / 5·75	5 / 5·42	6 / 4·44	7 / 3·79	8 / 3·47	8½ / 3·15	9 / 2·99	11 / 2·52	12½ / 2·22	13 / 2·16	13½ / 2·07	14½ / 1·92	15½ / 1·85	17½ / 1·64	145
40	3½ / 8·23	4½ / 6·25	5 / 5·59	5½ / 5·27	6½ / 4·29	8 / 3·64	8½ / 3·32	9½ / 3·01	10 / 2·85	12 / 2·39	14 / 2·09	14½ / 2·03	15 / 1·94	16½ / 1·80	17½ / 1·73	20 / 1·53	140
45	3½ / 8·06	4¾ / 6·08	5½ / 5·43	5¾ / 5·10	7 / 4·12	8¼ / 3·48	9 / 3·16	10¼ / 2·85	11 / 2·69	13½ / 2·24	15 / 1·94	16 / 1·89	17 / 1·80	18½ / 1·67	19½ / 1·60	22½ / 1·41	135
50	3½ / 7·89	5 / 5·91	5½ / 5·25	6 / 4·93	7 / 3·95	8½ / 3·31	9½ / 2·99	11 / 2·68	11½ / 2·53	14 / 2·07	16½ / 1·79	17½ / 1·73	18½ / 1·65	20 / 1·52	21 / 1·46	25 / 1·29	130
55	3½ / 7·72	4½ / 5·74	5½ / 5·08	5½ / 4·75	7 / 3·78	8½ / 3·14	9½ / 2·82	11 / 2·51	12 / 2·35	15 / 1·91	17½ / 1·62	18½ / 1·57	19½ / 1·49	21½ / 1·37	23 / 1·31	27½ / 1·15	125

60	30 1·0	24½ 1·15	23 1·20	20½ 1·32	19 1·40	18½ 1·45	15 1·73	11½ 2·18	11 2·33	9½ 2·65	8½ 2·96	7 3·61	5½ 4·58	5 4·91	4½ 5·57	3½ 7·55	120
65	32½ 0·85	26 0·98	24 1·03	21 1·15	19½ 1·23	18½ 1·28	14½ 1·56	11 2·01	10½ 2·16	9 2·48	8 2·80	6½ 3·44	5 4·42	4½ 4·75	4 5·41	3 7·40	115
70	35 0·68	26½ 0·80	24½ 0·86	20½ 0·98	19 1·05	18 1·11	14 1·39	10 1·85	9½ 2·01	8 2·32	7 2·65	5½ 3·30	4½ 4·28	4 4·61	3½ 5·27	2½ 7·26	110
75	37½ 0·52	26 0·63	23½ 0·68	19 0·81	17 0·89	16 0·94	12 1·24	8½ 1·71	8 1·87	6½ 2·19	5½ 2·52	4½ 3·17	3½ 4·16	3 4·50	3 5·16	2 7·15	105
80	40 0·35	24 0·46	20½ 0·52	15½ 0·66	13½ 0·74	12½ 0·80	9 1·11	6 1·60	5½ 1·76	4½ 2·09	4 2·42	3 3·08	2½ 4·07	2 4·41	2 5·07	1½ 7·07	100
85	42½ 0·17	16½ 0·32	13 0·39	9½ 0·54	8 0·64	7 0·70	5 1·03	3 1·53	3 1·69	2½ 2·02	2 2·35	1½ 3·02	1 4·02	1 4·35	1 5·02	½ 7·02	95
90	0 0	0 0·25	0 0·33	0 0·50	0 0·60	0 0·67	0 1·00	0 1·50	0 1·67	0 2·00	0 2·33	0 3·00	0 4·00	0 4·33	0 5·00	0 7·00	90
α°	1	1·25	1·33	1·5	1·6	1·67	2	2·5	2·67	3	3·33	4	4	5·33	6	8	α°

Values of $k = F_1/F_2$

F_1 = Stronger cylinder
F_2 = Weaker cylinder

$$k = \frac{F_1}{F_2}$$

α = Difference between cylinder axes of F_1 and F_2
A = Resultant cylinder axis. F_1 cylinder axis + θ when *a* is 0 to 90 or F_1 cylinder axis - θ when *a* is 91 to 180.
C = Resultant cylinder power. F_2 times lower numeral in the box.
θ = Upper numeral in the box.

* From Emsley: *Optical Tables and Other Data.* London, U.K.O. B & L, 1968.

3. Join the points plotted with a straight line.
4. Find the midpoint of this line. Draw a line from the midpoint to the center of the protractor. This is the axis of the new cylinder.
5. The length of the line from the center to the midpoint is (c), the actual (not doubled) power of the new cylinder.
6. The power of the sphere is found by the regular formula:

$$\frac{d_1 + d_2 - c}{2}$$

Combine the cylinders of these lenses:

R　+2.00 × 20
L　+1.50 × 80

As is plotted in Figure 71, the power and axis of the new cylinder is +1.80 × 43. The spherical element induced is

$$\frac{+2.00 + 1.50 - 1.80}{2} = \frac{1.70}{2} = +0.85$$

Thus the spherocylinder which represents these combined plano cylinders is +0.85 + 1.80 × 43

Mr. Emsley has also prepared the simplest of all methods for combining crossed cylinders. It is based upon Table V

EXAMPLE:　+2.50 × 90 ◯ +1.25 × 65

1. The power of the stronger cylinder is referred to as F_1 and the power of the weaker cylinder is referred to as F_2.
2. The ratio of these powers is always a whole number:

$$\frac{F_1}{F_2} = \kappa \text{ (Kappa)}$$

$$\frac{F_1}{F_2} = \frac{2.50}{1.25} = \kappa = 2$$

3. The separation in degrees of cyl axis of F_1 and cyl axis of F_2 is named α.

Axis F_1 − axis F_2 = α = 90 − 65 = 25

These differences are designated in the rows on the table:

α°	Value							
	1	1·25	1·33	1·5	1·6	1·67	2	2
0	0 2·0	0 2·25	0 2·33	0 2·50	0 2·60	0 2·67	0 3·00	3·
5	2½ 1·99	2 2·24	2 2·32	2 2·49	2 2·59	2 2·66	1½ 2·99	3·
10	5 1·97	4½ 2·22	4½ 2·30	4 2·46	4 2·56	3½ 2·63	3½ 2·96	3·
15	7½ 1·93	6½ 2·17	6½ 2·26	6 2·42	5½ 2·51	5½ 2·58	5 2·91	3·
20	10 1·88	9 2·12	8½ 2·20	8 2·36	7½ 2·45	7½ 2·52	6½ 2·84	3·
25	12½ 1·81	11 2·04	10½ 2·12	10 2·28	9½ 2·37	9 2·43	8 2·75	3·
30	15 1·73	13 1·95	12½ 2·03	11½ 2·18	11 2·27	11 2·33	9½ 2·65	3·

Figure 72. Example from table.

The upper number in the square indicates the amount to be subtracted from the axis of F_1 when α is 90° or less (and the amount to be added when the difference is more than 90°). The new axis is between F_1 and F_2.

Hence the new cylinder axis would be $90 - 8 = 82$. $F_2 \times 2.75 = 1.25 \times 2.75 = 3.44$. Thus the combination becomes $+3.44 \times 82$.

4. Across the top of the table $\kappa = F_1/F_2$ is shown.
5. The rows of the table (α) show the inclination between the axes of F_1 and F_2 in degrees.
6. The numerals in the box at the intersection of κ and solve the problem. The upper of the two numerals gives the amount the resultant axis varies from F_1 axis. The resultant cylinder power (C) is found by multiplying F_2 by the lower number.

What could be simpler? Somewhat mystifying to a layman but a neat exercise for a mathematician like Emsley.

Without doubt, with all of their artificiality, these are the simplest and easiest ways to plot and to recheck as compared with other methods of combining crossed cylinders.

The combining of obliquely crossed cylinders will be frequently done. Calculating lens power changes in the Provisional Plan for aphakic lenses and compensating certain asymmetric prescriptions require the procedure.

COMBINING AND RESOLVING OBLIQUE PRISMS

The rare case of combining oblique prisms can also be solved by this method of plotting. The procedure for prisms is also much simpler. The first step disappears, of course, because there is no transposition. The prisms are plotted precisely as prescribed. The diagonal found in step 4 gives the power of the resultant prism and the direction of the diagonal is the axis of the prism.

In actual practice this second procedure is seldom used. Diagonal deviations are usually resolved into horizontal and vertical components by present-day refracting methods and instruments. When the angle between the prisms becomes a right angle, or 90°, the parallelogram becomes rectangular and the diagonal is simply $c^2 = a^2 + b^2$, which is the hypotenuse of a right triangle. The axis of the resultant prism is the angle whose tangent is a/b.

Another instance is an oblique prism induced by decentration at the NVP in multifocals by cylinders at oblique axes. However this point in a lens has a simple prism when the cylinder axis is 90° or 180°. In the first instance there can be no vertical prism and an inconsequential prism is obtained by low power lenses from the 2 mm decentration caused by convergence. On the other

1·46	1·52	1·65	1·73	1·79	2·07	2·53	2·68	2·99	3·31	3
23 / 1·31	21½ / 1·37	19½ / 1·49	18½ / 1·57	17½ / 1·62	15 / 1·91	12 / 2·35	11 / 2·51	9½ / 2·82	8½ / 3·14	3
24½ / 1·15	23 / 1·20	20½ / 1·32	19 / 1·40	18½ / 1·45	15 / 1·73	11½ / 2·18	11 / 2·33	9½ / 2·65	8½ / 2·96	3
26 / 0·98	24 / 1·03	21 / 1·15	19½ / 1·23	18½ / 1·28	14½ / 1·56	11 / 2·01	10½ / 2·16	9 / 2·48	8 / 2·80	6 / 3
26½ / 0·80	24½ / 0·86	20½ / 0·98	19 / 1·05	18 / 1·11	14 / 1·39	10 / 1·85	9½ / 2·01	8 / 2·32	7 / 2·65	3
26 / 0·63	23½ / 0·68	19 / 0·81	17 / 0·89	16 / 0·94	12 / 1·24	8½ / 1·71	8 / 1·87	6½ / 2·19	5½ / 2·52	4 / 3
24 / 0·46	20½ / 0·52	15½ / 0·66	13½ / 0·74	12½ / 0·80	9 / 1·11	6 / 1·60	5½ / 1·76	4½ / 2·09	4 / 2·42	3
16½ / 0·32	13 / 0·39	9½ / 0·54	8 / 0·64	7 / 0·70	5 / 1·03	3 / 1·53	3 / 1·69	2½ / 2·02	2 / 2·35	1 / 3
0 / 0·25	0 / 0·33	0 / 0·50	0 / 0·60	0 / 0·67	0 / 1·00	0 / 1·50	0 / 1·67	0 / 2·00	0 / 2·33	3
1·25	1·33	1·5	1·6	1·67	2	2·5	2·67	3	3·33	4

Values of $k = F_1/F_2$

Figure 73. Example from table.

hand, cylinder axis 180° has its full power vertically and no power laterally; hence, convergence induces no decentration. Two examples of combined prism problems follow. They typify combining and separating a combined prism into its two simple prisms.

EXAMPLE

O.D. 3$^\triangle$ Base Out $\frown$ 2$^\triangle$ Base Down.
tan $\angle$ A = a/b = $\frac{2}{3}$ = 0.6667 = 33° 42′
This is the axis of the combined prisms.
The sine of angle A will provide the hypotenuse of $\angle$ A (the power of the combined prism).
sin $\angle$ A = a/c = sin 33° 42′ = 0.5548
1/c = .5548/a
c = a/.5548 = 2/.5548 = 3.6$^\triangle$
Hence the combined prisms become:
O.D. 3.6$^\triangle$ axis 34 Base Out and Down.

EXAMPLE

O.D. 5$^\triangle$ Base Up and In axis 65
a/c = sin 65 = 0.9063
a = 5 × sin 65 = 5 X .9063 = 4.5315 = 4.5$^\triangle$ Base Up
a/b = tan 65 = 2.1445
1/b = 2.1445/a
b = a/2.1445 = 4.5315/2.1445 = 2.109$^\triangle$ Base In
Hence the prism resolves into:
O.D. 4.5$^\triangle$ Base Up $\frown$ 2.1$^\triangle$ Base In

Figure 69 would seem to settle the erroneous concept that a cylinder at an oblique axis can be decentered to produce definite amounts of prism in any one direction in any other meridian than the axis or opposite principal meridian. The power meridian which intersects the center of the segment creates prism Up and Out *or* Down and In according to the sign of the cylinder and not Up or In exclusively.

When prescriptions are written for specific quantities Base In or Out and Up or Down, a surface-grinder ordinarily prefers to measure the prism effect in the two directions. For the purposes of producing a lens of proper edge- or mounting-thickness, the lens must be calipered on the horizontal line in most cases. It is convenient to make the thickness allowance for the prism at the same points.

The thickness of the glass blank required to produce a compound prism can be estimated only from the combined prism power. Occasionally the foregoing formula is necessary to calculate the lens thickness over a fused multifocal segment placed close to the apex of the prism.

A refracting procedure seldom used in which heterophorias were simultaneously measured by the displacement of a point source of light on a tangent screen (Maddox screen), this frequently produced lens prescriptions with diagonal prism such as O.D. + 1.00 + 75 × 90 $\subset$ 2$^\triangle$ Base Up at 20° Experience proves that it is more satisfactory to grind and inspect such a lens according to the prescription as written. Trial set prisms and lens-measuring instruments are calibrated in units of 0.5$^\triangle$. When a lens with an oblique base is resolved into vertical and horizontal components, small fractional values that can only be estimated are usually involved, and thus errors are easily introduced.

BIFOCALS

Many lens designs are available nowadays for the person who must supplement or replace his accommodation with spectacle lens power. Until 1784, it was necessary to have separate pairs of glasses when an individual's eyes required different focal powers for use at varied distances. In that year, Benjamin Franklin displayed his perspicacity when he requested his optician to split his framed distance and reading lenses and fit the halves used for near at the bottom. In his own words, "I have only to move my eyes up and down as I want to see distinctly far or near, the proper glasses being always ready."

The following pages will be a recitation of the development of bifocals and multifocals with some comment about the novelty or intention of each basic design. The reader is referred to the manufacturers' specification charts for up-to-the-minute information. Makers tend to change the sizes of lens blanks, position and size of segments, kinds of glass (absorption tints), base curves, and range of additions according to trends and demand. Likewise seldom used designs tend to lapse from factory stock to special orders, then discontinuance.

Another common procedure with a lens form that declines in popularity is for one or two manufacturers to make all of the lenses for the whole market and ship blanks to other makers to package the item as if it were produced by them. One-piece Ultex® lenses are going through that process at this time.

In an inventor's enthusiasm Franklin had not quite told the whole story. Nature, by the way of presbyopia, had deprived him of his previous ability to see clearly at all points with one pair of glasses. Now he was willing to concede the loss of the use of half of the field of either of his lenses and restrict his angle of fixation in order to escape inconvenience of two pairs of glasses. The development and application of this compromise (if it may be called a compromise) has been a boon to all persons of middle-age and has been a challenge to the optical profession and industry.

Comfortable use of bifocal or any multifocal lenses is dependent upon many factors. At this time the discussion will be limited to those of optical nature. Consideration of the individual application in which prescription, occupation, anatomy, and even the patient's psychology are involved will be left to the chapter on Multifocal Prescription Analysis.

Franklin's innovation required little adjustment from the optical aspects. As Figure 74 shows, the optical axes of the two parts still lie in the same line. As the eyes alternate from top to bottom, the projected fields are in their accustomed positions with the same prism displacement of extra-axial points for the distance or reading lenses. The seam across the middle made an unavoidable blurred line which must be tolerated. The angle subtended by this dividing line is determined by the pupillary diameter, that is, the blur does not completely disappear from the point of fixation

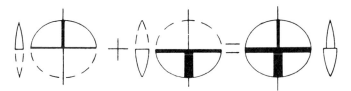

Figure 74. Split bifocal magnification.

until practically all of the light rays filling the pupil come from
either the distance or the reading portion of the lens. The exact
projection of the blur at the junction of the two focal powers cannot be calculated without consideration of the lens powers of both
distance and near. A lens at average distance from the eye projects
a blurred area almost fifteen times the width of the pupil at a near
point of 40 cm, that is, the zone of indistinct vision for a 3 mm
pupil is 45 mm (almost 2 inches) wide at the reading distance.

It would seem that the original idea for a bifocal lens had
minimum optical defects. Indeed the lens proved to be highly
satisfactory for many reasons. The fact that the two lenses were
independent permitted size, shape, or prescriptions to be varied
at will. Yet, there was one very important factor which could not
be disregarded. The ledge at the edge of the reading segment
margin collected dust and grime.

A hundred years later the idea of a thin lens cemented to the
distance glass was introduced. This cosmetic improvement increased the use of bifocals and simultaneously spurred inventors.
In the effort to improve the appearance, size, or shape of the
reading portions, some lens designs sacrificed part of the
optical advantages of the original idea. The reading segment of
the cemented bifocal contained the additional spherical power that
represented the difference between the distance and total reading
prescription. It was made sufficiently large to be split into halves
and thus serve for a pair of lenses (Fig. 75). The thin edge of the
reading segment was a distinct cosmetic advantage. The reduced
size of the reading area was an improvement over the original half
lens. An optical effect was introduced, however, that was quite
different from the split-type. Instead of a coincidence of optical
centers in the geometric center of the lens, the optical center of the

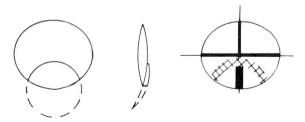

Figure 75. Round segment bifocal magnification.

reading segment was some distance below the edge of the lens. When the wearer's pupil crossed the dividing line into the reading portion there was an abrupt displacement or "jump" of the visual field.

The amount of the displacement at the segment margin is determined by the prism effect (Base Down) of the reading addition at that point added to the prism effect of the distance power at that point. Therefore the "jump" increases as the dioptric power of the addition increases. The distance of the optical center of the reading segment from the dividing line is equally significant.

When D_m = Dioptric power of distance (major) lens

D_s = Dioptric power of the reading segment

d = distance in centimeters from the optical axis (center) of distance portion to the segment margin

r = distance in centimeters of the optical axis (center) of the reading addition to the segment margin

The prism effect of "jump" at the periphery of the Ultex A reading segment in Figure 76 is (Jump + D_s × r).

EXAMPLE

+1.50D. Sphere for distance

+2.00D. Sphere addition for reading

Lens size 40 × 44 mm oval, segment size 38 mm wide × 15 mm high.

Segment Jump = 2.00 × 1.9 = 3.8$^\triangle$

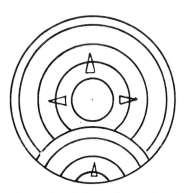

Figure 76. Prism isobars of one-piece bifocal.

Let the center of the reading segment be 19 mm below the edge of the segment. Let the distance prescription be 1.50D. Sphere and the segment be +2.00D. Boeder's graphs of the two elements are shown in Figure 76.

At the dividing line the distance lens is decentered.

$$+1.50 \times .5 = 0.75^\triangle \text{ Base Up}$$

At the margin of the reading segment the decentration is 19 mm:

$$+2.00 \times 1.9 = 3.8^\triangle \text{ Base Down}$$

Hence the jump is the total of the two prism effects:

$$3.8^\triangle - 0.75^\triangle = 3.05^\triangle \text{ Base Down}$$

Thus, at the point where the pupil crosses the dividing line, the prism Base Up effect is changed to prism Base Down. This gives the illusion of an abrupt upward displacement to the whole reading field. The unavoidable blurred area at the edge of the segment is further extended by the prismatic displacement of the "jump."

This "jump" is not as distracting as it might seem at first consideration. In practice the eyes are moved quickly through a rather large arc when fixation is changed from distance to near. The bifocal wearer's problem with "jump" arises when he wishes to see an object that is obscured in the "blind-spot" at the edge of the segment. He is put to the inconvenience of having to move his head the increased angle to compensate for the upward displacement from the Base Down prism.

Still another optical difference is found in a cemented bifocal. The *near-vision point* (N.V.P.) , a term introduced by L.W. Bugbee to describe the point through which the projection of the fixation axis passes in the act of near-point fixation, is usually about 8 mm below the center of the distance lens. At this point in Franklins' original idea, the wearer encounters the prismatic displacement characteristic of the whole reading prescription. The optical center of the reading segment in the cemented bifocal causes the prism effect (displacement) at the near-vision point to vary with each prescription and also with variations in the distances between the centers of the distance lens and reading segment in the same prescription.

The object displacement at the N.V.P. in Figure 77 is the total of the prism effects of the decentration of the distance lens added

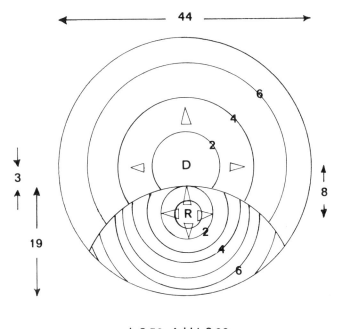

+ 3.50 Add+ 2.00

Figure 77.

to the prism effect from the decentration of the reading portion:

$\Delta_m \qquad = D_m \times c$

$\Delta_s \qquad = D_s \times d$

$\Delta NVP \qquad = \Delta_m \times \Delta_s$

Where $VN = c$

$RN \qquad = d$

R O.U $+3.50D$. Sphere

$\qquad +2.00$ add

Ultex A segment 3 below center

Reading position 8 below center

$\Delta_m = D_m \times c = +3.50 \times .8 = \quad 2.8^\triangle$ Base Up

$\Delta_s = D_s \times d = +2.00 \times 14 = \dfrac{2.8^\triangle \text{ Base Down}}{0.0}$

Hence there will be no prism at the desired reading position. The lenses are bicentric: a center in the distance portion and again a prism-free point in the reading segment.

A number of the lens manufacturers have spent much time in the development of the acceptance of this bicentric notion by the professions. They were able to show how their many different multifocal types were perfect solutions for this prism balancing caper and prepared much literature, many lectures, and some fitting table accessories to provide centered reading segments. In the end this concept is largely a drawing-board notion because balancing prescriptions for distance and near are required. Undesired very large or small segment sizes can be involved. Oblique cylinders can frustrate the whole effort.

From another approach, no individual has done so much as Virgil Hancock to follow up Bugbee's notion of producing an area (other than the axial zone of a lens) in which there was no prism. He began his research with Univis® Lens Company in Dayton in the days when he was doing multifocal designing and relentlessly followed up the subject at his own multifocal lens factory in Houston, Texas. In his publications and lectures he showed how prism could be ground Base Down on a minus lens to raise the center of this distance portion to a desired position. Then he calculated the prism Base Up required in a slab-off to set a new center in the reading position. His ultimate knowledge in the whole matter allowed him to go at a "rapid fire" pace that often caused his listeners to feel that they were incompetent to approach prescription analysis in his style. His procedure with a mirror to properly set the top edge of segment for regular or vocational lenses has never been matched, but it seems that its variation from other less precise methods has held back the acceptance it deserves. Since his retirement from the optical scene there has been no one to follow up the great work that he started.

The size of the original cemented bifocal reading portion has been found to be much larger than necessary for most purposes. As Percival* noted, reading or other near-point work is usually confined to an area not more than 6 inches wide and a height of about 4 inches and that we voluntarily turn our heads when fixation points are farther separated. This has been corroborated by

---

*Percival, A.S.: *The Prescribing of Spectacles.* New York, William Wood, 1910, pp. 54-55.

Fischer† in his statement that even emmetropic persons do not move their eyes in ordinary use more than 12° to right and left which at an average reading distance of 40 cm is 170 mm or $6\frac{3}{4}$ inches. When the spectacle lens plane is 27 mm from the center of rotation and the fixation distance is as close as 33 cm (13 inches), a rectangular segment, as Percival suggested, that is only 12.4 × 8.2 mm subtends the angle that covers that field of view. These segments, as well as 10 mm round (about 3 pupil diameters), are successfully worn only if the lenses are to be worn when the amount of reading is limited. At the other extreme, bifocals are available (Executive®) in which the reading portion covers more than half the area of the lens. When multifocals are carefully chosen to meet individual needs, the choice of the proper size and shape of the segments becomes extremely important. The variety of shapes and sizes now available, when combined with inverted segments and reversed lenses, meet almost any requirement. Progressive power lenses add further variety.

The inherent magnification of the distance lens prescription has been shown to have some effect upon the projected field. Therefore the formula to follow is an approximation. The vista through the reading segment at the assumed nearpoint is a projection of the triangle **UCT** in which the increase is more than fifteen times. The profile of the lens is usually curved and frequently point **T** is closer to the eye than the top of the segment. Therefore a slight variation in the position of the lens in front of the eye produces an important effect upon the conclusions. In Figure 78, the assumed reading distance is 40 cm **MW,** the pupillary diameter 3 mm, the width of the reading segment **UT** is 20 mm, and the distance of the segment to the center of rotation of the eye **WC** is 27 mm. As is shown in the drawing, the base of the cone of light subtended by the pupil has diminished slightly at the lens (about 3 percent); this small difference will not be taken into consideration because of the large number of other variables, including the variation in the diameter of the same pupil.

---

†Fischer, F.P.: Ueber die Verwendung von Kopfbewegungen beim Umhersehen. *Arch Ophthmol, 113:*394-416, 1924.

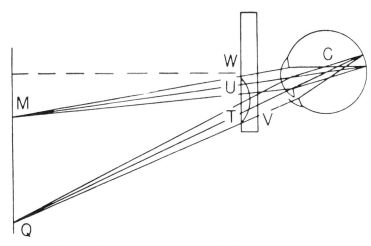

Figure 78.   Angular subtense of bifocal segment.

C   = Center of rotation
UT = Segment diameter
MQ = Vertical height of field of view
WC = Distance of segment from center of rotation

In practice, if the diameter of the pupil is subtracted from the width of the reading segment, the diameter of the useful field is found.   The field of view through the segment then is found by comparing the similar triangles **UCT** and **MCQ**, which in this case is:

$$\frac{MQ}{UT} = \frac{MC}{WC}$$

$$MQ = \frac{MC \times UT}{WC} = \frac{(400 + 27) \times (20 - 3)}{27}$$

$$= \frac{427 \times 17}{27} = 269 \text{ mm} = 10.6 \text{ inches.}$$

It is difficult to emphasize too much the effect of the distance of the lens from the eye in this calculation.   If the lens is set 5 mm closer to the eye the calculation becomes

$$\frac{422 \times 17}{22} = 326 \text{ mm} = 12.8 \text{ inches}$$

an increase of 21 percent.   Likewise, the diameter of the pupil assumes increasing importance as the size of the segment is reduced.

When the segment diameter is 20 mm, a fluctuation or error of 1 mm affects the calculation 1/20, or 5 percent, but the same deviation in the calculation of the intermediate segment of a trifocal 6 mm wide is a matter of $^1/_6$, or 16 percent, in the estimation. The pupillometer in Figure 79 suggested by Barkan* serves as a very convenient fitting-table accessory in estimating pupillary diameters when small segment areas are to be used.

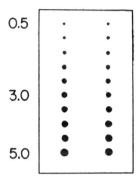

Figure 79. Barkan pupillometer.

Following cemented bifocals, the reading portion was made of denser glass (high refractive index) and fused into a depression ground into the major portion of the lens blank (Fig. 80). Again the use of bifocals was stimulated. The reading segments were so

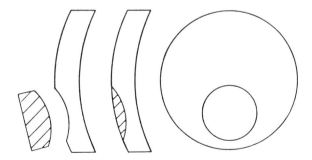

Figure 80. Fused bifocal construction.

---

*Barkan, Otto: Pupillometer and keratometer cards. *Am J Ophthmol, 32*:267, 1949.

unnoticeable as compared with previous lenses that the new Kryptok lenses were advertised as *invisible* bifocals. The width of these segments was standardized at 19 mm. Because the pole of the reading segment was closer to the dividing line, "jump" was reduced and thus the area of the small segment was more effective. A new defect was now encountered that marred the performance of this lens. The biconvex flint glass segment induced chromatic aberration* which induced red and/or blue color fringes around objects viewed through the reading portion. This aberration was not observed by many wearers and even many who did see the fringes at times still continued to wear the lenses because of their other advantages. Almost twenty years went by before research and glass technology had solved this problem. After the development of certain barium crown glasses, all first-quality fused multifocals are practically achromatic. The old flint glass Kryptok† is definitely a second-class lens.

In 1910, only a few years after the fused bifocal was invented, Conner‡ perfected a method of producing two different spherical curves on one surface of a lens. The optical effect of the original cemented lens was now available without a dirt-collecting segment edge and no Balsam cement to loosen and discolor (Fig. 81).

The large segment (32 mm wide) one-piece lens was quickly

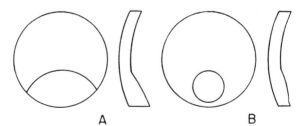

A   B

Figure 81.   One-piece bifocal cross sections.

*Obrig, T.E.:   *Modern Ophthalmic Lenses and Optical Glass.*   Philadelphia, Chilton, 1944, pp. 211-215.

Willmer, E.N.:   *Retinal Structure and Colour Vision.*   London, Cambridge U Pr, 1946, pp. 147-149.

†Spero, B.:   *A Scientific Corner.*   Chicago, House of Vision, May, 1943.

‡*Modern Lens Theory and Practice.*   Indianapolis, Continental Optical Company, 1941, pp. 46-50.

followed by the "B" size segment (22 mm round), which was only slightly larger than the fused bifocal. Undoubtedly these lenses had much to commend them. Under certain lighting conditions they are not quite as "invisible" as the fused bifocal but they are as achromatic as a single-vision lens. These lenses are more expensive to manufacture than Kryptoks. In their original form with the segment on the back surface, the plus based cylinder surfaces were more difficult to produce. The combination of these economic factors has limited the use of these very fine ophthalmic products. The introduction of photochromic glass which at first could not be heated to make fused bifocals temporarily made a windfall for one-piece bifocal products.

About 1926, Univis Lens Company produced a specially shaped fused bifocal with a rectangular reading portion which is the shape suggested by Percival* in 1910. At last a segment shape had been made in a fused bifocal that approximated the optical advantages of the original split-lens bifocal without the original unsightliness. In this and the several lens types to follow it, the pole of the reading portion is at or so near the top of the segment that "jump" at the dividing line practically disappears. The pole of the reading segment is also very close to the N.V.P. so that little or no prism effect is added to the displacement normal to the distance prescription at the same point. In the first form the segment was 9×19 mm (Fig. 82B), and the makers felt sure that the space below the segment would prove useful as a field of distance prescription for those who wished to see clearly at their shoe-tips. In practice, it was found that we seldom depress our eyes such large angles and that most multifocal wearers quickly learn to interpret the blurred image beyond the focal length of the segment. The lens was quickly followed by the D shape segment, which has a larger reading portion. Later the rectangular idea was produced in the R type segment 14×22 mm in which the pole is 7 mm below the dividing line. The grinding of the front surface of this lens type can be managed to set the pole of the segment at any point from the top to bottom edge and thereby produce prism effects Base Up

---

*Percival, A.S.: *The Prescribing of Spectacles.* New York, William Wood, 1910, p. 54.

or Base Down, thus affording the opportunity for moderate vertical prism to correct small amounts of prism induced by dissimilar lens powers in anisometropia (see Chap. 11). The lens is also available with prism up to $3^\triangle$ Base In or Out in the segment only.

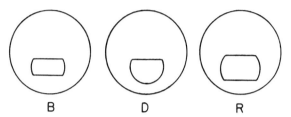

B   D   R

Figure 82. Univis bifocal segment shapes.

Similar flat-top lenses are also available from other major lens manufacturers. The Ful-Vue® bifocal has a slightly curved top that is tapered toward the front. The reading portion is 14×20 mm and the pole is 3.5 mm from the top edge. Bausch and Lomb, Inc., has presented a series of lenses called Panoptik® in which the segments all have slightly curved tops and rounded corners. The segments are 14.5×21.5 mm with the pole 3.5 mm below the margin and also 16×23 mm segments with the pole 4 mm down. Opticians choose this lens because it is identifiable and is obtainable in only one highest quality lens, therefore there is no cut-price competition.

Most recently, another lens producer has ingeniously conceived a method of making a flat-top Ultex bifocal K with a segment 14 $\times$ 19 mm. The pole of this reading section is $4\frac{1}{2}$ mm from the top edge of the segment. This lens has a slight shelf across the top. Like other one-piece lenses it is achromatic. However, all the new designs of fused flat-top multifocals from the major lens makers are now made with the new barium glasses that insure satisfactory color correction.

After World War II, American Optical Company announced a one-piece bifocal with a straight dividing line like the original Franklin lens. Different from all other bifocal forms, the relationship of the centers of the distance and reading portions of the lens is preset. In all other bifocals the center of the reading segment

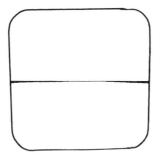

Figure 83. Executive bifocal segment shape.

is at some distance from the center of the distance portion and therefore can be decentered to have its optical center set in the path of the visual line as it turns nasalward for near vision.

The new lens is made with the center of the segment at the point of tangency of the distance and reading portions. If the point of tangency is moved nasalward, the optical center moves with it.

In 1961 American Optical Company's *Executive Bifocal Manual* simplified the matter by suggesting that segment inset be ignored altogether. It seems rather incongruous for one function of a lens factory to design a lens series to nullify very small power errors in lens margins for the benefit of *accommodation* while another section encourages a small Base Out prism error for the already exerted *convergence* of presbyopes.

The Executive®-type bifocal offers an opportunity not regularly possible with ordinary sized bifocal segments. Beginning with cemented bifocals in the past century, the horizontal center of the reading portion has been placed on the projected z-axis of the eye converged to the reading position. Scant mention has been made of the fact that although the *segment* was properly centered, the eyes were presented with some horizontal prism that varied with the power and sign of the distance prescription.

One of the most frequent references to this effect has been with lenses for aphakia. The classic statement has been +10.00 Distance, 2 mm inset produces $2^\triangle$ Base Out each eye. This is not inconsequential because the lensless eyes are already having to converge a total of about $20^\triangle$ to account for the loss of angle α. Referring to Chapter 12, you will note that aphakic lenses are centered for the reading centers for both distance and near in order to deliberately cause some prism Base In for distance and no prism in the reading segment. Because the convex distance and reading curve of Executive bifocals are tangent (minimum ledge thickness) very near the center of a 60 mm blank and because the seg ment extends the full width of the blank, the point of tangency which is directly above the center of the reading area can be decentered a very large amount to deliberately provide enough decentration (and prism) to offset the prism generated when the eyes look through the power of the distance lens at a distance less than the separation of lens centers. This procedure is usually impossible with 22 to 25 mm segments because the extra decentration required for low additions would virtually move the segments out of the reading field.

The only moves made to assist convergence have been prism segments (usually about $1.5^\triangle$ Base In) and Vision-Ease Cen-Cor® flat-top bifocal with a large segment decentered to the nasal side of the blank. Appearance and additional material cost seem to have retarded the acceptance of these notions.

Basically the solution to the problem is:

Distance ℞ (horizontal meridian $\times$ .2 $= +X^\triangle$

Additional reading add decentration $= - X^\triangle$
                                                     ———
                                                       0

FOR EXAMPLE

+2.50D. Sph.

+2.00   add

$+2.50 \times .2 = 0.5^\triangle$ Base Out

but the +2.00 addition segments must be decentered an additional 2.5 mm to create the neutralizing prism.

$+2.00 \times 2.5 = 0.5^\triangle$ Base In

Decenter segments 4.5 (2.0 for convergence +2.5 for prism).

In Form B-1070 Bausch and Lomb has presented a very simple formula to find the total inset: Total Inset equals Decentration plus (Distance power in the horizontal meridian times decentration. When the distance power is large and the addition power is small, the decentration could prevent a lens from being very large.

$$+5.00$$
$$+1.50$$

$$2 + \left(\frac{5. \times 2}{1.5}\right) = \frac{10}{1.5} = 6.7 + 2 = 8.7 \text{ mm}$$

This prescription would limit the lens length to about 42 mm. If the prescription order required a longer lens length and decentration had to be reduced, the lens would still have a better horizontal reading center than other bifocals down to the point that the decentration of the minimum ledge thickness (tangent point) was finally decentered only 2 mm.

Virgil Hancock, Shuron/Continental (nee Modern Optics), proposed that, after the minimum ledge thickness had been located by marking the blank where a vertical line appeared continuous, the appropriate amount of prism Base In for plus and Base Out for minus power be ground in the distance prescription to offset the prism in the horizontal meridian.

$$\text{R O.U. } +1.25 + 75 \times 90$$
$$+2.50 \text{ Add}$$
$$+2.00 \text{ (horizontal meridian) } \times .2 = 0.4^\Delta \text{ Prism Base In}$$

Forgetting technical accuracy in lens making and viewing the situation from the aspect of physiological optics, this discussion can be called a "tempest in a tea cup." The wearer of bifocal lenses in all probability was wearing substantially the same distance prescription until his first bifocals. He had accustomed himself to the small difference in convergence for all near-point fixations. For example:

Fixation 40 cm (16 inches) $= 2.50$D.

Interocular centers $60/56$

$2.50 \times 6 = 18^\Delta$ convergence

$(+2.50 \times 2$ mm decentration$) = 0.5^\Delta$ each eye

$18 + 1.0 = 19^\Delta$ through lenses (5.5% increase)

Possibly sliding the point of tangency over the customary distance (distance–reading) is adequate. Millions of other bifocals seem to have performed usefully with this calculable error.

The fact that the lens Franklin designed is monocentric is a boon to all bifocal wearers. There is no image "jump" or "blind

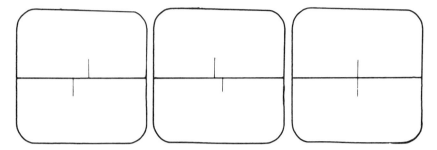

Figure 84.   Executive bifocal centering.

area" in the lens.   The ultimate is also accomplished for the
wearer who desires a wide reading area.   The lens also disposes of
the age-old effort to design an invisible bifocal.   The dividing
line with its overhanging ledge is easily visible but does not seem
to annoy lens wearers.   The lens deserves to be carefully handled
because small chips on the ledge sparkle like small stars.   This
could be bothersome to the wearer.   All in all, the lens is a good
lens and has been eagerly accepted by wearers.

At the other extreme a totally invisible segment dates back to a
low-priced one-piece bifocal made by Stead Optical Company in
1916 which, because of crude manufacturing methods, had a
blurred area between the distance and reading portions.   Stead
finally obtained a patent for this poor copy of an Ultex lens under
the name of Shock Absorber!

After the expiration of all of these patents a bifocal with a
small round segment with an "invisible" or blended margin between distance and reading was undertaken by several small manufacturers.   Younger Med-Optics® makes a high-quality lens of
this type in glass and CR39 plastic.   This lens is well received by
first and early bifocal wearers who wish to conceal their dependence upon bifocals.   The transitional curve becomes a manufacturing and optical problem in stronger additions (above 2.00D.).
Usually by this time the wearers are ready to capitulate to conventional lenses.

In France a totally different lens form was conceived.   Starting
in 1951 a continuing modification and development of the idea

has continued. In the beginning the progressive increase occurred through the whole vertical meridian of the lens which resulted in under correction in the upper distance area and over correction at the bottom of the lens. By their report the progression has been changed as follows:

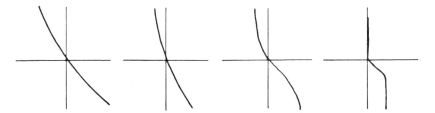

Figure 85. Development of the Varilux progressive curve lens.

In the last design the area above the datum (180°) line has little variation from the prescribed distance ℞. There is a neck about 3 to 5 mm wide through the transitional zone (12 mm long) that widens to more than 20 mm (segment width) in the full reading addition area.

This lens is called Varilux® and is being distributed in America by the manufacturer's agency. It is a progressive-surface lens in which a slightly tilted vertical strip through the center of the lens gradually increases from the power of the distance prescription to the total addition for reading. Although the continuing increase in power may suggest a poor lens effect, the small segment of the surface intercepted by a 3 mm pupil prevents this astigmatic surface from interfering with visual acuity. With a little practice the wearer finds the angle of depression that provides him with precisely the best additional power to obtain clear vision at any distance less than infinity. On either side of the central strip in the power portion of the lens are zones of degenerated curvature which are useless for critical seeing. The blurriness of these areas increases directly with the total power of the addition. It seems that it would behoove a prospective wearer to start with this lens design when his reading addition is weak and thereby learn to adapt to the lens even while his accommodative amplitude could meet the needs of intermediate distances.

A substantially improved design has been developed which is named Varilux II. The front surface, actually a series of surfaces, approaches incomprehensibility to an orthodox ophthalmic lens grinder. It is possible only by the calculations of a sophisticated computer (Figs. 86 and 87). In the distance area above the beginning of the progressive area, the curve is an oblate ellipse with its long axis across the lens which produces practically no lens change in curvature horizontally until it approaches the margins, where convexity gradually increases toward the end of the ellipse. This section gradually becomes a spherical curvature in the central zone of the lens, only to become a series of prolate ellipses as it moves into the near-point area, then to successively become prolate ellipses followed by parabolas and hyperbolas where the radii in the area for the reading addition must be shorter. The hitherto

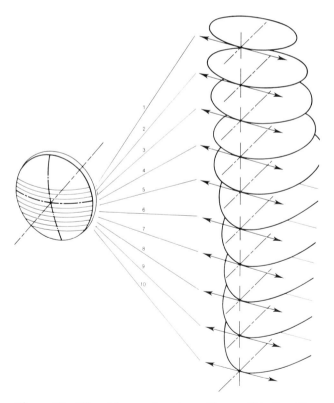

Figure 86. The oblate and prolate ellipses of Varilux II.

badly degenerated curves on each side of the reading area have been surprisingly lessened toward insignificance for medium additions up to +2.00. Figure 87 gives a graphical demonstration of the usefulness of the lens surfaces of different multifocal lens forms in which Varilux II demonstrates a vast improvement over the earlier designs. The improvements in Varilux II are a better shaped, progressive power zone and better treatment of the lens area on either side of the "reading segment." It was first offered to the professions in Europe where the acceptance and fitting could be closely observed. This approach in distribution has proved to be very important even if very expensive. Although sales of the new lens design is in the millions in Europe, cautiousness in fitting—lenses that the makers feel is at or near the ultimate design—is proving to be most rewarding.

VISION OF STATIONARY OBJECTS

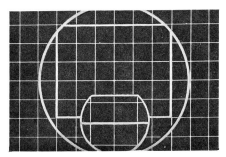

Bifocal lenses

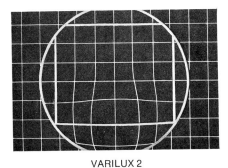

VARILUX 2

Figure 87. Plane view of Varilux II (left) and bifocal lenses (right).

Its introduction in the United States started in Oregon and Washington, where its distribution was limited to carefully selected optical firms. Among requirements for distributors, the head of the laboratories must visit the company's model laboratory near Chicago for instruction and actual experience in the fitting and grinding of the new lens. After months of experience in the Northwest, where doctors and dispensers were being detailed and instructed by factory representatives, distribution was started in California and again to a limited number of carefully selected optical firms. As the firm completes its intensive training campaign in each limited area, it proposes to add new areas of distribution. Distribution zones are religiously observed.

The American Optical Corporation lens designers have developed a progressive power multifocal which has been named Ultravue.® The lens is made of CR39® hard resin. It is being manufactured in one of their lens factories in Europe. This lens has a spherical surface in the distance portion and begins its pro-

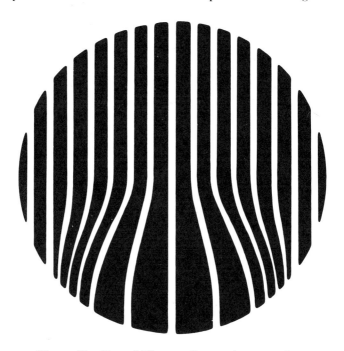

Figure 88. Plan of Ultravue Progressive power lens.

gressive power change from a straight line across the 75 mm lens blank. The progressive "'corridor" down the center of the lens is 12 mm from the top down to the full power of the reading addition. The width of the corridor varies with the power of the addition between 3 and 5 mm. The zones on either side of the reading area return to a spherical curvature.

To assure proper presentation and fitting of the lens, laboratory representatives of selected distributors receives instruction at specially prepared laboratories. Dispensers receive special instruction in small groups at seminars. Counsellors are available for problem cases. Everything possible is being done to give this radically different lens a proper presentation.

In 1954, David Volk, M.D., designed a series of lenses with aspheric surfaces for subnormal vision and followed with a progressively curved lens which he named Omnifocal®. It too provides a gradually increasing addition. House of Vision, Chicago, undertook the manufacturing and distribution of this lens but because the lens form is a bitoric and requires a great deal of accuracy in grinding this unusual lens form, production problems in the prescription laboratory have limited the acceptance of the lens.

In 1978 Younger Manufacturing Co., the makers of seamless bifocals, presented a progressive lens with several improvements. The degenerated curve on either side of the progressive corridor is rather like a bean shape rather than to extend straight across the lens. The lens power increase in the progressive corridor is not a straight line function. At the half-way point it has increased only one-half the power of the addition. As the trade-name indicates, the maximum width of the reading addition is 30 mm.

No one can accurately foretell the future of Varilux, Omnifocal, and Ultravue. Few such innovations are instant successes in the optical profession and industry because there is a rather long list of conservative (or reactionary?) individuals between the inventor and consumer who often hesitate to accept new products.

TRIFOCALS

To follow the bifocal for early presbyopia, there has always been a need for another lens design for all spectacle wearers from 50 to 55 years of age and for the remainder of their lives. This fact also has been very slowly accepted. A trifocal lens has a small area above the reading portion to provide clear vision at intermediate distances, particularly those distances at arm's length, 67 cm to about one meter. Hawkins* (1826) divided lenses (like Franklin) but into three portions. His efforts did not meet with much success for several reasons, among which were the small round lens sizes (1 inch or 25.4 mm) of that day and the selection of the power of the intermediate section. Hawkins corrected his eyes for 40 cm intermediate and 20 cm near (+1.50 add intermediate and +4.25 near). With the coming of cemented bifocals, other attempts at piling up segments was made. These, too, had scant acceptance.

Ultex lenses were made into a trifocal form but they had limited acceptance for some of the reasons of the nonsuccess of the former lens styles. The centers of the intermediate and reading portions of the lens are below the bottom edge of the lens, thus

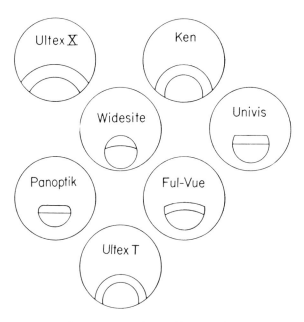

Figure 89. Various trifocal designs.

*Levene, J.R.: *Clinical Refraction and Visual Science.* London, Butterworth, 1977, pp. 181-186.

producing a large prism effect at the dividing lines. Further, a single intermediate addition of +1.37D. was used in all intermediates. When the wearer's accommodative amplitude is considered, the intermediate addition was much too strong for weak additions and not the proper power until +2.50D. or +2.75D. addition was required.

This problem was not solved until the advent of Virgil Hancock's Univis design for flat-top trifocals. These lenses have their segment centers close to the top edge of the segment which materially reduced or obliterated the "jump" and image displacement. Further, attention was paid to physiological optics and the intermediate addition was a percentage, usually about 50 percent of the total reading addition. Now the final stumbling block was the dispenser. The manufacturers offered to replace the lenses with bifocals if the wearers could not adapt. Much to the surprise of many fitters, a very high percentage of the lenses were retained by the wearers despite poorly located segments. Finally, when the resistance of fitters was broken, trifocals gradually assumed their rightful place in the market.

Not illustrated in Figure 89 are Executive trifocals with two lines across the lens. A CR39 lens has been made with the intermediate addition in the lower half of an Executive with a flat-top segment in it to produce the full reading addition.

There seems to be no limit to the ingenuity of the lens designers at the several factories. A wider selection of glasses and improved manufacturing methods have aided them materially. Some of their solutions to the problems of special occupational requirements will be discussed in the chapter on Vocational Glasses.

PROBLEM SOLVING

At the time this book is being read lens problems are simply solved, but as time passes, the technique will become cloudy and confused. There is a means to prevent this situation and always keep the knowledge alive.

Solve each problem by the same routine. Short cuts and separate note pages will add difficulty in the future.

1. Use millimeter cross-ruled paper*   It can be obtained with perforations for a notebook.
2. Identify the problem by page of book and problem number.
3. Make a sketch of the problem pretty well to scale.
4. List the known facts, such as object distance, focal length, and so on.
5. State what is to be found.
6. State the appropriate formula to solve the problem.
7. Rearrange the formula so that the item to be found is the only item on the left side of the equals sign.   For example:
   Given: Object size and magnification.
   What is the image size?
   $$\mathbf{M} = \mathbf{I/O}$$
   $$\mathbf{MO} = \mathbf{I}$$
   $$\mathbf{I} = \mathbf{MO}$$
8. When the quantities are filled in, this problem is lucid for a life-time.

REVIEW

1. Can a lens be classified without instruments?   Describe the methods fully.

2. Can spherical and cylindrical lenses be differentiated without equipment?   Describe the characteristics by which each is identified.

3. Name four uses for prisms.

4. Describe the difference between the optical center and vertex of a lens.

5. Explain why the focus of the correcting lens is at the far point of the eye.

6. If a +4.50 S. trial lens 14 mm from the cornea produces best vision, what is the vertex power of the spectacle lens placed 9 mm from the cornea which gives the same effect?

7. How much prism is generated 8 mm below the center of a lens?
   (a) +3.25 +0.75 × 90
   (b) − 1.50 − 1.25 × 45
   (c) − 1.25 +3.00 × 130

---

*Obtainable in any store selling draftsmen's supplies.

What is the direction of the Base of the prism in each instance.

8. If a $+6.00$ spherical lens is tilted to an angle of 15° with the line of vision, what is the change in the vertex power?

9. How much is the magnification of a $+3.00$ sphere with 3 mm center thickness altered when:
   a. the front surface is increased from $+5.00$ to $+9.50$?
   b. the lens is fitted 5 mm farther away from the eye?
   c. the lens is 1.5 mm thicker?

10. Discuss the intention of marginally corrected prescription lenses and how the desired effect is accomplished.

11. What is the approximate horizontal prism effect when $+2.50$ $+1.75 \times 30$ is decentered 6 mm nasalward? Make a sketch and show the work.

12. If -1.25 cyl. $\times 40$ is placed in front of $+10.00$ $+2.00 \times 160$, what is the vertex power of the combination? Solve by Emsley's table and confirm with his plotting method.

13. Find the amount of vertical prism at the N.V.P. 9 mm below the center in the reading portion of a 19 mm round fused bifocal when the segment is set 3 mm below the optical center of the distance portion and the power is $+1.75$ $+1.25$ ax 180, add $+2.25$.

ADDITIONAL REFERENCES

1. Prentice, Charles F.: *Ophthalmic Lenses.* Philadelphia, Keystone, 1900.
2. Fry, Glenn A.: The major reference point in a single vision lens. *Am J Optom, 24*:1-7, January 1947.
3. von Rohr, M.: *Die Brille als Optische Instrument.* Berlin, Springer, 1921.
4. Martin, L.C.: *Technical Optics,* Vol. I. New York, Pitman, 1948.
5. Ames, A., Glidden, G.H., and Ogle, K.N.: Size and shape of ocular images. *Arch Ophthal* (Chicago), 7:576, 1932.
6. Morgan, M. and Peters, H.B.: *The Optics of Ophthalmic Lenses.* Berkeley, U of Cal Pr, 1948.
7. Bennett, A.G.: *Graphical Methods of Solving Optical Problems.* London, Hatton, 1948.
8. Emsley, H.H. and Swayne, W.: *Ophthalmic Lenses.* London, Hatton, 1946.
9. Boeder, Paul: *Analysis of Prism Effects in Bifocal Lenses.* Southbridge, American Optical Company, 1939.
10. Jalie, M.: *The Principles of Ophthalmic Lenses,* 3 Vols. London, Assoc.

Dispensing Opticians, 1967.

11. Bennett, A.G.: *Ophthalmic Lenses.* London, Hatton Press, 1968.

12. Epting, J.B. and Morgret, F.C.: *Ophthalmic Mechanics and Dispensing.* Philadephia, Chilton, 1964.

13. Sasieni, L.S.: *Principles and Practice of Optical Dispensing and Fitting,* 3rd Ed. London, Butterworths, 1975.

14. Fry, Glenn A.: *Geometrical Optics.* Philadelphia, Chilton, 1969.

15. Sheard, Charles: *The Sheard Volume.* Philadelphia, Chilton, 1957.

16. Multi-Optics Corp.: *Varilux II.* Paris, 1974.

17. Reinecke, R.D. and Herm, R.J.: *Refraction.* New York, Appleton-Century, 1965.

18. Emsley, H.H.: *Ophthalmic Tables and Other Data.* London, Bausch & Lomb, 1969.

Chapter 6

EYE PLANES AND INTEROCULAR
DISTANCE

◆◆

A s discussed in Chapter 3, there is no displacement of objects
in visual space when the line of sight is coincident with the
optic axis of an ophthalmic lens. Since the macula is a very small
area on the retina, it follows that the rays of light from an object
in space to cover only this point are a very small bundle. Or to
reverse the notion, the line of sight is limited to a rather definite
direction.

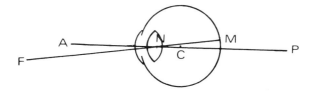

Figure 90. Axes of eye.

The center of curvature of the cornea and the centers of curvature of the crystalline lens and the center of the pupillary aperture
are very nearly in a straight line. Measurements made by many
physiologists have proved that the variations in normal eyes seldom exceed 1 mm. The straight line drawn normal to the pole of
the cornea, through the center of the pupil, and extending to the
posterior pole of the eye globe is defined by Gullstrand as the
optic axis of the eye. Like most physiological terminology with
reference to the eyes, more than one name will be found in the
literature for the same part or function. The *optic axis* is frequently called the *anterior-posterior axis* or *principal axis* of the
eye.

The center or rotation has been found to be a rather elusive

159

point. For the purposes of physiological and ophthalmic optics, it is convenient and in some instances necessary to assume a specific location of the center. Clinical observations by Donders and others reveal that the distance of the center from the corneal vertex varies with the axial length and refractive error. Verrijp* reported, in 1936, extensive research in which he shows that the eye has what he terms instantaneous centers of rotation which vary with monocular or binocular vision, the direction of vergence (vertical or horizontal), as well as the amount the eye may be turned from the primary position. The range of positions reported by all writers extends from 12.9 mm (Weiss, 1875) to 15.44 mm (Mauthner, 1876) with the greatest number averaging near 13.25 mm from the pole of the cornea and on or very near to the optic axis of the eye. In any event, it is generally agreed and should be remembered that the center of rotation is a hypothetical point.

In order to simplify the otherwise tedious and complicated optical calculations required to trace light through an eye, careful measurements of a number of normal eyes have been made and the average specifications have been accepted as the measurements of a schematic eye. The data for the schematic eye most commonly accepted and used are those established by Gullstrand in his appendix to Helmholtz's *Treatise on Physiological Optics.*

The macula of a normal eye is not at the posterior pole of the optic axis of the eye. It is taken to be 1.25 mm out and down on the temporal side. Therefore the line of sight is at a small angle to the optic axis. The nodal points of the eye are 7.078 and 7.332 behind the pole of the cornea. As we have seen, the mid-point between the nodal points of a lens is called the optical center. Because the nodal points are so very close together and because this schematic eye has a foundation in averages and assumptions, the nodal points are referred to as a single point in about the position of the first nodal point. Thus the line of sight from the macula crosses the optic axis at a point about 7.08 mm behind the cornea.

*Helmholtz, H. von: *Physiological Optics*, Vol. III. Menasha, Wis, Banta, 1924, pp. 127-136.
Berens, C.: *Diseases of the Eye.* Philadelphia, Saunders, 1936, pp. 109-114; 842-861.

The cornea is intercepted by this line of sight slightly nasalward of the pole (**A**) of the surface. The angle between the line of sight or visual axis **FM** (Fig. 91) and the optic axis **AP** at the point **N** forming angle **ANF** is called angle *alpha* (α). *The average size* of this angle is 5°, which would be computed as follows:

If **MP** is taken as 1.25 mm,
NM is 15 mm in the reduced eye.

$$\sin \alpha = \frac{MP}{NM} = \frac{1.25}{15} = .0833$$
$$\alpha = 4°47'$$

Consequently, when the eye is moved so that the fovea (central portion of the macula) is receiving rays of light from the fixation point **F**, the center of the pupil along with the optic axis is turned out (temporally) about 5°.

O. D.
Temporal

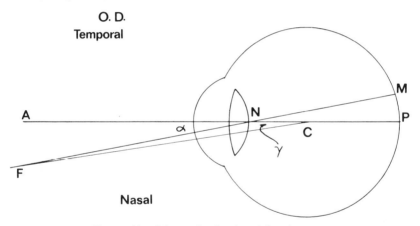

Nasal

Figure 91. Schematic visual and fixation axes.

The angles in Figure 91 have been exaggerated. In the figure, point **C** denotes the center of rotation around which the movements of the eye take place. Line **FC** joining this point with the point of fixation is called the *fixation axis* by Helmholtz. The angle between the optic axis **AP** and the fixation axis **FC** at point **C** is called angle gamma $\gamma = \angle$ ACF.

Angle alpha is a constant for any position of the fixation point **F** on line **FN** or its projection. When point **F** is at infinity, then lines **FN** and **FC** approach parallel and angles *alpha* and *gamma* become equal. It is only when the fixation point is quite close to the eye that angle *gamma* is found to be measurably less than angle *alpha*. At a reading distance of 33 cm, the difference is only $4°47' - 4°42' = 5'$.

If $\mathbf{AN} = 330 + 7.08$

   $\mathbf{AC} = 330 + 13.25$

Then $\mathbf{AF} = 337.08 \times \tan \alpha = 28.2$ mm

$$\tan \gamma = \frac{\mathbf{AF}}{\mathbf{AC}} = \frac{28.2}{343.25} = .08216 = 4°42'$$

Such a small difference is obviously inconsiderable under the circumstances. Therefore, although there has been considerable confusion over terminology in the literature, angles *alpha* and *gamma* can be used interchangeably as well as the terms "visual axis" and "fixation axis." By way of example, angle *alpha* (**ANF**) makes the correct geometric construction to compare object **AF** and the corresponding retinal image **PM**; angle *gamma* (**ACF**) with its vertex at **C**, the center of rotation, is used to describe an angle of vergence or rotation of the eye toward the periphery of a lens.

Point **C** in Figure 92, the hypothetical center of rotation, is also convenient to use as the origin, or point of intersection, of three primary axes perpendicular to each other which in turn describe some useful planes of reference of a lens.

This notion as presented by Fick (1854) conforms better to present-day usage when the letters are altered. Let the eye be fixed in the position illustrated in Figure 92. A plane is erected which is perpendicular to the fixation axis (z-axis) through the center of rotation marked *C;* this plane can be described by the horizontal (180) axis, shown as the x-axis, and the axis perpendicular to it (90) designated as the y-axis. This particular frontal plane is known as *Listing's* (1844) *plane.* It is a fixed plane with regard to the head and usually parallel with the face plane. In the illustration, it practically corresponds with the equatorial plane of the eye, but of course it does not move when the eye rotates to any new position.

The eyes are said to be in *primary position* when they are looking straight in front with the head vertical and the fixation axes parallel and perpendicular to Listing's (and the face) plane. When the eyes look upward or downward from this position, that

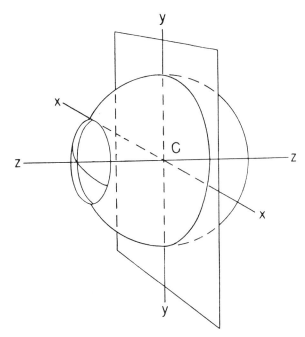

Figure 92. Listing's plane.

is, when they rotate on the x-axis, the angle is called an *angle of altitude*. When the eyes are turned to the right or left and rotate on the y-axis, the angle generated is described as an *angle of azimuth*. Eye movements that involve rotation on only one of these axes are referred to as *cardinal movements* and the new positions are *secondary positions*.

It is observed that the movements of the eyes on the x-axes and y-axes are voluntary and that they may be made through wide angles of vergence. Rotation of the eyes on the z-axis is not voluntary and is comparatively limited. The eyes do make compensatory movements on inclination of the head.* When the head is inclined to the right, the eyes roll to the left and vice versa owing to the control of the vestibular apparatus over the oblique extraocular muscles.

---

*Helmholtz, H. von: *Physiological Optics*, Vol. I. Menasha, Wis, Banta, 1924, pp. 350-358, 392.

When the eyes are moved obliquely from the *primary position,* this is designated as *tertiary position.* The movement of the eye, in this case, involves a simultaneous rotation around both the x-axes and y-axes. It was for the purpose of investigating the geometry of these complicated movements that the Listing plane of reference was conceived. Prolonged research since Fick (1838) has demonstrated that the eye *wheels, rolls,* or *inclines* in definite, calculable amounts of torsion when it is turned in any *tertiary position.*

Proof is simple by the use of afterimages.* Cover one eye, fatigue the open eye thoroughly with an *AO* (or similar) after Image Test. Immediately cover the fatigued eye, turn the lamp 90°, to thoroughly fatigue the second eye. Now when both eyes are opened and directed in primary position to a blank wall, a symmetrical cross will be seen as in Figure 93.

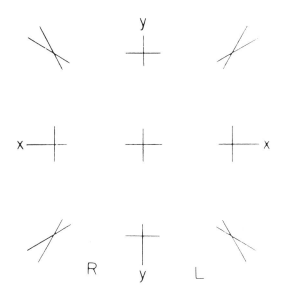

Figure 93. Distortion in projected frontal plane.

---

*Bielschowsky, A.: *Lectures on Motor Anomalies.* Hanover, Dartmouth College Publications, 1940, pp. 2-3.

Duke-Elder, Sir W.S.: *Text-Book of Ophthalmology.* St. Louis, Mosby, 1949, pp. 3883-3885.

Now verge the eyes strongly right, left, up, and down, secondary positions; since these are movements on only one axis at a time there is no torsion. The cross is slightly distorted because the image is projected obliquely on the frontal plane (the wall) that is not perpendicular to the z-axis in the *secondary position*. In the corners, the crosses are not only distorted, they are also tilted. Thus it is proved that the eye has rotated on the fixation axis (z-axis) which is referred to as torsion. Using the Listing reference plane, Shubert (1820) derived a trigonometric formula for the angle of torsion, but Table VI (devised by Maddox*) provides an opportunity for the evaluation of the angles generated. It will be noted that the deviation is small for the first 20° but that each 5° thereafter shows a rapidly increasing rotation.

TABLE VI
TORSION INVOLVED IN ROTATING ABOUT AN AXIS 45° FROM THE HORIZONTAL

Degrees of Rotation	5	10	15	20	25	30	35	40	45
Angle of Torsion	6.5′	26′	1°	1°47′	2°49′	4°6′	5°40′	7°33′	9°44′

As a consequence, it is now apparent that horizontal and vertical lines in the object space do not form the same retinal images associated with the eyes in primary position as when the eyes are moved into a tertiary position. Nevertheless, if such lines give the impression of still being vertical or horizontal, this is effected by a so-called *sensory revaluation* of the retina (Shoda, 1928). However, such compensation requires points of contact or projection previously experienced.†

The relation of the eyeplanes, frontal plane in the object space, and ophthalmic lens plane can now be discussed. When the eye is in primary position, a test-chart is perpendicular to the fixation axis (z-axis) and the plane of the chart is parallel to the

*Maddox, E.E.: *Tests & Studies of the Ocular Muscles.* Bristol, John Wright and Company, 1898, p. 57.

†Van Wien, S.: Influence of torsional movements on axis of astigmatism. *Am J Ophthmol, 31*:1251-1260, Oct., 1948.

Luneburg, R.K.: *Mathematical Analysis of Binocular Vision.* Princeton, Princeton U Pr, 1947, pp. 1-9; 40-49.

Listing plane and also the equatorial plane of the eye. If a lens
is placed before the eye with its optical axis coincident with the
fixation axis and, therefore, its focal points lie on the z-axis of the
eye, the plane of the lens will also be parallel with both the test
chart and the eye planes (Fig. 94b); it shows some derangement of
the original positions. Since Listing's plane is fixed with regard
to the head, the top of the plane is tipped back with the plane of
the face. The extraocular muscles have made the proper compensation and the equatorial plane of the eye containing the x-
axis and y-axis is still vertical and the z-axis, of course, has not
moved. The spectacle lens (or trial lens in a trial frame) is
attached to the head and therefore moves with the head and the
lens plane continues to be parallel to Listing's plane. The optical
axis of the lens is intercepted at an angle of 15° below the
previous position of the lens and the optical center is raised 15°
above the fixation axis. Unless the lens has been corrected for
marginal astigmatism, the effectivity of the lens at this extra-axial
point is somewhat different from the axial power. Displacement
generated by the prism effect of decentration is also introduced at
this new point of intersection of the z-axis, unless the lens axis
intersects the center of rotation of the eye.

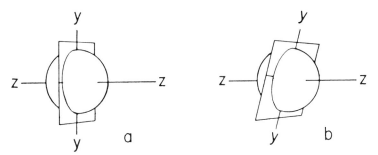

Figure 94. Tilt of Listing's plane in extra central fixation.

The lens is also tilted. This generates a spherocylindrical error.
If the cylinder axis of the trial lens is not vertical or horizontal,
the cylinder power generated by the tilt presents an obliquely
crossed cylinder. Aside from the lens power change, the induced
cylinder causes a change in the axis of the trial lens.

The plane of the test chart is still perpendicular to the fixation axis, and therefore, no distortion from obliquity is introduced. Thus, at a secondary position of the eye that involves a rotation around only one axis, in this instance the x-axis, the axial effectivity of a spectacle lens at the marginal point is altered by prism displacement Base Up or Down and uncorrected marginal aberration.

When the eye is moved to a tertiary position such as a point 45° above the horizontal and an azimuth angle of 30° away from the primary position as is shown in Figure 95, another set of variations is found. This time the head is not moved, so Listing's plane remains fixed. The equatorial plane of the eye is turned 30° on the line QQ' in Listing's plane. The lens axis continues to intersect the center of rotation of the eye, but the z-axis of the eye now intersects the lens at a point up and to the right of the optical center. The plane of the test chart is no longer perpendicular to the fixation axis, which of itself causes some obliquity to the image. According to Maddox's Chart, the eye develops 4°6' of torsion from the oblique fixation. Again, prism effect is generated because the lens center is below and to the left of the intersection of the z-axis. Uncorrected marginal aberration at this point alters the effectivity of the lens. A new element is introduced if the eye requires an astigmatic correction. The eye has rotated more than 4° on the z-axis for which the correcting cylindrical

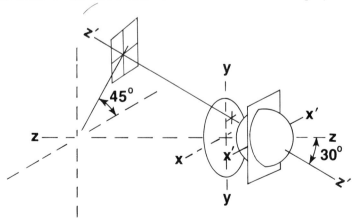

Figure 95. Tertiary fixation.

lens makes no compensation. In the weaker astigmatic errors, this is only an error of axis. Strong cylinders must be treated as obliquely crossed to estimate the error created.

A common activity of the eyes is the act of reading in which the z-axes intersect at the point of fixation. This requires opposing angles of azimuth or rotation on the y-axes of the two eyes. Like most other near-point activities, reading matter is usually held below the horizon which induces an angle of altitude or rotation on the x-axis. But when the eyes are turned in these opposite tertiary positions the torsions are opposite. That is, they tend to assume the projections in lower corners of Figure 93 marked R for the right eye and L for the left. In practice, the effect of torsion in the reading position (even in the case of multifocals when the eyes must be turned away from the lens axis) is negligible. Each eye is turned little more than 5' in the act of convergence for reading, which develops a very small rotational error. The angle of altitude, a cardinal movement, is the greater portion of the reading angle and it has no torsional effect.

Since the two eyes are ordinarily fixed upon the same point in the object space, the z-axes converge to the fixation point. The lines of fixation form two sides of a triangle and the line that connects the centers of rotation, Helmholtz Base Line, forms the other side. The plane in which this triangle C_LFC_R lies is the *plane of fixation.** It becomes obvious that since it contains both the centers of rotation of the eyes and the fixation point, binocular vision is impossible without it. When fixation is at infinity, the angles at C_L and C_R approach 90° as the fixation lines become more nearly parallel, yet it is not difficult to still think of the fixation triangle. Another variation develops when the visual axis of one eye is not turned toward the fixation point and the direction of the light rays must be corrected with a prism. In this instance one side of the triangle is not a straight line. The fixation line is deviated at the prism through the fixation center.

It is remarkable that, with an almost unremitting research by physiologists throughout the world, who more than a hundred

---

*Duke-Elder, Sir. W.S.: *Text-Book of Ophthalmology.* St. Louis, Mosby, 1934, pp. 582-584.

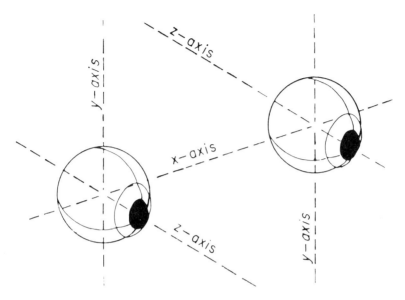

Figure 96. Axes of eyes.

years ago established the fixation plane and fixation triangle described above, until comparatively recent times it has been ignored in ophthalmic dispensing. A large part of the early literature has used some anatomical feature such as the brow-line or side of the face as the landmark to establish the "straightness" of a pair of ophthalmic lenses.

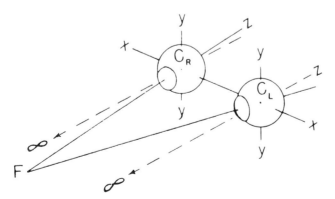

Figure 97. Axes with converged eyes.

Until about 1925, the vast majority of refracting was done with trial lenses and a trial frame. Practically all trial frames had an end piece and temple construction similar to an ordinary metal frame. Because there was no vertical adjustment to the temples, the position of the patient's ears and the crest of his nose became the three points to describe a horizontal triangle that set the planes of the lens cells of the trial frame. If one ear were lower than the other the frame tipped to that side, and if the error were not pronounced, it might go unnoticed. If the tilt were noticeable and eyes were not centered in the lens cells, one temple would have to be raised above one ear to that point where the trial frame seemed centered before the eyes. The best trial lens sets contained plain lenses etched with cross lines to assist the doctor in this improvisation. On other occasions the ears might seem to be the same height, but still the eyes could not be centered with respect to the lens cells. From this latter condition there grew a repeated reference to one eye being "higher" than the other. At least one manufacturer attempted to cope with this point of view by designing a trial frame in which one cell was vertically adjustable.

The optician who attempted to make glasses for these patients was "at sea" unless he knew the refracting habits of the prescribing doctor. Many heated discussions have been held while "line through pupil centers," "line perpendicular to sides of head," "real horizontal line," "high eye," etcetera, were being attacked or defended. Nor was all this confusion without foundation. The change in cylinder axis or prism base affects the lens prescription for both eyes if the $180°$ line used by the doctor, optician, and laboratory do not agree.

In 1920, Sidney L. Olsho, M.D., presented a simple and workable basis to provide uniformity. His text, published in 1928, entitled *The Coordination of Refraction with Spectacle and Eye Glass Fitting*, shows how the understanding between doctor and optician cannot be confused if a line connecting the outer canthi (corners of the eyes) is used as the base or $180°$ line. To be able to set a trial frame so that it would fit the face in this manner, he induced a manufacturer to make a frame with angularly adjustable temples. Nowadays all trial frames have this adjustment.

It is interesting to note that this ophthalmologist still relied on

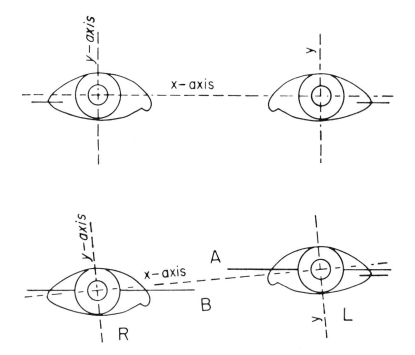

Figure 98. Tilt of Helmholtz base line (x-axis) for misaligned eyes.

an external feature for his landmark. Without doubt, the relationship of the outer canthi to the fixation lines (projected z-axes)
is found to be more consistent than other more remote features.
If, however, one deals in absolutes, it can be seen in Figure 98 that
the line between the outer canthi is not quite the same as the line
through the centers of the pupils in some rare cases of facial
asymmetry. This exception does not invalidate the use of easily
visible landmarks in a dimly lighted refracting room.

The choice of the line connecting the canthi had an immediate
advantage. It promoted the thought of a single continuous line
representing the x-axes of the two eyes. Hitherto any decision
that one eye was higher than the other immediately led to a seg-
mented line in which the separation of the horizontal lines represented the difference in height. It can be seen at once that a rather
large discrepancy can develop between the two line segments and

the x-axis. For example, when RL = 60 mm and AB = 3 mm, the angle between the x-axis connecting the centers of rotation and the "horizontal" lines is

$$\frac{AB}{RL/2} = \frac{3}{30} = 0.1000 = 5° \ 43'$$

For small differences in height and average separation of eyes (Fig. 99), the error in each cylinder axis is approximately 2 degrees per millimeter of difference in height. The datum line (180°) of the lenses in the illustration is rotating on the cyclopean center.

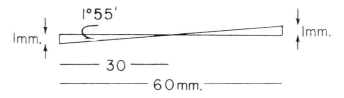

Figure 99. Angle of tilted base line.

The choice of this line (Olsho's base line) which is an external representation of Helmholtz's base line (the line between centers of rotation) immediately disposes of any discussion as to whether and how much one eye may be above or below the other. Despite the fact physiologists have regularly accepted Helmholtz's triangle for more than a hundred years, some writers, mostly optometrists, continue to discuss the intricacies of lens fitting, especially bifocals, when one eye is a "high eye." The widespread use of phoropters and refractors present the line connecting the centers of rotation as the patient peers through the apertures of the lens batteries of these refracting instruments. The natural position for the patient's eyes is at the centers of the tubular effect so that he can have his eyes set for the maximum field of view. The whole refraction, involving cylinder axis, prism base, and all muscle measurements, is made from this position. It follows that the 180° line of the glasses must be in the plane of fixation, that is, the same plane that connects the visual axes.

This discussion is not a denial that some faces do have one eye higher than the other when the sides of the face, the median line of the head, or the line perpendicular to the nose are used as reference points. Frequently the distance from the center of one pupil to the brow-line of one eye is markedly less than the other. Occasionally one eye is radically lower than the other because of a head injury.* For cosmetic, not optical reasons, it is sometimes necessary to modify the glasses. This can be done and the glasses can be checked for fitting by the doctor or adjusted by an optician without reference to the prescription or record, if the idea of base line is not neglected.

In many styles of glasses, the cosmetic effect is not improved by setting one lens higher than the other. Little can be done to modern metal frames that does not involve resetting (welding) the eye-wire. Such practice is not recommended because it destroys the temper and rigidity of the frame. Rimless glasses offer the greatest opportunity for asymmetric lens sizes and shapes. Some lightweight plastic frames can be modified.

Experience teaches that the fitter should proceed on these asymmetric cases by choosing a lens shape that fits nicely to the higher brow. The lens pattern should be slightly wider than the shape finally desired. The glasses should be finished and adjusted in the routine manner. If a plastic frame is used, the laboratory should be instructed to use the eye size next smaller than regular so that it will be easy to shrink the frame. After the glasses are adjusted for centers, and so forth, ink lines should be drawn on the lenses to show the areas about to be cut off to reset the brow-line lower on one side and if necessary remove some of the lens to obtain clearance from the cheek on the other side (Fig. 100). Since the glasses have been put in proper optical adjustment first and are in complete agreement with the doctor's prescription, the matter of how the lenses are reshaped is a matter of the optician's judgment and the patient's wishes. It is good practice here to let the patient see what is going to be done (ink-lines) and have his understanding and cooperation before the glasses are recut. It is much better to do too little and let him decide later that he wishes to have another modification than to be too rash and have to make a new pair of lenses. Further, there is a point past which the odd-

---

*Lyle, T.K. and Jackson, S.: *Practical Orthoptics*. Philadelphia, The Blakiston Company, 1949, p. 174.

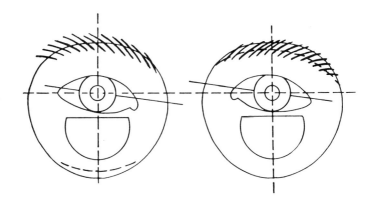

Figure 100. Segment position with tilted base line.

shaped lenses or frame become more conspicuous than the original defect.

After the lenses have been recut and while they are still out of the frame, a pencil should be run around the edges of them on the back of the record. Even if it is not too precise, it will have some value when a duplication is made. This pair of glasses can be easily reproduced because it *was* a regular order in the laboratory and was derived from a regular shape. The handwork was done *after* the glasses were finished.

Modification of regular lens shapes is often desirable in cases of broken or asymmetric noses. If a metal frame is used, a pair of fitting model lenses should be cut to the frame to confirm the fitting before the prescription lenses are made. If the deviation is not too great, a great deal of fitting can be done with a file on plastic frames. When the nose pads are removed, there are two or more millimeters of stock available for contouring. It is much better to make all the correction possible without involving the lens shape.

INTEROCULAR DISTANCE

The secondary focal point of the ophthalmic lens used to correct ametropia must fall on the far point of the uncorrected eye. This point is on the fixation line or its projection. It follows that the optical axis of the correcting lens must be coincident with the z-axis of the eye. When a pair of eyes is fixing upon a point infinitely distant, the z-axes are parallel and separated by the distance between visual axes at the centers of rotation (Fig. 101*a* and *c*). For this fixation distance, the maculas, far points of the uncorrected and corrected eyes: the poles, centers, and focal points of the ophthalmic lenses are precisely the same distance apart. Since the z-axes arc parallel, the separation of the lens centers must be the same regardless of the distance between the poles of the eyes.

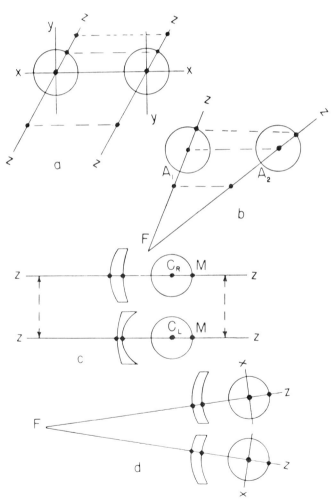

Figure 101. Projected visual axes.

When the eyes are fixed at some finite distance the arrangement of the points must be altered as shown in Figure 101*b* and *d*, if the optical requirements continue to be met. The z-axes converge and intersect at point **F**. The centers of rotation are still the same distance apart, but the x-axes of the individual eyes and the equatorial planes make a small angle (approximately 5° for reading distance) with the base line. The points on the corneas (A_1 and A_2) where the z-axes intersect are somewhat closer and the poles of the ophthalmic lenses are still closer. It is apparent that the proper position for the poles of the correcting lenses depends not only upon the length of the base line ($C_R C_L$), but also upon the fixation distance and, quite importantly, upon the distance between the lens and center of rotation (or more conveniently, the apex of the cornea).

This measurement (called "pupillary distance") is one of the early measurements made by an ophthalmic dispenser at the time a lens prescription is filled. Much has been written and several rather complicated instruments have been produced to make this measurement. In most instances, the device is designed to measure accurately the separation of the centers of the pupils or the distances of the centers of the pupils from a midline established by resting an arch or bridge on the nose. The patient's fixation is not always controlled with these special rules.

The project in hand is to set the optical centers of a pair of lenses at the points where the z-axes of the corrected eyes intersect the lens planes when the eyes are fixed at the distance for which the lenses are prescribed. In its truest sense, the separation of the centers of the pupils or the "pupillary distance" is not the required information. The misnomer will probably continue, through usage, as the term that describes the distance between the centers of rotation for distant fixation. "Near pupillary distance" will likely continue to refer to the separation of the centers of the pupils when the eyes are fixed at near and to add to the confusion (a) the distance between the fixation axes (z-axes) in the lens plane, (b) the separation of the centers of reading lenses, or (c) the centers of multifocal segments!

At the risk of censure, it is suggested that the term *"optical centers"* (O.C.) be substituted to designate the required separation of centers for a particular pair of lenses. When the O.C. distance for infinite fixation is given, the length of the base line, the interocular distance (I.O.D.) between the centers of rotation, is known. The separation of the optical centers for any finite fixation distance can then be easily computed for any fixation distance and spectacle lens plane. Conversely, with the same information for near point, the distance between the centers of rotation or the I.O.D. for infinity can be found.

Recently the frame manufacturers have taken the term *"pupillary distance"* (P.D.) to indicate the total length of the bridge (distance between lenses) plus the "A" length of the lens. It is suggested that the frame manufacturers continue to use P.D. and that the lens laboratories use the initials in the same way to indicate the total length of a pair of glasses across the 180 line without reference to the position of the optical centers.

The use of O.C. to denote the desired position of optical centers can be conveniently used when decentration is desired to create prism effect. When the present convention of P.D. is used there is a possibility of confusion between doctor, dispenser, and laboratory. For example, a certain amount of prism Base In effect is desired for a myopic patient. Doctor adds 5 mm to the measurement of the z-axis separation for distant fixation and writes on his prescription, O.C. 70 mm. When the dispenser measures for near-point O.C., he finds a reading of 61 mm, and although he will set the centers of the multifocal segments as measured, the lens centers will be ground to be 5 mm wider as prescribed and thereby induce the desired prism. If the prescription read P.D., the optician would face the dilemma of setting the segment centers as apparently desired and risk the loss of a pair of lenses, or of setting the lenses where the measurements indicated and risk undesired results. The use of O.C. refers to an optical measurement and is not an anatomical or physiological term appropriated for optical usage.

Figure 101 shows the requirements for two planes of fixation— that is, infinity and a certain near-point. It is obvious that the lenses cannot be precisely correct for more than one fixation distance. If the centers are set for a distant fixation point, the lens centers are too widely separated for near-point fixation; and conversely, a pair of lenses properly centered for reading distance have the centers closer together than the z-axes when the eyes are fixed at a point more remote.

Lateral decentration of meniscus or toric lenses is a radial movement and causes the lens axes to be tilted in the direction of the decentration. Since the optical centers are moved in opposite directions—that is, toward or away from one another—the tilted effect cannot be overcome or reduced by vergence as in the vertical meridian. When the eyes turn toward the normal for one lens, the tilted effect is increased in the other. Because these meniscus prism lenses are actually the peripheral portions of large lenses, they present the marginal errors (astigmatism) in their central areas. The tilt can be corrected for lenses to be used for distant fixation by bending the endpieces slightly behind the plane of the bridge.

The tilt of decentered lenses can be reduced by bending the endpieces forward until the inner and outer ends of the lenses are in a straight line. This small rotation of the lenses on the y-axis resets the z-axis. It is also apparent that the converging visual

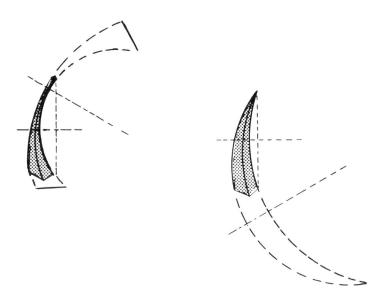

Figure 102. Astigmatism of meniscue prisms.

TABLE VII
TILT FROM DECENTRATION OF 6.00D. BASE LENS

2 mm	1°18′
4	2°36′
6	3°54′
8	5°12′

axes would be coincident with the z-axes of the reading lenses in Figure 101d, only if the lenses were centered about 7 mm each eye (angle ZFZ = 60/400 or approximately 9°). Such drastic treatment is unnecessary, but the principle involved does suggest that nasalward decentration of lenses to be used at finite distances is advantageous.

Probably the earliest attempt to measure the intervisual axis distance as distinct from the anatomical measurement of the separation of pupillary centers was undertaken with the device designed and made by J. I. Hawkins* (c. 1802). It consisted of a pair of angularly adjustable pinhole discs. When the patient looked through them at a distant object, he saw two brightly lighted spots, which were the shadows of his pupillary margins on his retinas. When the pinholes were adjusted to superimpose the spots, the distance between the visual axes was measured. The method has been abandoned because it is sometimes difficult to otbain dependable patient cooperation in this subjective test. However, it is still readily available by using the refractor pinholes and a muscle light.

In 1932 H.A. Lambert-Smith† presented a reflex Inter-Pupillary Gauge based on the physiological principle that the corneal images of a viewed luminous object denote the exact position of the visual axes when they are observed from the point of fixation. A retinoscope mirror was attached to one end of a 33 cm rod with a notched bar with apertures for the patient's eyes at the other end. A small light reflected from the mirror, and the optician viewed the corneal reflections through the hole. The scales above

---

*Taylor, H.L.: *The Manipulation and Fitting of Ophthalmic Frames.* Birmingham, J., & H. Taylor, 1907, pp. 29-31.

†Sasieni, L.S.: *Spectacle Fitting and Optical Dispensing,* London, Hammond, Hammond & Co., 1950, p. 92.

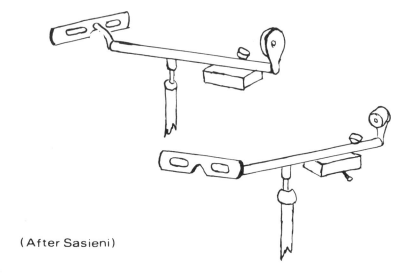

(After Sasieni)

Figure 103.   Intervisual axis measuring device.

and below the apertures showed the near point and distance measurements. It is regrettable that the use of this instrument has not been more widespread.

INTEROCULAR DISTANCE MEASUREMENT

A quite accurate measurement of the separation of the z-axes can be made in the following manner, which is a slight modification of the method described by Guibor.[‡] A light source such as a flashlight is held vertically against the face so that the lighted tip is below the optician's open eye. The lamp tip is covered except for a vertical slit on the side about 1 cm long and 2 to 3 mm wide. The patient is directed to look at the light source. The corneal reflections of the light are two small vertical lines usually on the nasal sides of the centers of the pupils (Fig. 107). A millimeter rule is laid on the patient's nose in such a position that the zero of the rule is below the reflection in the right eye while the optician keeps one of his eyes closed. With the eye still closed and without moving his head, the optician looks over to the patient's

---

[‡]Guibor, G.P.:   *The Interpupillary or Pupillary Distance, Geometric or Physiologic.*   Guildcraft, Guild of Prescription Opticians, January, 1943.

left eye and notes the point on the scale over which he sees the corneal reflection in the left eye. This is the measurement of the separation of the fixation lines (z-axes) in the plane of the rule, that is the crest of the nose, when the patient's fixation is at the distance of the light held by the optician.

The rechargeable flashlight made by Oculus in Germany is most satisfactory. The lamp is bright and can be partially covered with black lacquer to produce a vertical slit of light to increase the accuracy in alignment of the corneal image with millimeter scale.

In the discussion of angle alpha (α), Figure 104 shows that the path of the visual axis is not through the *absolute* center of the pupil nor the pole of the cornea. However, at the plane of the pupil the nasalward decentration is very small.

First nodal point $7.08 - 3.60$ iris plane $= 3.48$ mm
$\tan (5°) = .08749 \times 3.48 = .3045$ mm

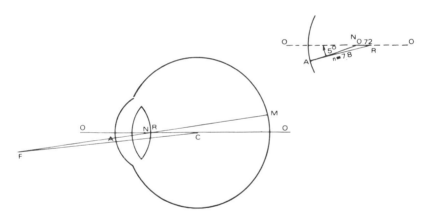

Figure 104. Corneal reflection analysis.

FM = fixation line (visual axis)
N = first nodal point $- 7.08$ mm
OO = optic axis
R = center of curvature of cornea, AR = 7.8 mm
M = macula
A = corneal apex

It would be senseless quibbling to discuss this disparity. Since the pupil is frequently set slightly nasalward from the center of the iris, it may actually denote the point intersected by the visual axis. Using the iris margin or the limbus, both of which may be indistinct or blurred, is certainly more difficult than the landmarks of corneal reflections by Guibor's technique. This corneal reflection technique for near, plus a measurement for distance, is described by Reinecke in the programmed text *Refraction*.[*]

Because the corneal image does not fall precisely upon the visual axis, the possible error is reviewed. The fact that the point of incidence of the light from the flashlight is not upon a normal (radius) of the surface causes the image to be slightly displaced. The center of curvature of the cornea is slightly behind the first nodal point from which the visual axis proceeds to the object (flashlight). In the $\triangle$ ONA, the angle at N will be the angle of the incident ray:

$\angle$ ONA $= \angle \alpha = 5°$
$\angle$ ANR, the external angle to $\triangle$ ONA $= 175°$
AR $=$ opposite $\angle$ N $=$ n $= 7.8$
AN $=$ opposite $\angle$ R $=$ r $= 7.08$
NR $=$ opposite $\angle$ A $=$ a $= 7.8 - 7.08 = 0.72$

By the law of sines

$$\frac{\sin A}{a} = \frac{\sin N}{n}$$

$$\sin A = \frac{\sin N \times a}{n}$$

$$\begin{aligned}
&= \log \sin N &= 8.94030 \\
&+ \log a &= 9.85733 \\
&+ \operatorname{colog} n &= 9.10791 \\
\hline
&7.90554 &= 27'13''
\end{aligned}$$

The image is located slightly behind the focal distance of the 7.8 mm radius convex mirror, say 4 mm behind the surface of the cornea. The angle of the object is so very small that the sine and tangent of the angle are equal.

$$\begin{aligned}
\log \tan 27'13'' &= 7.90554 \\
+ \log \text{(image distance) } 4 &= 0.60206 \\
\hline
8.50760 &= .03218 \text{ mm}
\end{aligned}$$

Thus we see that the error (0.03 mm) is the displacement of the

*Reinecke, R.D. and Herm, R.J.: *Refraction*. New York, Appleton-Century-Crofts, 1965, p. 205.

image of the corneal reflection from the fixation line. This is caused by the fact that the center of curvature of the cornea is not precisely on the fixation line. It is altogether too small for consideration. The symmetric parallactic displacement of the images due to the fact that the light-source is not always precisely in the optician's line of vision still does not increase this error to the point of any importance.

A second error arises from the fact that the rule does not always lie on the nose in exactly the same plane in which the spectacle lenses may be finally fitted. If the measurement is made at near point of 400 mm (16 inches), a difference of as much as 5 mm between the plane of the crest of the nose and the final distance of the lenses from the cornea becomes 400 : 60 : : 5 : *x*, or .75 mm. Such a large difference as 5 mm could not go unnoticed. That is, it would be in the instance of a very prominent nose or a shallow bridge with prominent eyes. It follows that when the measurement is made at a greater distance from the eyes than the final position of the spectacle lenses, the measurement is too short. The proper allowance is easily estimated.

No attempt is made to measure the separation of the axes with fixation at infinity because the distance can be computed more accurately than it can be measured. Table VIII shows the distance between the centers of rotation when the rule is 12 mm from the cornea and fixation is at 25, 33, or 40 cm from the rule.

TABLE VIII
DIFFERENCE BETWEEN INTEROCULAR DISTANCE FOR INFINITY
AND OPTICAL CENTERS FOR NEAR POINT

Fixation Distance (cm)	Optical Centers for Near							
	54	*56*	*58*	*60*	*62*	*64*	*66*	*68*
25	59.4	61.6	63.8	66.0	68.2	70.4	72.6	74.8
33	58.1	60.2	62.4	64.5	66.7	68.8	71.0	73.2
40	67.4	59.5	61.6	63.8	65.9	68.0	70.1	72.3

ESSEL CORNEAL REFLECTION PUPILLOMETER

It would seem that Essel of Paris has approached the ultimate with their Corneal Reflection Pupillometer. An internal light provides a distance fixation point for the patient and also the corneal reflection by which the measurement is made. A vertical hairline is superimposed upon the pin-point corneal reflection.

Detachable rubber nose-piece pads support the instrument similarly to an eyeframe. When the device is turned over, both the monocular distances and the sum can be read on the three scales. A knob has the effect of bringing the fixation target nearer, upon which the patient converges. A reading can be taken for any distance from infinity to 35 cm.

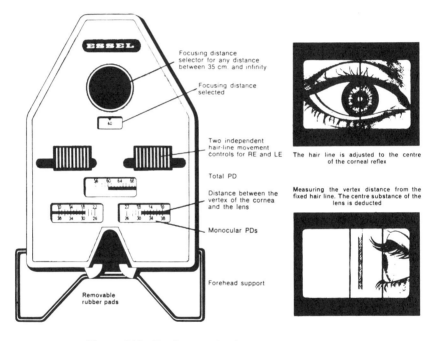

Focusing distance
selector for any distance
between 35 cm. and infinity

Focusing distance
selected

Two independent
hair-line movement
controls for RE and LE

Total PD

Distance between the
vertex of the cornea
and the lens

Monocular PDs

Forehead support

Removable
rubber pads

The hair line is adjusted to the centre
of the corneal reflex

Measuring the vertex distance from the
fixed hair line. The centre substance of the
lens is deducted

Figure 105. Essel corneal reflection pupillometer.

If binocular vision is faulty (strabismus) there is a right and left eye shutter which occludes one eye while the other is measured.

The instrument also measures vertex distance without touching the lens or eye lid. A hairline is moved to a position tangent with the corneal apex, then a movable hairline is adjusted tangent to the front vertex of the lens. Deduction of the lens thickness gives an exact measurement.

Recent measuring instruments that employ a split-image range-finder method of measurement offer a precise means to find interocular separation using the pupil center and facial details for criteria.

Several charts and tables have been made to show the amount that bifocal segments should be inset. The factors to be considered are (a) the optical centers for infinity; (b) the fixation distance; (c) the distance of the reading segment from the spectacle lens plane (or center of rotation) ; and (d) the decentration of the distance lens. Four variables provide the chart maker with a real problem. Some of them do not materially affect the amount in many cases and therefore most tables or charts have made some assumptions, such as a fixed vertex (posterior pole to cornea) distance.

One of the most widely used tables is the one prepared by Sterling* in which a 40 cm near-point is taken and distance lens prescriptions from +15.00 to − 22.00 are figured with optical centers for infinity ranging from a total of 54 to 72 mm. Boeder[†] has prepared a series of charts which, used successively, take most of the variables into account.

Fixation at near-point for reading and most manual tasks is a rather fixed distance. Physical height and arm length are ordinarily the determining factors; sometimes subnormal vision may have some effect. The depth of field with most reading glasses is definitely limited. If, then, the fixation light is held at the correct fixation distance, a remarkably accurate measurement is made.

All methods and instruments used in measuring the proper position for lens centers in the horizontal meridian for near-point fixation are measured with fixation on the median line. Remembering the lens fitting procedures of some dispensers, in which decentration of multifocal segments has been assymetric for near according to handedness, a research project was set up at Ferris State College under the observation of Doctor Ernest Bahnsen.

---

*Rayton, W.B.: *Ophthalmic Lenses. Their History and Application.* Rochester, NY Bausch & Lomb, 1945, p. 79.

[†] Boeder, P.: *Analysis of Prismatic Effects in Bifocal Lenses.* Southbridge, Mass., American Optical Company, 1939.

Near emmetropic college students who were not wearing glasses were selected. The subjects wore a headband upon which a small rod was fitted to represent the median line. Below it, another lightweight rod was fitted which could be turned to represent the fixation axis. A protractor was fixed on the headband to measure the angle the fixation axis deviated from median for different size and weight pieces of reading matter.

The subject's handedness and dominant eyedness were ascertained. A small magazine, *Reader's Digest* size, was given to the subject on the side of his handedness. After he had read a page for awhile, the fixation rod was turned to be over his visual axis and the protractor was read. Second, a heavier magazine, which was held with two hands, was used and the protractor reading recorded. Third, a small book was placed in the hand opposite the handedness. Again, the angle of the fixation axis rod was recorded.

After an elapse of more than a week, the test was repeated and again recorded. Several groups of students had this complete test during a whole semester. The final results were very interesting. The individuals were not consistent on which side or how far away from the median line the reading matter was·held. Handedness and dominant eyedness were not consistently correlated.

The conclusion was that all readers tended to converge toward the median line more than elsewhere, thus demonstrating that symmetrically decentered reading lenses and multifocal segments are in the best position. These findings do not eliminate those whose activity requires a particular posture with near-point attention in a special position. A dispensing optician should be ever alert for these instances.

One variable is the difference in the plane of the back surface of the spectacle lens as compared with the position of the millimeter rule used for measuring. As previously shown, the error is 1 mm for about 6 mm disparity in planes. If the optician is about the same height (and therefore about the same arm length) as the patient, the comfortable reading distance of both will be about the same. Hence, the position the optician assumes to read his millimeter scale will closely approximate the distance the patient uses for reading, and the fixation distance to the light source is correct. If there is a considerable difference in heights, allowance for the variance in reading distance must be made. When for some special reason (vocational or otherwise) the patient is fitted for a specific distance, he is asked to hold the light source while the optician corrects the distance with a tape-line. The measurement can then be made while the patient continues to hold the light. In no instance should the reading distance measurement be taken at a greater distance from the eyes than the focal distance of the reading addition. If doctor has prescribed + 4.00 addition for near, move in to 25 cm (10 inches) to take the O.C.

Accuracy in the near-point measurement is much more important in most cases than the distance O.C. Most patients are hypermetropic and wear stronger lenses for near than for distance. Larger prism values are generated in the reading prescription from decentration than those in the distance correction. Second, the distance from the eyes to the reading matter will not vary more than a few inches by the very prescription of the lenses. The triangle between the eye centers and the reading fixation point is almost a constant.

As previously discussed, the distance measurement is incorrect (too wide) for all intermediate points, such as within a room, and is correct only when the eyes are fixed at a distance of 20 feet or more. When glasses are intended for general use, it is better to err on the side of a slightly short measurement for distance vision because most wearers of such glasses spend much of their time indoors where the fixation distances are ten feet or less.

This measuring routine can be accurately used on heterotropic (crossed or diverging) eyes. No difficulty is experienced with children. Lens centers which are too close for convergent squint or too wide for divergent squint are disadvantageous to the patient. Make sure the measurement for binocular vision at distance is accurate! The light provides a good fixation point and even in uncorrected or amblyopic eyes it is adequate to hold attention. The modification of the procedure for those patients without binocular fixation is to hold the rule slightly tilted so that while the zero is under the pupil of the right eye, the rule is *in front of* the pupil of the left eye. After the rule is properly set for zero, tilt the rule to cover the right pupil and uncover the left. The deviating eye will now look at the light, and the corneal reflection will give the reading for the near point O.C. that the eyes will assume when they are straightened and have binocular vision. It will be observed that eyes with very large errors of refraction, including aphakia, will fix steadily on the light source without correction when it would otherwise be difficult to make the measurement without glasses.

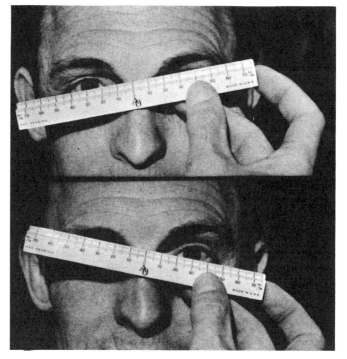

Figure 106.   Mm scale used as an occluder and measuring device.

Another justification for the use of the corneal reflection as a bench-mark is that the location of the pupillary center is not relevant to the image-forming system of the eye. Proof of this fact is simple: (A) Set two + 3.00D. uncut meniscus lenses on an optical bench about 3 inches apart with the concave sides facing. This is the general design of a 6 inch anastigmatic camera lens. Set a lamp house with an arrow or cross target on it. Place the lamp about 12 inches from this lens combination. Set up a card screen to receive the image at about 12 inches behind the lenses. Put cross-lines on the card to identify the position of the image. Take a 6 by 6 piece of cardboard and cut a $\frac{1}{2}$ inch round aperture in it. Hold this stop at mid-distance between the lenses. Move the aperture off center in all directions. The image does not move. (B) Remove the +3.00D. lenses and replace them with a +6.00D. lens in the first bracket. Now you have simulated cataract surgery and *all* of the power is on front of the pupil. Again move the aperture about. Again the image does not move.

If you had stood behind the lamp box at the end of the bench, the surface reflection (corneal reflection) of the front lens would not have moved through the whole experiment.

The placement of the optical center of the correction lens before the eye of a patient who has vision in only one eye involves more than the measurement of the distance from the corneal reflection to the midline of the nose. The patient must be carefully observed to learn his habitual reading position, including the head position. Some of these patients compensate for the unbalanced visual field by turning the head toward the eye with defective vision. They have found that when the nose is turned out of the field of view, the width of the visual field is increased. A satisfactory method of making the proper estimation is to approach the solution by trial and error with ink marks on the plano lens in a fitting-model frame of the proper size and type.

Thus far, the measurement of the position of optical centers for distance or near has been the total distance between centers of rotation of the intercepts of the z-axis at the lens plane. In clinical application the weight of most spectacles is borne by the patient's nose. Although it is obvious that the nose is in no way related to the centers of rotation or the eye movements, it is normal because of its function as the support of the lenses that it is used as a reference point. Theoretically, a more accurate choice might be a point in the median plane of the skull if it could be established. Practically, the crest of the nasal bone is the accepted reference line.

The individual distances of the two eyes are measured by any of the several P.D. rules which read right and left from zero in the

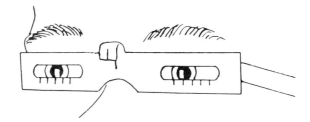

Figure 107. Guibor interocular measuring device.

center. The patient's fixation point is highly significant in this measurement. If the light is not held very close to the median plane at the crest of the nose, the patient's eyes must move conjugately to the right or left. As is shown in the discussion, an error in the fixation plane of about 15 mm will add or subtract 1 mm in the plane of the scale. The P.D.-Meter made by Precision-Cosmet Co. (Fig. 107) is designed to elude this difficulty.

A projection on the upper side of the frame has a vertical white line. When it is aligned with a similar line on the bridge of the frame, the optician's eye is precisely in the median plane of the scale. The slightest lateral movement breaks the alignment of the white lines. The device is also convenient because it rests on the face somewhat like a trial frame. The temples can be bent to align the plane of the rule parallel with the patient's corneal vertices. Much of the extraneous light that may reach the patient's corneas is intercepted by the slotted strip and thereby the reflection of the fixation light is enhanced. The differences between optical centers for near point and the distance lenses are shown in Table IX. The centers of the lenses for distance vision

TABLE IX
DISTANCE FROM CENTER OF NOSE TO FIXATION LINE
(Center of Rotation of Lens Plane 25 mm)

Fixation Distance (cm)	Optical Centers for Near									
	25	26	27	28	29	30	31	32	33	34
25	27.5	28.6	29.7	30.8	31.9	33.0	34.1	35.2	36.3	37.4
33	26.9	28.0	29.0	30.1	31.2	32.3	33.3	34.4	35.5	36.6
40	26.6	27.6	28.7	29.7	30.8	31.9	32.9	34.0	35.1	36.1

are correctly placed when they agree with the individual differences. Other considerations which will be subsequently discussed often enter into the placement of the optical centers when the eyes are used at near-point.

In the days of saddle-bridges and assembled hoop-spring eyeglasses, opticians routinely corrected the fitting of the glasses at the time of delivery. Unbalanced features in which "one eye was farther from the nose than the other" presented no great problem because the shanks of the bridge or the studs of the eyeglasses could be managed to set either lens very close to the nose and the other a considerable distance away from it as required. Even the adjusting screw for the pupillary distance of trial frames altered the positions of the lenses symmetrically. It was only when plastic frames with fixed bridge shapes grew in popularity that attention was attracted to the high percentage of asymmetric faces. Many opticians find that a high percent of all persons have one eye or the other closer to the nose than its mate. It has been noted that the left eye is the closer in the majority of cases.

Many devices have been designed to measure this asymmetry. Trial frames were made with individual adjustments for pupillary distance. With a pair of crossline lenses the separate distances to the pupil centers could be found. Several interpupillary gauges followed, in some of which lenses and double scales were used to reduce errors from parallax. In all instances, like the trial frame, the gauge rested on the crest of the nose. As frame and mounting designs developed, the weight of the glasses was more frequently placed on pads that rest on the sides of the nose. It would follow that unless the slopes of the sides of the nose were nearly the same, the accuracy of the measurement made from the ridge of the nasal bone would be invalidated to some degree. Adjustment of the pad arms would compensate many metal bridges, but a plastic frame would come to rest according to the contour of the nasal bone.

It is shown in Chapter 10 that lens centers must not only be separated by the total distance between the centers of rotation for distance fixation, but that, unless the lens powers are identical, decentration (as prism) is present unless both lens centers are intersected by the z-axes (fixation lines) when the eyes are fixed at distance. The amount of prism may be negligible in very weak lenses but the decentration may displace the *area of comfortable binocular vision* in some of these cases. It is good practice to routinely measure the distances of the two eyes separately.

A large part of the discussion of this subject of "asymmetric pupillary distances" has been directed toward the proper placement of multifocal segments. Many formulas and tables have been presented to show the necessary compensation for those lenses fitted to persons whose eyes were not symmetric with reference to the crest of the nose. The premise in all of these calculations is that the point of fixation is on the median line directly in front of the nose. The Ferris State College research on convergence habits for reading allays much of the concern on asymmetric convergence habits for reading position. However, in the act of writing, most individuals tend to converge in the side of the field that agrees with handedness.

No one has ever researched vocational eyewear fitting as well as Clark Holmes in his *Guide to Occupational and Other Visual Needs* (Los Angeles, Anderson, Ritchie & Simon, 1958). The industry is indebted to Vision Ease Corporation, St. Cloud, Minnesota, for continuing the project.

The violinist and typist look down and to the right, the right-handed artist works straight ahead and looks down and to the left at his pallette. Machine operators often have widely separated points of fixation. A typist who wears bifocals and copies from notes at the right side of a typewriter is a classical case. Several questions are posed: Shall the reading portions of a pair of vocational bifocals (a) be set for right vergence in proper position for the notes, (b) have the position compromised and have the eyes rotate slightly to the right of center for the notes and left to the typewriter, or (c) be set in the regular balanced position and let the wearer move from one field to the other by head movements? It has been found a successful practice to hand a test-type book to a patient and, while he reads it, carefully note whether he rotates his head to one side while he reads. One should be careful not to draw an erroneous conclusion from a patient's demonstration through a poorly fitted (or adjusted) pair of bifocals.

It would follow that symmetric decentration of the reading portions even for those persons who have symmetric faces forces some

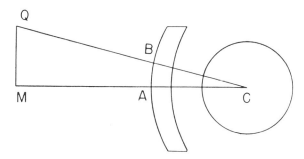

Figure 108. Fixation alteration referred to lens.

multifocal wearers to modify their previous habits of near-point fixation. Referring to the similar triangle formulas in the discussion of the usable area of a reading portion, several interesting observations can be made. In Figure 108, when the center of the segment **AC** is 25 mm from the center of rotation and the distance of fixation **MC** is 40 cm (400 mm) the distance **MQ** is to **AB** as **MC** is to **AC**.

$$\frac{\mathbf{MQ}}{\mathbf{AB}} = \frac{\mathbf{MC}}{\mathbf{AC}} = \frac{400}{25} = \frac{16}{1}$$

Therefore, if the distance **MQ** is 16 mm, the excursion of the eye is 1 mm at the lens.

If the individual measurements of a patient reveal that the intersection of the z-axis of the right eye in the plane of the lenses is 4 mm farther from the nose than the left, it would seem in (Fig. 109) that the centers of the segments should reflect the asymmetry.

RM = 32, **ML** = 28, **RL** = 60

The assumption, of course, is based upon the patient's fixation at point **F**. It is seen above that if the fixation point were moved to **F**₁, a distance of, 32 mm, the eyes would rotate toward the right 2 mm in the plane of the lenses as demonstrated above and the distance **RM** would be increased to 34 mm while **LM** would reduce to 26 mm. If it were assumed that this patient habitually favored the field of his left eye for fixation and **F**₂, a distance of 48 mm from **F** was the point of fixation, the measured asymmetry would be reversed. The distance of 48 mm would cause a vergence that

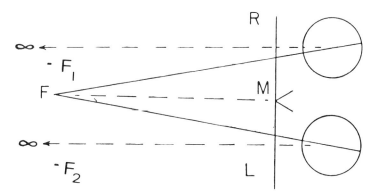

Figure 109.   Fixation point alteration.

would measure 3 mm at the distance of the spectacle lenses. Then

$$RM = 32 - 3 = 29$$
$$LM = 28 + 3 = 31$$

It becomes immediately apparent that the *point of fixation* is the decisive consideration. Despite the fact the centers of rotation are not equidistant from the median line of the skull, the centers of reading lenses or segments of multifocals will not always reflect the precise asymmetry as measured. Conversely, proper placement of near-point centers for some persons with balanced centers of rotation may require dissimilar decentration.

Sheard emphasizes the effect of ocular dominance upon the reading position. The research on convergence at Ferris State College does not agree with Doctor Sheard's observations.

If an Essel Corneal Reflection Pupillometer is used, the following paragraphs referring to the use of a mm scale and a pen light are irrelevant.

In practice, when an unbalanced measurement is noted, the position of the patient's face-plane and the fixation light must be carefully checked and the measurement repeated. When the positions of the optical centers are decided, the lenses in a fitting-model frame of appropriate size or his own spectacle lenses are marked with vertical ink-lines according to the measurements found. The ink-lines should extend up from the bottoms of the

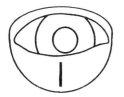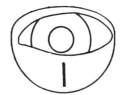

Figure 110.   Lines to verify lens accuracy.

lenses to the lower lid as shown in Figure 110. The position of the lines with respect to the pupils is observed for a few moments while the patient uses his eyes for near-point fixation. The dispenser closes one eye to remove parallax and makes his observations from a point directly in front of the patient's fixation point.

The size of the segment in the multifocal also enters into the consideration. A pair of golf glasses with 10 mm round segments that are only three pupil diameters wide must be very accurately set in order to be of any use, while a pair of Executive bifocal segments are as wide as the lenses.

For obvious reasons, this observation must not be made through the patient's bifocals. Unless the patient tells of difficulty that unquestionably suggests trouble that might arise from asymmetric decentration or convergence, it is not wise to alter a bifocal wearer's habits once they are established unless requested.

The ink-line observation is equally valuable when a decision is to be made about the optical centers for distance lenses. The asymmetry connected with fixation at near-point may be altogether different for infinity. Most persons set the x-axis (the line between the centers of rotation) parallel to the plane of distant fixation. Thereupon, the unequal distances between the midline and the z-axes of the two eyes become increasingly significant when the dioptric power of the two lenses is different in the horizontal meridian. To illustrate

O.D. + 1.00D.
O.S. + 3.00D.
RM = 34 mm, **ML** = 30 mm, Total 64 mm

If the optical centers of the lenses are set equidistant from center

(32 mm), the z-axis of the right eye intersects the lens, 2 mm to the right of the center

$+ 1.00 \times 0.2 = 0.2^{\triangle}$ Base In (toward the nose)

and the left eye looks through a point 2 mm to the right of the center

$+ 1.00 \times 0.2 = 0.2^{\triangle}$ Base In

and the left eye also looks through a point 2 mm to the right of the optical center but because the lens is stronger

$+ 3.00 \times 0.2 = 0.6^{\triangle}$ Base Out.

The total effect is $0.4^{\triangle}$ Base Out or, because the difference in lens powers in the horizontal meridian gives the effect of the total separation of the lens centers, is too narrow. Of course, the prism can be compensated by turning the eyes 2 mm into the left field to intersect the optical axes of the lenses.

A multifocal wearer may experience some confusion under these circumstances, because the segments are rotated into the left field when the head is turned. Many persons have sufficient fusion amplitude to overcome the small prismatic effect in the primary position and have reconciled projection to compensate for the slight displacement of all objects to the left. On the other hand, this small inaccuracy may contribute to the difficulty a patient experiences in "learning to get used to his new prescription."

Added to this are those instances when extra wide reading segments cover errors in indifferently measured I.O.D.

A special group among those whose habitual near-point fixation points are not on the median line are persons who have the use of only one hand or who are otherwise crippled. The time spent in the observation of the postural habits of these individuals is more than repaid. Occasionally the reading segment should be decentered out to permit the patient to continue his habits that compensate for his deficiency.

To summarize:

1. The z-axis fixation line can be conveniently located by the use of a light source and its corneal reflection.

2. The position or separation of optical centers of prescription lenses is dictated by the intersections of the z-axes.

3. The patient's posture and habitual fixation points must be

carefully observed and discussed to approach proper placement of lens and segment centers.

REVIEW

1. Why is the *line of sight* not the same as the *optic axis* of a normal eye? What is the average deviation? Describe the angles between these two axes.

2. Describe the primary position of the eyes; secondary position; tertiary position.

3. If an eye turns to view an object on a diagonal at an angle of 40°, according to Table VI, the eye rotates 7.5° on the z-axis. If the ℞ is + 0.75 + 2.25 × 90, how much is the effect of the prescription changed because of the crossed cylinders?

4. Define the plane of fixation. Make a sketch to describe it.

5. Why is it difficult to describe or define "which eye is higher or lower than the other?"

6. If the refraction is made with a trial frame adjusted to the Base Line and the spectacles are adjusted to "compensate" for a condition in which one eye seems to be 3 mm above the other when the distance between the eyes is 65 mm, what is the discrepancy in the cylinder axes in the lenses?

7. Name five of the points of eyes and their correcting lenses that are equidistant when the eyes look at a test chart at 20 feet (optical infinity) .

8. Make a sketch showing how lenses are tilted, as described in Table VII, when they are decentered.

9. If the centers of rotation are 65 mm apart (I.O.D.) at what distance should the centers of reading lenses be spaced when the lenses are 12 mm from the corneas and the reading distance is 40 cm? 33 cm? 25 cm?

10. If the eyes are symmetric with reference to the midline but the patient holds reading matter 75 mm to the right of the midline when he reads at 40 cm, how much would the placement of bifocal segments be affected? Make a sketch.

11. Discuss the fallacy of "high eye."

12. What is the cylinder axis error per millimeter of disagreement in reference points between doctor and optician about how "high" an eye is measured?

ADDITIONAL REFERENCES

1. Helmholtz, H. von: *Physiological Optics,* Vol. III. Menasha, Banta, 1924.
2. Duke-Elder, W.S.: *Text-book of Ophthalmology.* St. Louis, Mosby, 1949.
3. Maddox, E.E.: *Tests and Studies of Ocular Muscles.* Bristol, Wright. 1898.
4. Olsho, S.L.: *The Coordination of Refraction with Spectacle and Eyeglass Fitting.* Philadelphia, Pelham, 1928.

Chapter 7

FITTING TRIANGLE

◆◆◆

I t is interesting to think of the simple geometry involved in the support of a spectacle frame. The bridge of the nose and the tops of the two ears are the apices of a triangle that sets in or very near to the horizontal plane when the head and eyes are in primary position. This triangle is usually rather close to an isosceles triangle because the nose is very near the midpoint of the base line between the ear tops. Mostly outside of this triangle near the nasal apex, and in a plane nearly perpendicular to the triangle, is the plane of the spectacle lenses and Listing's plane.

Now with these observations, we have completed the outline for ophthalmic frame fitting. The centers of rotation have been designated as points of origin for a three-dimensional space in which the line connecting the centers of rotation is the x-axis. Perpendicular to it in the same plane (90°) is the y-axis. The fixation line which is normal (perpendicular) to the x-y plane becomes the z-axis of the eye. The horizontal (180°) line of the spectacle lens is parallel to the x-axis of the eyes. The y-axis of the lens is at a right angle to the x-axis (90°) and in the same plane. The optical axis of the lens, the line through the centers of curvature of the lens, is the z-axis. The fitting triangle (Fig. 111), described above, is the support that establishes and maintains the relationship between the planes of the eyes and lenses.

The straight bow frame of colonial times had a saddle or an "X" bridge that rested on the crest of the nose and the straight bows rested in the notches at the tops of the ears. When the head was erect, most of the weight of the glasses was borne upon the contact point on the nose. If the nose of the wearer was sufficiently prominent, the front of the frame with the lenses could be balanced on the wearer's nose if the head were held quietly in the primary position. In this particular case, the temples served to

199

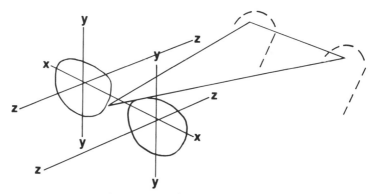

Figure 111. Fitting triangle.

steady the front of the glasses and prevent it from listing to either side. The three contact points, nose and ear tops, completed the horizontal *fitting triangle* that controlled the planes of the lenses.

If the plane of the wearer's face is elevated, to look up, the weight of the glasses still remains on the nose and again the temples are needed merely to stabilize the glasses. It is when the head is tilted forward that the support of the glasses is radically changed. The head is tilted 15° to 45° forward in practically all near-point activities, especially those involving the use of the hands. Therefore, the support of the lenses and the fitting of the frame for this position of the head are worthy of examination.

Table X is a comparison of four pairs of glasses. The lenses are identical in size, shape, and weight. The bridge measurements are the same and the temples are the appropriate lengths for the same head size *(fitting-triangle)*. The first mounting is a Numont® with comfort cable temples. The second pair is a standard gold-filled Ful-Vue frame. The third is a regular 150 weight Ful-Vue plastic frame with 5½ inch skull temples. The last frame is a 200 weight library frame with semiskull temples. The comparison of the weights of the spectacles with the same lenses set in the different frames is interesting. For example, the library glasses (38.0 gm) are about twice the weight of the rimless glasses (19.5 gm). The weight of the glasses as borne by the pads on the bridge and the temples at the ear top is compared in three positions—that is,

TABLE X
EFFECT OF INCLINATION UPON DISTRIBUTION OF WEIGHT OF
GLASSES

	Numont Rimless	Ful-Vue G.F. Frame	Ful-Vue 150 Weight Plastic	Library 200 Weight Plastic
Total weight	19.5 gm	22.1 gm	26.0 gm	38.0 gm
Distance				
Center of mass				
behind pads	6.3 mm	8.7 mm	13.2 mm	27.6 mm
Horizontal				
Pads	18.2 gm	19.8 gm	22.7 gm	27.3 gm
Temples	1.4	2.3	3.3	10.7
15° Inclination				
Pads	17.4	15.6	25.1	28.2
Temples		6.4	1.0	9.8
30° Inclination	2.0			
Pads	3.9	5.9	20.0	20.0
Temples	15.6	16.1	6.0	18.0

with the temples horizontal, inclined forward 15°, and again at 30°. The weights given do not consider the support of the glasses that may be carried by temple pressure on the skull. This is regarded as a constant.

It is interesting to note that the weight on the pads of the plastic frames increases at 15° shifts to the temples at 30°. This is apparently due to the position of the center of mass (center of gravity). The temples of the metal frames do not receive more than 10 percent of the total weight in the horizontal position. The centers of mass are consequently very close to the plane of the pads and the weight of the glasses rapidly transfers to the temples as the glasses are tipped forward.

Study of the weight at the pads and the ratio of weights immediately provokes some thought with reference to the square area of contact. The library frame exerts about 50 percent more pressure on the nose than the rimless glasses when the temples are horizontal and inclined 15°. If the contact area is half again as large, the comfort should be comparable. If a pair of adjustable pads is attached to the library frame and the contact points are thrust farther behind the lens plane and closer to the center of mass, the pressure per square millimeter is rapidly increased. In this instance, a much larger contact area is required to distribute the increased weight on the pads over a larger area of the nose.

As the head tips forward and the ridge of the nose approaches a vertical position, less and less of the weight of the glasses bears on the contact point on the crest of the nose. If the temples do not extend beyond the ear tops, the glasses would begin to slide forward almost as soon as the head tilts forward and finally fall from the face.

Fleck et al.* have delved more deeply into the mechanics of weight-bearing by frame pads than others. Figure 112 suggests their thoroughness. Their assumption, however, is that the nose carries the whole weight of the eyewear. Table X shows that most of the weight is upon the nose but that the percentage of weight

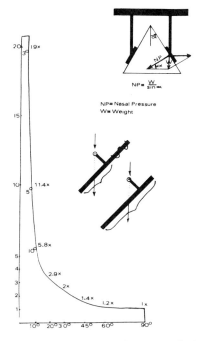

Figure 112.   Frame pad stress analysis.

*Fleck, et al.:   *Die Praxis der Brillenanpassung.*   Leipzig, VEB Fachbuchverlag, 1960, pp. 44-46.

borne by the nose varies greatly both from posture and style of frame. Experienced dispensers have learned empirically that a thin narrow nose has more difficulty from the depression of pads into tissue, but hitherto it has not been demonstrated how the pressure increases so radically with the alteration of angle. From the low limit of 1 $\times$ when the pad faces are parallel to the lenses for an Ethiopian or Oriental nose, the increase is to 19 $\times$ for a nose that has only 3° of slope.

The point in the length of a pad where the weight is exerted is very important, too. When the downward thrust is applied to a pad which is pivoted at the center, the upper part of the pad is almost valueless. The same length of pad pivoted nearer the top accepts the thrust nearer the center and thereby distributes the weight over the whole square area of the pad.

Friction between the bridge and the tissue on the crest of the nose and the temples against the sides of the head offers the only restraint. Support from the slope of the nose disappears quickly. In fact, many noses are so nearly vertical that, even when the head is in primary position, little support is offered. The tissue of the bridge of the nose is often sufficiently compressible for a groove or depressed area to be formed after the glasses are worn for a period of time. The bridge of the frame becomes seated in this position and thus friction is increased.

In more recent times, the weight of the glasses has also been placed on the sides of the nose. Oftentimes the design of the bridge is intended to place the whole weight of the glasses at points on the sides of the nose slightly below the eyes. Several advantages are immediately evident. The weight of the glasses is spread over a larger square area and thereby the pressure per square millimeter on the skin surface is reduced. The placement of the pads is under greater control and frequently better slopes can be found on the sides of the nose than on the crest.

The temples of the glasses in the case above were assumed to stop at the ear tops and not exert pressure against the sides of the head. Therefore the glasses immediately responded to the force of gravity. In clinical practice it is found that the sides of a large number of heads are nearly parallel at the point above the ear tops. A sufficient pressure against the head to support the glasses

is tolerated by many spectacle wearers. The line of force is between points **A** and **B** in Figure 113. Sufficient tension can be
generated at this point with wide plastic temples to accept the
entire weight of the glasses, but such pressure is rapidly fatiguing
to most individuals. However, a pair of "on and off" reading
glasses can frequently be satisfactorily fitted with this frame type.
The notion of a contact point or apex of triangle becomes obscured when the glasses are held in place by head pressure. In
fact, when spectacles are secured to the head by the clamping pressure of temples alone, the mechanics of the fitting is similar to that
used in the fitting of eyeglasses (pincenez).

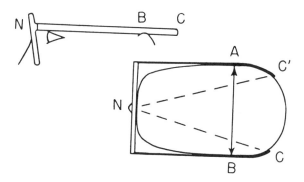

Figure 113.   Frame pressure analysis.

At some point close to the top of the ear, most skulls begin to
slope to the back. If the temples are made slightly longer and
follow the shape of the head to points **CC'**, the *fitting triangle* is
developed again **CNC'**). When the head is in primary position,
most of the weight of the glasses is at **N**. As the head is tilted forward, the weight is transferred to points **C** and **C'**. Finally when
the plane of the face is parallel to the floor, the entire weight of
the glasses in on the tips of the temples.

The sides of many heads tend to remain rather parallel for some
distance behind the ear at the level of the top of the ear. A very
long temple would be required to reach the point where the tip of
the temple might be best as described above. Behind the ear in
the area of the mastoid process, the skull tapers in toward the

neck. Temples should be bent down slightly spaced from the backs of the ears at the tops and contoured to follow the shape of the mastoid process until *locks* at points **C** and **C**¹ are established. Most temples as supplied on frames by the manufacturers are too short. With small complaint from purchasers they save material, have a frame that folds prettily, and packs more easily. When I see a speaker distracting his audience by constantly pushing his eyeframe back into place I sympathize with him and wish I could tell him to go back to his optician to have the job of fitting completed. *The temples of the speaker's frame are too short.* The ends are in front of points **C** and **C'**. This cardinal point in frame fitting will be repeated.

The "length to bend" (LTB), that is, the length of the temple from the joint to where a sharp bend down is made, is a specification as important as the bridge fitting, yet, few dispensers show this on their laboratory orders. Anything less than a sharp bend promotes a fitting that lets the eyewear slide down the nose. If the proper bend is not at the right length, it causes poor fitting. When the length is too short, the temples crawl up with the normal movement of the flesh at the ear tops which is caused by muscle movements under the facial flesh in the acts of speaking, laughing, or eating. As the temples rise from the ear tops, the bridge slides down the face. On the other hand, if the length to the bend is too long, the bend must be 90° or more to prevent the glasses from sliding forward. The bend should be just a little behind the back of the crotch at the top of the ear as it extends to the back of the ear. This lets the first contact of the temple with the ear be near the center of the back of the ear. From this point, pressure against the head is *down* and *in* which secures the temple in the crotch at the top of the ear and establishes two of the apices of the fitting triangle. It assures the lines of force from points **C** and **C'** and secures the eyewear in its proper position. This ideal fitting requires temples long enough to reach these points.

At the time of the selection of the frame, a dispenser must determine if the temples on the frame are sufficiently long for a proper fitting. He must also know whether different length temples are available. There is nothing so disastrous as a good looking pair of glasses that will not stay in place because of the improper length of temples. They wear out the customer's patience by requiring frequent returns for temple adjustments and assure a dispenser's undoing if the customer visits a competitor for help.

Before the bent or skull-fitting temple was invented, straight temple frames had extensible or hinged ends so that the temples almost encircled the wearer's head. Equestrians who had to wear glasses frequently fastened a cord or ribbon to the temples and tied it behind the head. Some unrecorded English inventor conceived the idea of encircling the ear by following the crotch between the ear and head to the lower lobe of the ear. He publicized the innovation as a "riding-bow." All temples that follow the shape of the back of the ear are still known by that name.

In its first form the riding-bow temple was made of wire, and it served satisfactorily with the small lightweight glasses of that day. As the size and weight of glasses increased, it became necessary that a softer and more comfortable tip for the temple be produced. The improvement was a temple made of a cable of several smaller wires. Finally a heavy shank or side-piece was used with a still heavier cable section to fit behind the ear. These temples are called *comfort cable* (C.C.) temples. Another solution of the problem of discomfort from wire temples is a cover for the end of the temple where it contacts the ear. The bulk of the temple is increased and the material used is softer than metal. Rubber, plastic, and varnished tubing are also used. A disadvantage of some of the covers is the effect upon the elasticity and pliability of the temple. For example, a plastic sleeve is rather soft and adjustable when the temples are new. Later, when the material has dried out, the temple becomes quite rigid.

While the comfort cable temple lends itself to a more simple adjustment, it is much less efficient in retaining a permanent shape than the wire-core plastic covered type called pearl tip riding-bow. When this style temple is carefully formed to the contour of the back of the ear, the adjustment lasts indefinitely.

The shape of the crotch behind the ear assumes a great deal of importance when the fitting of riding-bow temples is undertaken. Most ears are set closely enough to the head to provide a definite crotch into which the temple can be fitted. In occasional cases, the ears protrude from the head, or the shape of the external ear is such that the back of the ear is perpendicular to the head (Fig. 114*b*). Riding-bow temples should be avoided in these instances because they will have a tendency to crawl away from the head and press painfully against the back of the ear. Particular attention must be paid to this condition with small children. Deformity of the ears can definitely be exaggerated by ill-fitting temples.

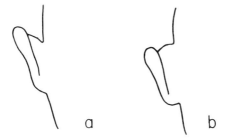

Figure 114. Ear crotch differences.

The contour of the crotch between head and external ear falls into one of three general shape types illustrated in Figure 115. The shape of the external ear does not seem to suggest which shape of crotch may be found behind it.

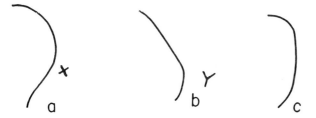

Figure 115. Back of ear variation.

Type *a* is found in the majority of cases. If the temple follows the shape of the ear from the middle of the back of the ear at the point marked "x," it locks itself to the ear and holds the temple securely down against the top of the ear.

Type *b* is a more difficult shape to fit. The long straight slope offers no place for the temple to obtain a purchase. It is necessary that the temple be long enough to pass point "y" so that a hook can be bent on the tip to hold the temple against the ear top.

Type *c* also presents a difficult fitting problem. The temple must be bent at a right angle at the top and, much like the fitting of a skull-fit temple, it should not exert any pressure until the last 10 or 15 mm of the temple at the tip. In that way the line of force will tend to hold the temple against the ear top. It takes very little handling of this temple after it is adjusted to lose some of the bend at the top. If the temple is straightened only slightly, the glasses are loosened very much.

Skull-fit temples are frequently fitted rather close to the back of the ear like a riding-bow temple. Type *a* offers the opportunity for an easy and satisfactory fitting if the temple is long enough to pass point "x." Skull-fit temples adjusted in the crotch behind the ear of type *b* must be very long. If the temples do not pass "y," they will slide up when the head is moved and thereby tilt the lenses and loosen the fitting on the nose. Type *c* is more difficult for a "riding-bow adjustment" of skull-fit temples. The bend at the top of the ear controls the performance of the fitting. Skull-fit temples can be adjusted to this type case, but the temples will require frequent attention if the glasses are to stay in place on the nose.

It is now apparent that an optician must have an unobstructed view of the backs of the ears and the mastoid processes before he ventures an opinion either to himself or to the patient about the possibilities of fitting *any* type of temple. This observation is quite simple with short-haired patients. It is merely necessary for the optician to stand up at the fitting table and look down over the top of the patient's head and be able to see either or both of the areas. A hat and hair-dress often obstruct the view of a patient's ears. The patient's assistance may be necessary, but in no circumstances should an optician depend upon guesses or palpation. The crotches back of the ears and the mastoid processes must be *seen*. Omission of this small detail has ended in many hours of wasted time, disappointed patients, and unsatisfactory fittings.

Most present-day glasses do not rest on the crest of the nose.

the weight is carried by pads on the sides of the nose. Therefore the *fitting triangle* has four contact points and it appears to have become a quadrilateral. In Figure 116, it can be seen that the triangle has not disappeared. The line of force from the right temple has its terminus in the pad on the opposite (left) side. Conversely, the right pad and left temple are related in the same way. The intersection of these lines, which is somewhat behind the plane of the lenses, is the new apex formerly on the crest of the nose. It follows that a temple that is too tight gives symptoms to the ear on the same side and the nose pad on the opposite side.

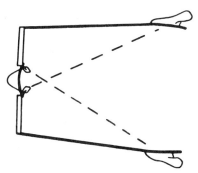

Figure 116. Temple stress analysis.

It has been shown that the first purpose of the temples of a pair of glasses is to establish two of the apices of the *fitting triangle* and thereby fix the lens planes. This is accomplished when two particular points on the temples are maintained at the ear tops. The function of that part of the temple that extends beyond these points is to accomplish either or both of two purposes: (a) hold the temple securely against the top of the ear or (b) keep the temple from sliding forward. The length of the temple from end piece to ear top and the angle to which the temples spread control the plane of the lenses. If either temple is too short or the temple joint opens too widely, the frame will rotate on the y-axis and the lens on that side will be too close to the eye while the vertex distance of the other lens increases. No pair of spectacles can be correctly positioned if this relationship is not strictly observed.

When the positions of the vertices of the *fitting triangle* are altered by the adjustment of the glasses, the patient can be expected to have discomfort. Figure 117 shows two common maladjustments of spectacles. In the first instance, *a,* the temples press against the head some distance in front of the ears. This tends to set the base of the *fitting triangle* forward of the normal position at the ear tops. Therefore the lines of force between the pads and temples are shorter and the triangle is much flatter. The advantage of the resiliency of the temple is lost. Most heads are wider at the ear tops than the temporal area. The snug-fitting temples taper toward the front. Like squeezing on the sides of an equilateral triangle, the harder the squeeze the quicker the fingers meet at the apex. Extra pressure is thus placed on the temples behind the ears. If the temples loosen behind the ears, the glasses slide down the nose, but the fact that the temples fit tightly in front of the ears causes them still to keep tension on the temples behind the ears. Truly the patient's honest complaint is paradoxical, "My glasses are tight and uncomfortable behind my ears, but my lenses are sliding down my nose!" The patient will be relieved and the glasses will assume their normal suspension when the pressure of the temples in front of the ears is relieved.

In the second case, *b,* the pressure in front of the ears is on only one side. The normal isoceles triangle with equal legs and equal tension has been destroyed. The resiliency of the tight temple is

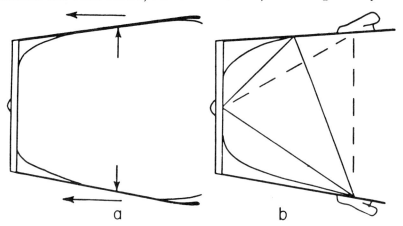

Figure 117. Temple pressure before the ears.

not effective. Most of the weight of the glasses is forced upon the pad on the opposite side. Comfortable adjustment is not effected until both ear tops are the vertices of the *fitting triangle*.

Eyeglasses cannot be discussed quite the same as spectacles. The French name and definition is quite complete: "Pince-nez. Eyeglasses kept in place on the nose by means of a spring." The hoop-spring type, including oxfords, is held in place by the effect of a spring wound around a horizontal axis. The distance between the lenses and likewise the tension of the spring is increased by the act of placing the glasses on the nose. The *finger-piece* type of eyeglass has two movable pads that turn on a vertical axis. The distance between the pads is increased when the eyeglasses are attached to the nose. It is possible to place the glasses on the nose in a silghtly different position each time they are applied. Eyeglass wearers, however, develop a sense of touch, coupled with feeling of security and satisfactory optical performance that altogether causes them to clamp the glasses on their noses in approximately the same position at all times, if the primary adjustment is made consistent with the peculiarities of each patient's method of applying the eyeglasses to his nose.* This can be attained only by careful observation on the part of the optician and the precision of the compensating adjustments made.

REVIEW

1. Name the points of contact of the fitting triangle. Discuss the exception in the case of the two points of contact of a pad bridge.

2. From Table X which type of frame would be most desirable for reading glasses if one wished to place the most of the weight on the nose?

3. Why must a dispenser make a visual inspection of the area behind the patient's ears? How can ear and skull shape affect choice of frame?

4. Discuss the effects of fitting upon comfort of frames when points of contact or pressure are not equally distributed at ear

---

*Waters, E.H.: *Ophthalmic Mechanics*, Vol. I. Ann Arbor, Mich., Edwards Brothers, 1947, pp. 298-301.

tops and behind ears.

5. Name and discuss x-, y-, and z-axes of individual lenses, also a pair of lenses in an eyeframe.

6. Discuss importance of constant projection of lens axis through the center of rotation.

Chapter 8

VISUAL ACUITY AND CORRECTING
LENSES

◆◆◆

V isual acuity, or rather the lack of it, is one of the primary causes of the ophthalmic professions and the arts that deal with lenses. The subject is carefully discussed in all texts on the subjects of physiological optics and refraction. An ophthalmic dispenser should have a clear concept of visual acuity and the effect of lens powers upon it. A practical demonstration upon one's own eyes is probably the best way to impress indelibly the effects of lenses upon the eye. Little equipment is necessary and surely the material in any textbook will be measurably more lucid after the demonstrations and experiments. A standard Snellen chart, a Jaeger reading chart, and a trial-lens set are all that are necessary. These items can be found in any ophthalmic laboratory as well as in a doctor's refracting room. The time and effort spent in conducting the suggested personal demonstration will more than repay the experimenter. By the use of trial lenses, a methodical investigation of many of the common errors of refraction can be made without any ill effects aside from the incidental blurred and/or confused vision during the demonstrations.

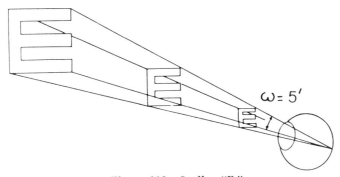

Figure 118. Snellen "E."

213

Most Snellen charts have about ten rows of letters. When the eye is 20 feet from the chart, there are two or more lines of letters smaller than normal eyes can see. The line marked 20 is the line seen by normal eyes at 20 feet away from it. This is called 20/20 vision. The letters on this line are 8.87 mm high. At 20 feet they subtend an angle of 5' at the eye. This is considered normal acuity.* The letter "E" in Figure 118 is a typical test letter. It will be noted that it is composed of three lines and two intervening spaces. Therefore each line or space subtends an angle of only 1' of arc at the eye. An eye that is able to resolve (see separately) lines and spaces this size has normal vision. It follows that visual acuity is inversely proportional to the resolving power of the eye as measured by angle ω.

$$\text{V.A.} = \frac{k}{\omega}$$

where the constant k equals 1 and when ω is measured in minutes of arc or 0.000291 when measured in radians.

Upon inspection, it will be noted that the Snellen letters increase in size in direct proportion to the number of feet at which they should be seen. The 40 foot letters are twice the height of normal letters. The largest letter at the top of the card which should be seen at 200 feet is ten times as high (88.67 mm) as the normal line. Figure 118 shows how the same angle at the eye confronts gradually larger letters as the distance increases.

When the smallest size letters discernible are larger than normal, the accepted method of recording the acuity shows the number of feet between the chart and eye, and the smallest size letters seen at that distance. For example, 20/60 indicates at the normal distance of 20 feet, the eye could not resolve the letters smaller than those normally seen at 60 feet in which the individual legs of the letters are 3 minutes wide and the whole letter is 15 minutes high. If the fraction 20/60 is expressed by the formula above

$$\text{V.A.} = \frac{k}{\omega} = \frac{1}{3} = 33\%$$

This is called the International Acuity Rating. Table XI compares the notations most commonly seen.

*Southall, P.C.: *Introduction to Physiological Optics*. London, Oxford U Pr, 1937, pp. 75-79.

TABLE XI

International Acuity Rating	A.M.A. Efficiency Rating	Navy Notation Equivalent
20/20	100%	100%	20/20
20/25	80%	95.6%	16/20
20/30	67%	91.4%	13/20
20/40	50%	83.6%	10/20
20/50	40%	76.3%	8/20
20/60	33%	69.9%	7/20
20/100	20%	48.9%	4/20
20/200	10%		2/20

ACUITY DEMONSTRATION

Place the Snellen chart 20 feet away under good illumination and keep the general illumination of the room lower than normal, but not necessarily dark. Take a seat near the trial set. If the experimenter wears glasses, he should remove them and as he occludes first one eye and then the other he should find his own visual acuity without lenses. When the glasses are replaced, it will be instructive to note the difference, if any. If the refractive error is hyperopia of low degree, there may be scarcely any difference. Even if there is some difference, it will frequently be instructive to *not* put on the lenses some morning and note whether the eyes do not have better acuity than they had directly after removing the correction on another occasion. If the experimenter is myopic, there will be a reduction in acuity that is almost directly proportional to the lens power; the experiment of an overnight rest may not demonstrate quite the same as in the case of hyperopia.

One of the most common methods of subjective refraction is called the "fogging" method. It is described in all texts on refraction. The principle of the procedure is to increase systematically the plus lens power before the patient's eyes until he is overcorrected. Too much plus lens makes the patient artificially myopic, fogs his distance vision, and places his far point in front of his eye inside of infinity. The careful reduction of plus (addition of minus) lens power to the amount that moves the artificial far point to the patient's own far point measures the refractive error. Assuming that lenses needed for distance are being worn, the use of the "fogging" technique demonstrates the effect of each lens on visual acuity. It is well to perform the procedure slowly in order to get the effect of the lenses involved. The method is simple. Cover one eye in such a way that it cannot see and thereby confuse the impressions. Wear the normal distance prescription, if any. Hold a +0.25D. sphere before the eye and note any diminution in vision. Record on a piece of paper what effect this lens has made. For instance, 20/25 − 2 means that all but two letters on the 25 foot line were read. Continue with the report through the series. Take a +0.50D. sphere from the trial set and hold it up in front of the +0.25D. before the first lens is removed. Now remove the +0.25D. sphere, leaving the +0.50D. in place. It is one of the conditions of this procedure that the eye continue to have stronger plus lenses added without an opportunity to use accommodation in the habitual manner. After the effect of the +0.50D. sphere has been observed and recorded, the power is increased to +0.75D. Finally after the lens power has been increased by quarter diopter intervals to +2.00D. or +2.50D. visual acuity should be so poor that the top letter is visible but it should hardly be legible.

This demonstration should not be too uncomfortable because accommodation is being relaxed, not stimulated, throughout the procedure. In the course of the discussion of acuity, texts on refraction make reference to depth of focus and how it is increased by small pupils. The experimenter should confirm this phenomenon. Keep the illumination on the chart as before but raise the general illumination of the room to normal and set a desk lamp about three feet away with the reflector turned so that the full effect of the lamp is toward the right eye. Comparison of the new finding should be made with the previous finding. The increased illumination will cause the pupil to contract and a smaller pupillary diameter reduces the size of the blur circles as the eye approaches the effect of a pinhole camera. The plus lenses should not blur vision so quickly. Begin at +0.25 as before and increase to the point where the 20/200 "E" at the top of the chart is blurred as much as before. It is possible that more lens power may be required. This experiment explains why some eyes see better in sunlight than indoors.

Concave spheres are used to show the effect of image size reduction, which is caused by accommodation and the fact that the trial lens is not held at the anterior focal distance of the eye. These tests and the ones to follow should all be made in the subdued lighting setup for the first experiment. Stronger minus lenses can be overcome than were used in the plus lens experiments, but the effect of the accommodative effort is sometimes unpleasant.

This series of experiments and observations is not complete without some inquiry into the effect of cylindrical lenses upon visual acuity. Only plus cylinders will be necessary. Begin with a +0.25D. cylinder and hold it at both axis 90 and 180. Vision should not be affected as much in either of these positions as it was with +0.25D. sphere. When the lens is rotated, however, the letters will be twisted and distorted and it is possible that the same lens may cause a more serious disturbance than the sphere of the same power. Although it will be unnecessary to go through the whole routine of the plus spheres, it is highly instructive to find out at what lens power vision is reduced to 20/200 with a cylinder at horizontal, vertical, and oblique positions.

These observations should be followed with an investigation of the effect of crossed-cylinders—that is, a lens combination in which the sphere and cylinder are of opposite signs and the power of the cylinder is precisely twice the power of the sphere, for example: −0.37 +0.75. The transposition of this lens is, of course, +0.37 −0.75. When this lens is diagrammed in the way the interval of Sturm is illustrated in texts on refraction, the two focal lines shown in Figure 119 are equal distances from the screen or retina. In other words, the circle of least confusion is at the retina; therefore, the clarity of the image is not improved by accommodation. In fact, when the eye accommodates by 0.37D., the line behind the retina is brought forward, but the one already in front of the retina is moved farther away.

Another way to consider this type of lens is to reduce it to its spherical equivalent—that is, the dioptric power at the circle of least confusion. The rule for this transformation is to add half of

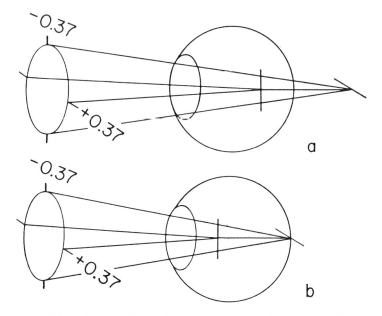

Figure 119.   Schematic focus: demonstration of Jackson cross cylinders.

the power of the cylinder to the power of the sphere $(+0.37 - 0.75/2 = 0)$. Since a cylinder has no power in the direction of its axis but has the full power at a right angle to the axis and between these two meridians has varying curves of more than zero and less than the marked power of the lens, one might say that the average power of any cylindrical lens is half its marked power. A proof of this might be given by placing two plus cylinders of equal power at right angles to one another and then neutralizing the lenses with a minus sphere of equal strength, or setting two equal power cylinders at right angles to one another in a lensometer and noting that the target acts as if a spherical lens were in place and that the combination measures as a sphere of the same strength. Thus it may be said that either of the cylinders is half of the effect of a sphere of the same marked power.

When the $+0.50$ cylinder has a -0.25 sphere placed against it (making the effect of crossed-cylinders) and the combination is held at either axis 90 or 180, visual acuity should not be greatly disturbed. Some letters may look slightly blurred in some meridians, but one should expect to see practically all of the letters seen without the lens in place. If there is a radical difference in acuity when the lens is changed from one axis to the other, the observer's own lens prescription is not likely the best one he could wear for distance acuity. When the lens combination is slowly rotated, all horizontal and vertical lines in the letters are slightly distorted and blurred. This is much the same effect as turning one's own astigmatic prescription lens off axis. It is instructive to try stronger crossed-cylinder effects and again relate them to distance acuity. It is surprising to note what strength of these combinations can be tolerated. In bright light when the pupil is contracted, fairly good acuity is maintained through even stronger lenses.

As a last experiment, take a minus cylinder that corresponds to the plus cylinder of one of the stronger combinations and hold it in the same positions of the crossed-cylinder. There should be a very similar effect. When the eye has accommodated to precisely half the strength of the cylinder, which it will automatically do in the effort for best vision, this will bring the circle of confusion to the retina and produce the visual effect of a crossed-cylinder. Again, as in the experiments with minus spheres, the image size is slightly reduced and overall visual acuity suffers somewhat.

There are also a few observations that should be made in the near-point field. It is important to have an appreciation of the effects of subnormal distance vision on reading ability as well as the effect of the several refractive errors on near vision. If the plus sphere, minus sphere, plus cylinder, crossed-cylinder effect, and minus cylinder that previously produced 20/100 vision are compared on the Jaeger card held at the normal reading distance, the effects of myopia, hyperopia, and combinations of astigmatism will be observed. As in all the tests above, it will be advantageous to keep a careful record of the effect of each lens.

One of the limitations of presbyopia should be demonstrated. In succession, use +1.00, +1.50, +2.00, +2.50, +3.00 before the eye. Have a yardstick or tape measure available for this demonstration. With the +1.00 before the eye, distance vision will have depreciated to 20/80 to 20/100 but the reading area will be clear and slightly magnified. Objects past the focal distance, that is, more than a meter away, show an "against" motion when the head is moved. Blurriness is not noticeable at your feet when you stand, but there is some fuzziness farther out on the floor. This is much the same effect of a presbyope's first reading glasses. As the stronger lenses are used, the Jaeger card should be held in normal reading position and slowly moved away from the eyes to the focal distance of the lens. For example, the +1.50D. sphere lens has a focal length of 67 cm (26 inches). Past that point acuity diminishes.

As the stronger lenses are used in succession, it will be noted that the shorter focal lengths bring the blurred area closer and closer to the eye until finally the +3.00D. sphere sets a spherical space of about 13 inches radius in front of the eye as the limit of clear vision. Reference to Table XII of presbyopic additions for 33 cm also shows another important development. Demonstration has now proved that objects are blurred at very short distances beyond the focal length of the reading addition. The table shows that the rapidly declining accommodative amplitude finally hampers the use of the eyes at distances beyond the reading distance. When the reading addition +2.00D. sphere is prescribed, the total ability is in the order of 1.00D. amplitude. That is, the limit of the patient's use of accommodation is to see clearly for a moment at a distance of 1 meter (40 inches). The test also implies that this limit of exertion cannot be sustained. It becomes self-evident that a weaker addition is also required for intermediate distances (60 to 80 cm) if the patient is to have clear vision at all points. Thus the decline in accommodative function makes trifocal lenses a necessity when the reading addition becomes +2.00D. or more, if the wearer wishes to continue to see clearly at all distances with one pair of lenses. Until the advent of recent improvements in trifocal lens design, the blurred intermediate field was considered part of the "presbyope's burden" and nothing much could be done about it. At the present time, there is little excuse for any person to be deprived of satisfactory "arm's length" vision at the same time his distance and reading vision are corrected. New progressive power lenses such as Varilux II or Ultravue Younger 10/30 present a gradual power change that supercedes the two distinct additions of trifocals.

In all these experiments in which there has been an attempt to simulate refractive errors and their correcting lenses, there exists the disadvantages of artificially produced conditions. In all instances, the observations were made monocularly to relieve the complications of the involvement of convergence. When the plus lenses were used, it might have been better to be able to continue to hold fixation at infinity rather than to use accommodation intermittently to choose new lenses or make the record, but these observations are intended to give only the general effects and are not scientific research. If, in the end, there is a better understanding of what lenses do and what defenses or compensations are made by the eyes in an attempt to offset the effect of refractive errors, much has been gained.

OPTOMETERS

The first instrument by which the refractive error could be subjectively measured had its principle in Scheiner's double aperture disc (1619).* W. Porterfield named his device (1637) *optometer*. It had two narrow slits instead of round apertures. In 1696, De La Hire used trial lenses in conjunction with Scheiner's disc to measure the refractive error. Thomas Young made an optometer using slits; it is in the Museum of the Royal Institution, London. Badal (1840-1929) designed an optometer using a target at the focus of a lens usually +10.00. It became very popular with peripatetic opticians in the second half of the nineteenth century.

The optometers of the following era were represented by objective instruments such as Gullstrand's Parallax Refractionometer, the Finchham Coincidence Optometer, and Rodenstock Refractionometer. After a pause of about fifty years, a third era emerged with electronic instruments based upon lasers and computers made by Bausch & Lomb, Rochester, New York; Coherent Radiations, Inc., Palo Alto, California; and Acuity Systems, Inc., Reston, Virginia. A short subjective test based upon the instrument findings produces a satisfactory refraction in a very few

*Levene, J.R.: *Clinical Refraction & Visual Science.* London, Butterworth, 1977.

minutes. Thus the progress of almost 360 years from Scheiner's disc has been traced.

IDEAL EYE

The ophthalmic lens prescription is the patient's card of introduction to the dispensing optician. Under the ℞ sign there may be no more than three numbers for each eye to describe sphere, cylinder, and axis, but even this brief message can tell a definite story about the patient's eye problem. With the added information of the patient's apparent age, and the character of his activities both vocational and avocational, an optician should have some appreciation of the patient's probable inconvenience or discomfort without the prescribed lenses, as well as the intended use of them. With this impression he should be ready to discuss with the patient the various glasses suitable for his purposes.

It is necessary to have some superficial knowledge of physiological optics and refractive errors in order to make such deductions. In this chapter, some parts of these subjects as they apply to prescription reading will be discussed. This sketchy treatment of the extensive and profound subject of the practice of refraction is not to be construed as more than reference to some of the rudiments.

It is hoped that the reader's curiosity about this phase of the subject will lead him into the enjoyment of other texts.* The subject of children's eyes as an extensive research project at the Clinic of Child Development at Yale University by a group headed by Gesell has been reported.

First, let us discuss the growth and decline of a pair of "ideal"†

---

*Cowan, A.: *Refraction of the Eye.* Philadelphia, Lea & Febiger, 1945.

Berens, C. and Zuckerman, J.: *Diagnostic Examination of the Eye.* Philadelphia, Lippincott, 1946, pp. 293-320; 347-357.

Emsley, H.H.: *Visual Optics.* London, Hatton Pr, 1948.

Borish, M.: *Clinical Refraction.* Chicago, Prof Press, 1949.

†Gesell. A., Ilg, F., and Bullis, G.E.: *Vision: Its Development in Infant and Child.* New York, Paul B. Hoeber, Inc., 1949.

Parsons, J.H. and Duke-Elder, Sir W.S.: *Diseases of the Eye.* New York, Macmillan, 1948, p. 523.

Duke-Elder, Sir W.S.: *The Practice of Refraction.* St. Louis, Mosby, 1949, pp. 67-68.

eyes. With some information about the *norms,* comparisons of the pathologic or other conditions that are relieved by spectacles can be better understood.

Normal eyes in a newborn child are somewhat smaller than their size at maturity. The curves of the crystalline lens, as well as its position in the eye, change with growth. For these reasons the far points of the baby's eyes (see Chap. 5) are behind the retina. The eyes are hyperopic and will require +2.00D. to +3.00D. spherical lenses to see clearly at distance without accommodative (focussing) effort. This refractive error slowly reduces until the child is about 10 to 12 years of age. At that time his "ideal" pair of eyes will no longer accept convex lenses for distant vision. The far points of his eyes will have approached infinity and he will for all practical purposes have emmetropia. That is, his eyes will need no lenses for best vision without accommodative effort. This condition, with slight variation, maintains for distant vision until very late in life when the eyes may again become somewhat hyperopic.

In childhood, the accommodative mechanism is very active. From Figure 120 it is seen that at eight years of age about 14.00 diopters of accommodation are available. This means that the child has the ability to focus his eyes so that he can see clearly up to a point as close as 70 mm (the focal length of 14.00D.) from his eyes. A further study of the chart shows that accommodation slowly deteriorates through the years. At about age 44, for this "ideal" case, there is a more rapid loss of this function for a few years until about the age of 52, when the rate reduces and becomes a gradual decline for the remainder of life. In the later years, the total power is about 1.00D.—that is, with maximum effort, the closest distance at which objects can be clearly focussed is one meter. Loss of accommodation is seldom noticed by a person whose eyes are nearly emmetropic until he is 40 to 50 years of age.

Reinecke, R. and Hern, R.: *Refraction: A programmed Text,* 2nd. ed. New York, Appleton-Century-Croft, 1976.

Tait, E.F.: *Textbook of Refraction.* Philadelphia, Saunders, 1951.

Michaels, D.D.: *Visual Optics and Refraction.* St. Louis, Mosby, 1975.

Thorington, Jas.: *Refraction of the Human Eye.* Philadelphia, Blackiston Co., 1947.

This condition, called presbyopia, is the first occasion when a normal (probably better named, "ideal") pair of eyes will need the assistance of a pair of spectacle lenses to provide clear vision at near.

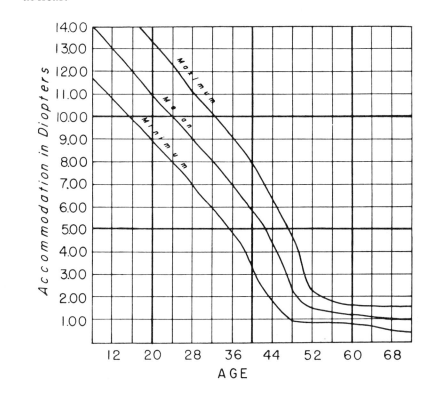

Figure 120. Duane accommodative amplitude chart.

The measurement of accommodative amplitude is made by slowly moving some small test type toward the patient's eyes to the point where vision is blurred. This determines the maximum accomplishment for a moment. The eyes would not be expected to be able to continue to see at this extreme near point very long. Experience has proved, however, that a pair of eyes can continue to use one-half to two-thirds of the total amplitude over long periods of time. If this formula is applied to the mean line in the chart for a person who wishes to use his eyes at 33 cm (13 inches) and therefore have 3.00D. of his accommodation in use, he reaches the limit (threshold of discomfort) at 40 to 45 years of age. That is, if a reserve of half of his accommodation is to be maintained, his difficulties do not start until he passes age 40, when the amplitude is 6.00D., or twice the amount required. If a reserve of only one-third is considered adequate, then the limiting age is age 44, when the total accommodation is 4.50D. (4.50 $\times$ $\frac{2}{3}$ = 3.00D.). Table XII, calculated from Doctor Duane's chart, shows the additional spherical lens power required to provide sustained comfortable vision at 33 cm when only one-half of the measurable ability is in use and the other half is a reserve to account for fatigue. The second calculation is figured with two-thirds of the amplitude in use and only one-third as a reserve for fatigue.

TABLE XII
PRESBYOPIC ADDITION REQUIRED

Age	Accommo- dative Amplitude	Near- Point*	Fixation at 40 cm 2.50D.		Fixation at 33 cm 3.00D.	
			50% Reserve	33% Reserve	50% Reserve	33% Reserve
40	6.00D.	17 cm	Threshold	Adequate	Adequate	Adequate
44	4.25D.	24 cm	+0.87	Threshold	+0.37	Adequate
48	2.50D.	40 cm	+1.75	+1.37	+1.25	+0.87
52	1.50D.	67 cm	+2.25	+2.00	+1.75	+1.50
56	1.25D.	80 cm	+2.37	+2.12	+1.87	+1.62
60	1.12D.	89 cm	+2.37	+2.12	+1.87	+1.62
64	1.12D.	89 cm	+2.37	+2.12	+1.87	+1.62
68	1.00D.	100 cm	+2.50	+2.37	+2.00	+1.87
72	1.00D.	100 cm	+2.50	+2.37	+2.00	+1.87

*From median line of Duane accommodative amplitude chart.

Nothing, however, could be more unsatisfactory than reading glasses fitted by rule. Different from distance glasses in which eyes are fitted to have accommodation completely relaxed at one distance, that is, for infinite distance (20 feet), the lenses for near point use must be individually considered. When the Duane chart is studied again, one notes that the age range for 6.00D. amplitude, for example, is 32 years for minimum to 45 years for maximum. Some individuals lose this ability to focus the eyes for near much younger and more rapidly than others. Another consideration is when the individual's eyes are incapable of normal vision at distance. The fixation distance also varies within wide limits for different individuals. The near-point fixation distance for a baby after congenital cataract surgery is not more than 20 cm because of his short arms. The reading position of a six-foot adult may be 40 to 45 cm. Then, too, because the near-point glasses may be intended to include other purposes than reading, the strength of the plus lens addition may be made weaker to accommodate the distance from eye to ironing board, kitchen sink, workbench, or desk top. For a fixation as close as 33 cm the first prescription of +1.00D. spheres is written at some time between the ages of 40 and 45 and increased from time to time until the addition finally becomes +2.50 to +2.75D. sphere when the minimum of 0.50D. accommodation is available at age 72.

Even with these slight variations for presbyopic prescriptions, the so-called "ideal" eyes have very simple requirements throughout a whole lifetime. No glasses at all until some time past 40 years of age, then a gradual increase through the years to a limit of +2.50D. to +3.00D. spheres. All in all, three to five changes in reading glasses (or bifocals with plano distance) suffice. The vast majority of all eyes, however, do not present these ideal findings. Long before the complications of presbyopia, large numbers of eyes will have had difficulty. The premise for the "ideal" case has been emmetropia for distance. According to DeSchweinitz, "Emmetropia is comparatively uncommon, occurring in not more than 1.5 to 2 percent of properly examined eyes."

Despite refractive errors, the accommodative amplitude in nonpathologic eyes closely follows the Duane chart except in rare instances. Therefore when refractive errors are discussed it is necessary to keep in mind the fact that the error is superimposed upon the available accommodation.

In much the same seven age groupings that Shakespeare gave us in Jacques' speech in *As You Like It* (Act II, Scene 7), we shall now consider man's need for spectacles. The earliest prescription that is likely to be presented to an ophthalmic dispenser is the correction of bilateral congenital cataracts after surgery. These lenses are in the order of +10.00D. to +15.00D. spheres and may be fitted before the baby's first birthday. The power of these

lenses may not be changed for several years, but it will be necessary to replace the eyewear from time to time as the child outgrows
the frame and lens size. The doctor will have impressed upon
the parent the importance of these lenses. It is well, however, to
repeat his orders that the baby wear the glasses regularly. The
eyes fail to develop best vision if lenses are not worn to provide
the eyes with clear retinal images.

A reasonably rare disease of babyhood is *buphthalmos* in which
the drainage of the eyes is defective and the eyes become enlarged
from internal pressure. Unless surgical relief is obtained very
early, this condition produces seriously reduced vision or blindness. The distension of the globe produces myopia.

After two years of age, the most common prescription is for the
correction of eyes with strabismus (crossed-eyes) and is ordinarily
for +4.00D. to +8.00D. spherical lenses. Occasionally a dispenser has a dramatic experience when he puts a pair of convex
lenses before the eyes of a child and sees a pair of badly turned
eyes straighten out completely and smile at him!

In most cases, however, the doctor prescribes convex lenses to
correct the hyperopia and reduce the stress on accommodation.
As in the congenital cataract case, it is important to present sharply focussed images on the retinas. It was previously stated that the
macula is not developed at birth* and that it does not fully
mature for several years. A condition called *amblyopia exanopsia*
develops rapidly in young eyes when, because of blurred images or
lack of fixation, the macular areas are not used. Vision deteriorates to 20/200 or worse in a short time and if it does not have
prompt attention, normal vision is seldom regained with or without glasses. Therefore, though the glasses may not cure the
squint, they are serving an important service to the eyes until
such time as surgery and/or orthoptics bring the eyes into alignment.

Another variation from the normal is the child with hereditary
or racial myopia (nearsightedness). Usually at least one parent
has moderate to high myopia and therefore is sympathetic with
the child's problem. In the lower degrees, there may have been

---

*Duke-Elder, Sir W.S.: *Text-Book of Ophthalmology*, Vol. I. St. Louis, Mosby, 1934, pp. 332-334.

no symptoms and the child may have been taken to the doctor only because of the prevalence of myopia in the family and the parents wish to do everything possible to prevent a high error. Most of these cases that require lenses when the child is very young progress through childhood during the time when the eyes of the "ideal" case are becoming less hyperopic. Knowing this, the doctor uses every known device to thwart the progressive tendency. Separate prescriptions for distance and near and, in some instances, bifocals are ordered for these children to check the course of the condition.

Visual acuity tests which are repeated several times before and through a child's school life screen out those with subnormal vision and these are the doctors' patients seen between the ages of six and twelve. A test of acuity on a standard Snellen card placed at twenty feet detects those children who are myopic or highly astigmatic. It also calls attention to those who have poor vision in one eye only. The amplitude of accommodation in children of these ages occasionally covers up even rather high degrees of hypermetropia. Hence, children needing plus lenses, and they are in the majority as previously noted, usually have their eyes examined after symptoms of asthenopia (fatigue, discomfort). The child's pediatrician or parents ordinarily decide that difficulty with studies or other signs are symptoms of ocular conditions. The prescriptions for this group of patients vary from small astigmatic corrections to spherical corrections of two or three diopters with cylinders.

The prescriptions for early adolescents who have not previously worn glasses tend to be weaker plus lenses and in some cases weak minus lenses. The great majority of them have corrections for varying degrees of astigmatism. Prescriptions of this type continue to be written as first glasses for adults up to the beginning of presbyopia. For a large part, these prescriptions are not written for persons with a complaint of poor vision. As a matter of fact, despite small degrees of astigmatism, some of these patients seem to see as well without the lenses as they do with them. Usually the symptoms are from discomforts related to prolonged visual efforts in the near-point field. Reference to the accommodative amplitude chart discourages the thought that the extra accommodative effort required to correct the refractive error should be the cause of discomfort. The majority of these prescriptions is less than 1.50D. and this amount of error represents a small percentage of the available accommodation for individuals in this age group. In any event, these adults are using less than 50 percent of their available accommodative amplitude and do not fall in the category of those who have similar symptoms from presbyopia. Practically all of these individuals are having discomfort or fatigue after reading or doing other close work in which the act of converging the eyes is involved. Donders (1864)* and Percival (1891) † made some investigations that lead to the explanation of the difficulties of these patients. That part of his work which is of interest to a ophthalmic dispenser is concerned with what Percival calls the "area of comfort."

The functions of accommodation and convergence are closely interrelated. For example, if the eyes are focussed on an object at 40 cm, the two visual axes are directed to the same point. When this physiologic act is reduced to ophthalmic units, it is described as +2.50D. accommodation in use and if the separation of the centers of rotation of the patient is 60 mm, there are 15 Prism Diopters of convergence in use.

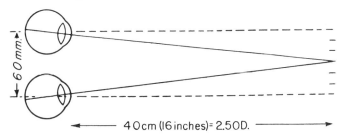

Figure 121. Accommodation and prism convergence in use.

The rule by which this conversion is made is

Accommodation $\times$ Distance I.O.D. in cm $=$ Prism Diopters of convergence

*Donders, F.C.: *Accommodation and Refraction of the Eye*. London, New Sydenham Society, 1864, pp. 110-115.

†Percival, A.S.: *The Prescribing of Spectacles*. New York, William Wood and Company, 1910, pp. 97-108.

Thus it is seen that when the separation of the centers of rotation (I.O.D.) is an average distance of 60 mm, it could be said that the relationship of convergence to accommodation is 6 to 1 (15 : 2.5 :: 6 : 1).‡ Further investigation shows, however, that this association between the functions is not fixed. In fact, it is normally quite elastic and either accommodation or convergence can be exercised or suppressed to a sufficient extent to alter the above ratio materially.* Lenses with progressive addition such as Varilux II, Ultravue and Younger 10/30 solve these problems of considerably reduced accommodative amplitude, because the gradual increase in the power of the addition provides the proper lens power for each distance inside infinity. They are thus superior to any limited number of specific additions. The looseness of the association between accommodation and convergence can be readily demonstrated. For example, if +0.50D. spheres are held before the eyes while fixation is held at 40 cm, some accommodation is replaced by the plus lenses (2.50D. − 0.50D. = 2.00D.), but convergence is not changed because the z-axes are still directed to the same fixation point. The ratio is changed to 15 : 2 :: 7.5 : 1. In the same manner, if when −0.50D. spheres are held before both eyes the eyes can make the extra effort still to see clearly at 40 cm, the ratio is changed in the opposite direction. It regularly takes 2:50D. accommodation to see clearly at 40 cm, but when −0.50D. must be overcome, 3.00D. accommodation is active while the eyes are still converged the same amount. Therefore, 15 : 3.00 :: 5 : 1.

The relationship can also be investigated by altering the amount of convergence in use. We have seen that if prisms are placed before the eyes, light is deviated and the eyes must overcome the effect of the prism to continue to fix at the same point. If 3^Δ Base Out is placed before the eyes the eyes must converge a

---

‡Sheard, Chas.: *The Sheard Volume.* Philadelphia, Chilton, 1957. ,
*Southall, J.P.C.: *Introduction to Physiological Optics.* London, Oxford U Pr, 1937, pp. 214-221.
Dvorine, L.: *Analytical Refraction and Orthoptics.* Baltimore (published by the author), 1948, pp. 55-62.
Jaques, L.: *Fundamental Refraction and Orthoptics.* Los Angeles (published by the author), 1936, pp. 100-113.
Gibson, H.W.: *Clinical Orthoptics.* London, Hatton Pr, 1947, pp. 22-29.

greater amount. If the accommodation changed in precise ratio with convergence, the eyes would be focussed at this closer point. In practice, the eyes can be forced to converge slightly more or less than normal while accommodation is not altered. Thus if 3^Δ Base Out can be overcome and the eyes still see clearly and singly, the ratio is

$$15^\Delta + 3^\Delta = 18^\Delta \qquad 18 : 2.50 :: 7.2 : 1.$$

On the other hand, if 2^Δ Base In is placed before the eyes, part of the convergence effort is replaced by prism. In these circumstances, since accommodation cannot be reduced if clear vision is maintained, the ratio is changed oppositely. Now accommodation is stimulated more and convergence less than the habitual amounts.

$$15^\Delta - 2^\Delta = 13^\Delta \qquad 13 : 2.5 :: 5.2 : 1$$

A classical instance of derangement of the accommodative-convergence relationship came to my attention at Folsom Prison, California, in 1926. An inmate who had been excused from the customary work activities was spending practically all of his waking hours reading in the bunk in his cell. The very low light level had caused him to become convinced that he needed reading glasses although he was only about thirty years old. Not being able to have an eye examination promptly by the visiting ophthalmologist, he chose a pair of $+1.00$D. spheres from some ready-made glasses in the infirmary. Subsequently over a period of time he exchanged the glasses for stronger lenses until by the time the doctor saw him he was using $+4.00$D. spheres to read. This meant that he was reading at 25 cm (10 inches). This act required about 25 of convergence and *no accommodation at all!* An eye examination revealed that he needed no ℞ for distance. Doctor's prescription was that he reverse his self-imposed "orthoptics" and start on the long road back to normal function by gradually reducing the power of his reading glasses while he continued to read in good light, preferably out of doors. Thus he would gradually increase the amount of accommodation in use and also reduce the amount of convergence by slowly increasing his reading distance.

Ordinarily, derangement of the relationship of the functions is limited. The amount by which the functions can be dissociated varies widely between different individuals. It reflects fatigue and, therefore, varies with the same individual on different occasions. The effort to overcome an imbalance to the normal ratio, such as may be necessary when either greater or lesser amounts of accommodation or convergence are required, may be the cause of asthenopia and severe ocular symptoms with some persons. Measurements suggested by Percival reveal the amounts by which these functions can be dissociated in a particular instance and suggest to the doctor the effect of the correcting lenses.

The amount by which accommodation can be stimulated or inhibited without affecting convergence is termed *Relative Accommodation;* and conversely, the amount by which convergence can be increased or decreased while accommodation remains fixed is called *Relative Convergence.* The criterion by which this test is made is blurred vision.

If a pair of eyes is fixed on small type at 40 cm and increasingly stronger minus lenses are added before both eyes, accommodation is stimulated. When the type blurs, it is evident that accommodation can no longer be stimulated without affecting convergence. This is the measurement of *Positive Relative Accommodation.* When plus lenses are used to replace or inhibit accommodation, the limiting lens value is called the amount of *Negative Relative Accommodation.* Figure 122 is a diagrammatic construction of the test.

When prism Base Out is placed before the eyes, convergence is stimulated and the eyes turn farther in. This can be tolerated to a certain limit, but finally accommodation is likewise stimulated and the reading type blurs. The amount of prism tolerated is referred to as the amount of *Positive Relative Convergence* available for the test. The effect of the prisms is shown in Figure 123. Again, when this test is reversed and prism Base In is introduced, it does the work of convergence. When the eyes have turned toward parallel to that point where the limit of dissociation inhibits accommodation and the type becomes blurred, the test for *Negative Relative Convergence* is completed.

Figure 124 from Percival's text is a graph that diagrams the relationship of the functions in the excellent range of convergence for Campbell. The amount of accommodation active in these

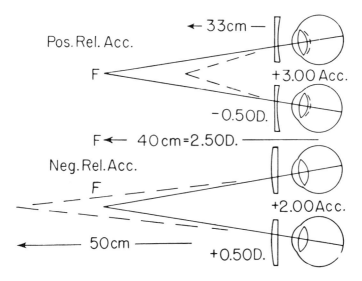

Figure 122.   Positive and Negative Relative Accommodation.

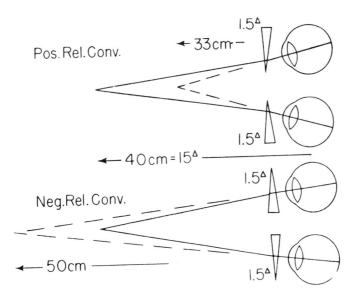

Figure 123.   Positive and Negative Relative Convergence.

near-point tests is shown at the left and convergence is shown in
Meter Angles which are converted into Prism Diopters for an
interocular distance of 60 mm. The dotted line in the shaded
area shows the normal association of 6 Prism Diopters of convergence for each diopter of accommodation. At several fixation
distances, prisms Base Out were used to measure the total Positive
Relative Covergence and prism Base In was introducted to measure the Negative Reserve. The dotted line shows the results of
these measurements. When the convergence required for binocular function is subtracted from the total measurement, the Relative Convergence is found. For example, at 3.00D. accommoda-
tion the Positive Reserve is $48^\triangle - 18^\triangle = 30^\triangle$. On the other side,
convergence could be inhibited until there was no convergence
while accommodation could still be maintained active. Therefore, the Negative Relative Convergence for this accommodative
distance was $18^\triangle$.

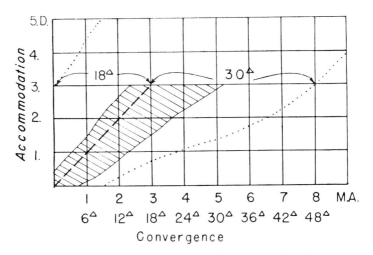

Figure 124. Percival's (after Donders) zone of comfort.

Percival found that if no more than the middle one third of the
measureable reserve was in constant use, the patient would have
comfort. In this case, the patient had a range of $16^\triangle$ ($30 + 18 =$
$48^\triangle \times \frac{1}{3} = 16^\triangle$) which he named the "area of comfort." The
shaded zone on the graph describes this area. It will be noted

that the diagonal line is enclosed within the shaded area—that is, some reserve or tolerance is available to compensate for the effects of fatigue of either accommodation or convergence.

Figure 125 diagrammatically describes another of his patients. This man, aged 29, with accommodative amplitude of 7.00D., showed a manifest refractive error of +0.50 but use of his eyes for reading caused symptoms. When +1.00 spheres were added to his distance prescription the patient was comfortable.

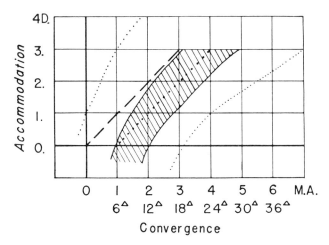

Figure 125. Unbalanced zone of comfort.

Referring to the graph, the normal relationship of binocular vision shown by the broken line is outside of the "area of comfort" at all points. The patient has a large positive reserve but Negative Relative Convergence is inadequate. When less accommodation is required after the +1.00D. lenses have been added, the heavy dotted line which shows the new relationship between accommodation and convergence now bisects the shaded area. Percival remarks that the patient was completely satisfied with the correction.

For an ancillary worker, Percival's diagrammatic presentation based upon Donders' original findings is undoubtedly the finest presentation conceived. Become familiar with it, review your personal experiments with Base Out and Base In prisms. If you have access to a refracting instrument, repeat the experiments using a Risley prism. Learn about the accommodative-convergence reflex. It is the essence of most of the near point problems of the doctors' patients for whom you work.

In many cases, all the relative measurements are much lower than those in the illustrations. Obviously the balancing of functions is more sensitive in such instances and smaller refractive errors give distress and so-called "eyestrain." It is among these last described cases that many individuals who can demonstrate good distant vision without glasses find great relief in prescriptions of less than 1.00D. sphere. These patients with functional imbalances seldom have symptoms with casual use of the eyes. Difficulties arise only after protracted effort. A classic example of these conditions was the case of the workers in war plants. A great number of housewives and others who were not accustomed to the demands of sustained critical vision quickly got out the glasses they had worn in school days to operate drill presses or to work for hours at a time with their eyes intently focussed upon some small object at some fixed distance. The power of the lenses was often reasonably small, but it was the required amount to balance up the "area of comfort," so they could proceed with their daily work. With the war finished and their return to domestic lives or to work that required less precise vision, many of these individuals put their glasses aside.

At the other extreme, when the functions of accommodation and convergence are closely associated and the tolerances of the "area of comfort" are small, one finds extremely sensitive persons for whom prescriptions of less than 1.00D. are the difference between comfort and distress that approaches the severity of migraine. An unusual sensitivity to pupillary distance or cylinder axis that seems all out of proportion to the dioptric effect of the lenses is frequently seen in these cases. Experiment will often prove, however, that the patient's reaction is quite real and in no way a psychoneurosis. Frequently these rather insignificant prescriptions (from the aspect of lens power) have extended the professional skill of the doctor. These patients who are oftentimes on the brink of nervous exhaustion deserve the utmost care and consideration from an ophthalmic dispenser.

Later in adult life and before the onset of presbyopia, there is another group of hyperopes of 1.00D. to 2.00D. spherical equivalent who begin to have symptoms at the theatre and blurred vision after a short time at reading. Among these individuals, who are usually healthy and robust, accommodative amplitude is lessening to a point that visual fatigue sets in quickly when the eyes are taxed with the necessity of accurate vision. Some of this group are persons who are proud of their ability to do without glasses. Even the reference to dependence upon glasses is unpleasant or even obnoxious to some of them. This attitude is found among both men and women and an ophthalmic dispenser can easily create a difficult situation with tactlessness. Any reference to lack of acuity without the lenses or remark about the delay in coming to an important prescription is completely out of place. For these persons the prescriptions often read "Rest glasses" or "For near only."

Finally at some point between 40 and 50 years of age, the scene shifts to what Shakespeare calls the sixth age "With spectacles on nose and pouch on side" and presbyopia enters. Different lens powers will then be necessary for distance and near vision. Hyperopic patients usually are the first to require extra plus power for near. Myopes of low degree who do not regularly wear their glasses and therefore willingly tolerate slightly blurred vision, and who have learned the tricks that assist a person with lowered acuity, will often approach age 50 before they feel the necessity for a prescription for reading. If the distance correction approximates—1.00D. spherical equivalent, the first reading lens total is near plano. Experience teaches a dispenser to be very cautious with these people. Distaste for glasses may be expressed in complaints about the weight, size, or shape of the eyewear. Surface reflections can be a problem. It is wise to not order any part of the eyewear that has not been demonstrated to the wearer. A bifocal demonstration lens is a "must." Tact and patience are indispensable. These individuals must have a real need, usually vocational, for clear vision at *both* distance and near to be successful with bifocals at this time. These persons often seem to have a difficult time to forget consciously and unconsciously that they can do quite well without any glasses at all for reading.

Later, when the addition has increased, the acceptance of bifocals is much improved.

Aside from some specialized vocations, there are three distances at which all persons need discriminating vision. Because the act of accommodation is suspended at or beyond the hyperfocal distance of 20 feet (6 meters), distance vision has been used as the base for the measurement and discussion of vision. From the standpoint of physiological optics, this approach is quite justifiable. Aviators, railroad engineers, motion-picture projectionists, and others must have keen vision for great distance. Automobile drivers must demonstrate 20/40 to 20/50 vision in most states. In ordinary living, however, rather reduced visual acuity at distance is tolerated by a great number of persons. There are others to whom very clear vision at distance is a psychological necessity, aside from possible economic or social requirements.

There are two other distances that are easily as important. The first is called *reading distance,* that is, an average of 40 cm (16 inches). The precise distance varies with the individual. A person near five feet tall may read, write, or do other manual acts at 33 cm (13 inches), while a person over six feet tall may be more comfortable with his eyes 17 or 18 inches away from near point subject matter. Sometimes the habitual distance may be established somewhat closer to the eyes because of the habit formed with an uncorrected myopia.

The second distance, called *intermediate distance,* may also be referred to as arm's-length distance. It is that distance across a desk-top, to music on a piano or stand, to the dummy hand in bridge, to an ironing board or sink, to one's reflection in a mirror, to the instrument board in an automobile, or to the dishes surrounding one's plate at dinner. For these and many other activities, highly discriminating vision is required at this middle distance of 26 to 32 inches where 1.25D. to 1.50D. accommodation is required. Until quite recently there has not been any good solution to the problem. Such lenses as were available had shortcomings that discouraged their wide acceptance.

If this intermediate distance is assumed at 67 cm (26 inches), the presbyopic patient can no longer see objects clearly at that distance through the reading prescription when his addition exceeds +1.50D., the lens that focusses at that distance. Further reference to Duane's accommodation amplitude chart, and the compilation of Table XIII for this intermediate distance, emphasizes several very important considerations.

TABLE XIII
PRESBYOPIC ADDITIONS FOR INTERMEDIATE AND READING
DISTANCES WHEN 50% OF AMPLITUDE IS HELD IN RESERVE
AT BOTH DISTANCES

Age	Total Accommodative Amplitude	Reading Distance 33 cm = 3:00D. Accommodation in Use	Reading Addition	Intermediate 67 cm = 1.50D. Intermediate Addition
50	2.00D.	1.00D.	+2.00D.	+0.50D.
52	1.50D.	0.75D.	+2.25D.	+0.75D.
56	1.25D.	0.62D.	+2.37D.	+0.87D.
60	1.12D.	0.62D.	+2.37D.	+0.87D.
64	1.12D.	0.62D.	+2.37D.	+0.87D.
68	1.00D.	0.50D.	+2.50D.	+1.00D.

To allow one-half of the available accommodation to remain in reserve, at age 50 when the total amplitude is 2.00, use of one-half of the function would require the assistance of +0.50D. sphere to see clearly at a distance of two-thirds of a meter. There is a slight fallacy to this reasoning. The patient is making just as much accommodative effort to see at this distance as he is for reading distance because 50 percent of the available amplitude is used in each case. However, the patient does not converge his eyes as much for the intermediate distance and, therefore, it is a change of habit or accommodation—convergence (A.C.A.) ratio to converge a different amount along with the same accommodative effort. This can be corrected by a slight increase in the addition at the intermediate distance and thereby partially relieve the function of accommodation while convergence is also reduced. A fuller discussion of this phase of fitting will be made in Chapter 11 when trifocal lenses are examined.

For the moment it is important to realize the presbyope's dilemma at middle distance. Some time shortly after age 50, his momentary near-point (the limit of his accommodative power) will have receded to 67 cm and the focal length of the addition of his bifocal addition, +2.00D., is only 50 cm; therefore the area between 50 and 67 cm is blurred. As the days go by, this area of indistinct vision increases. The focal length of the addition grows shorter and the patient's near point recedes until, at age 68, all objects between 16 and 40 inches are out of focus unless additional lens power is made available for intermediate distance vision. Nature's redeeming compensation is that in those instances where the media are clear (not cataractous), the reduced size of the pupils in advanced life becomes useful. The admittance of only the central rays of light lengthens the depth of focus of the eyes (see Fig. 246), and when adequate light is available, the blurred area described above is somewhat reduced.

With the passing of time, improvements in ophthalmic surgery have greatly ameliorated conditions for those who reach the last stage, so it is no longer, as Jaques' lines read, "sans eyes, sans teeth, sans everything." Cataract surgery has prolonged useful vision for the vast majority of all sufferers of this disease of senility. In that period of time (and frequently it is prolonged) while the patient waits for the proper development of conditions for cataract surgery to be undertaken, the doctor may make several changes to the lens prescription. On some occasions, the doctor may not have told his patient the precise cause of his failing vision for any of several good reasons. It is, therefore, incumbent upon a dispenser never to speculate or as much as refer to any eye disease in such a way that the patient can imagine that what has been said is a diagnosis.

Spectacle lens prescriptions at this time are usually disappointing to the patient. Despite the fact that the doctor will have told the patient that the change may not show any marked improvement in vision, he usually forgets what has been said by his doctor and hopes for greatly increased acuity. In some of these pathological cases there are alternating days or periods when vision improves or recedes. If the refraction was made on the "good" day and the glasses are delivered on a "bad" day, everyone is in for difficulty. This same "uphill, downhill" course frequently affects the patient's feelings about opticians and especially doctor's assistants. If an optician services a pair of glasses on a "good" day, his reputation is often made and will last through several "bad" days. On the other hand, if after the most painstaking care on a "bad" day no improvement in vision is accomplished, the patient is frequently not much impressed. This is a moment for much diplomacy on the part of the dispenser. Unending patience and sympathy are essential.

During the maturation of cataracts, the crystalline lenses sometimes swell and reduce the hypermetropic prescription for distance or increase the minus lens prescription in myopia. Accommodation is almost nil in these cases and, because of the dimness of vision, the doctor may increase the addition to as much as +4.00D., so that the reading distance is less than regular and the closeness provides larger retinal images. Even with these optical devices, vision is often very unsatisfactory and repeated assurances should be given the patient that the doctor is to be relied upon to do everything possible for his eyes. The location of the opacity varies greatly in the many different types of cataract. If the opacity is nuclear, that is, in the center of the pupil, the patient may see better in reduced illumination where his pupil size is larger and light can get in around the dense area in the lens. In other cases the center of the lens is clearer and the patient sees best in very bright light. There is only one way for an optician to find out what type of light serves the patient best; ask him, then try to find the kind of light in which his eyes perform the best. Some of these cases are helped by a typoscope, designed by C.F. Prentice.* The device is a rectangle of dull black material in which a slot about 8 mm high and 15 cm long is cut. When this is laid on a white page, only two or three lines of type are visible. The benefit of the device is derived from the reduction of scattered or dazzling light on the retinal area that surrounds the point of fixation.

REVIEW

1. What does the notation 20/50 vision mean?
2. What is the power of the + sphere (− sphere; + cyl × 90; + cyl × 180; and cross cyl.) that reduces your vision to 20/50?

---

*Prentice, C.F.: *Ophthalmic Lenses.* Philadelphia, Keystone Press, 1900.

Stimson, R.L.: *Optical Aids for Low Acuity.* Los Angeles, Braille Institute of America, 1957, p. 18.

3. What is a cross-cylinder? Where is the circle of least confusion?

4. To read comfortably at 40 cm, how many diopters of accommodative amplitude should be available? Why?

5. Make a list of common types of lens prescriptions at different ages.

6. Define "Positive Relative Accommodation," "Negative Relative Accommodation," "Positive Relative Convergence," and "Negative Relative Convergence."

7. Explain why Percival's "area of comfort" indicates satisfactory vision with the prescribed lenses.

8. When a person needs and is wearing + 2.25 addition for reading, at what distances between infinity and his nearest point of clear vision does he (she) have blurred vision when bifocals are worn? Make a diagram.

9. Why may an individual's prescription for plus lenses slowly change to minus lenses?

ADDITIONAL REFERENCES

1. Southall, J.P.C.: *Introduction to Physiological Optics.* London, Oxford, 1937.
2. Emsley, H.H.: *Visual Optics.* London, Hatton, 1948.
3. Borish, M.: *Clinical Refraction.* Chicago, Professional Press, 1970.
4. Duke-Elder, Sir W.S.: *The Practice of Refraction.* St. Louis, Mosby, 1949.
5. Donders, F.C.: *Accommodation and Refraction of the Eye.* London, Sydenham, 1864.
6. Percival, A.S.: *The Prescribing of Spectacles.* New York, Wood, 1910.
7. Sheard, C.: *The Sheard Volume.* Philadelphia, Chilton, 1957.

Chapter 9

EYEWEAR DISPENSING

◆◆◆

EYEWEAR MATERIALS

Since the brief reference to eyeframes in Chapter 7, no further mention has been made. Now that a discussion of dispensing of eyewear is being made, it is appropriate that the materials from which eyeframes are currently made should be discussed.

As optical museums confirm, in ancient times eyeframes have been made of wood, leather, tortoise shell, iron, steel, nickel alloy, aluminum alloy, silver alloy, gold, gold alloy, gold-filled, gold plate, cellulose nitrate, cellulose acetate, Lucite®, nylon, and Optyl®. At the beginning of this century, solid gold in 10K and 14K were the finest quality metal frames. Higher karat such as 18K would have had too little alloy to make the metal sufficiently hard and elastic for eyeframes. With the world price of gold varying from about $100 to about $200 per ounce in recent years, the price of solid gold frames would be priced in the area of fine jewelry. No metal frame maker is producing or cataloging solid gold today.

For many years, most of the ophthalmic metal frames were gold-filled, 1/10 12 K. This metal had all of the benefits of solid gold in appearance, noncorrosiveness, and hardness, but it did not have the elasticity of gold and therefore was not as satisfactory for eyeglass springs.

This material was made by drawing a tube of 12K gold with a wall thickness 5 percent of the outside diameter. A base metal (brass) rod was produced to have a diameter which made a "slip fit" in the tube when covered with a thin coat of solder. The rod was forced into the tube and heated to solder the base metal to the tube. From this gold-coated rod, wire is reduced in size by draw-plates to the diameter to be usable for the parts of an eyeframe. It is interesting to note that the ratio of gold to base metal remains constant even if a large rod is drawn down to small wire. This is confirmed by sections cut from the wire to demonstrate the gold content for government analysis. Even the small percentage of gold by weight in this material has substantially priced gold-filled eyeframes out of the market. The next cheaper, but still serviceable, metal frame is gold plate. These frames do not have the useful life of gold-filled metal because the actual thickness of gold on the base metal is not controlled or known to the purchaser. Frame wearers with high acid content in their perspiration have corroded the eyewires of plated frames to the point they are useless in a very short period of time. The high class frame factories do make heavily plated frames that are more serviceable but which cost about as much as solid gold in the 1920s.

The world decline in the population of tortoises has raised the price of these frames enormously. They are still made by hand in Italy virtually on a custom basis. It is difficult to fit lenses into these frames or to bend the temples unless the shell is very fresh. Along with the brittleness comes elasticity which makes the frames very comfortable with temples that hold by head pressure and with small bends behind the ears. Some real shell frames are still sold in Europe, but rarely in the United States.

Since 1910, there has been an increasing percentage of plastic frames sold. These were first made of cellulose nitrate (celluloid) and called imitation shell. Although this material is flammable and the recorded cases of injuries from ignited nitrate frames have been small, it is nevertheless hazardous. The FDA has rated nitrate frames as unsalable—hence, plastic frames are now cellulose acetate. A practical example of the use of these materials is found in commercial and amateur (home) motion picture film. The danger in the flammability of nitrate motion picture film is demonstrated in theatres where the projection booths are made fireproof by law, and projectionists must be educated and licensed to operate the projectors. The nonflammable acetate film for 16 and 8 mm cameras and projectors requires no special handling. This same material for eyeframes is equally safe. Evidence of its versatility is demonstrated in the wide variety of colors and designs in which it is made for eyeframes and sunglasses.

Nylon is used for eyeframes, but it has had limited acceptance. The material is not available in a wide variety of colors. It requires greater heat to make it sufficiently soft to insert lenses. It is more difficult to soften to adjust temples. This great heat requirement and the stiffness of the material interfere with the insertion of CR39 lenses and specially coated lenses. The material is very durable and is difficult to break.

Optyl

The first plastic material specifically designed for eyeframes, Optyl, conceived and produced in Austria, has proved to be an unusually acceptable product; it is an epoxy resin. Because eyeframes made from it are die-cast, there is no objectionable tendency for the material to gradually flatten to the original flatness of sheet stock from which all other plastic frames are made. In the trade this is called "plastic memory." Another feature is that the material does not bend easily until it approaches its softening point (176°F). This characteristic makes it especially desirable for use with the CR39 lenses. It does not create warping of the lenses by the "creeping" of cellulose acetate.

In its original state, Optyl is slightly translucent. It is not dyed in the process of manufacture as is cellulose acetate. The die-cast frames are colored by a vacuum process after being formed. By this method an almost limitless variety of color combinations can be offered. The dyed frames are coated with firm clear coating that enhances the beautiful pastel coloring. Although major frame manufacturers have not thus far prepared to offer Optyl eyeframes, the material continues to grow in popularity on its merits.

DISPENSING TO CHILDREN

In the case of the child, the notion of eyewear does not originate with the wearer. Like the hardware supplied by the orthodontist, the lenses and eyeframe follow the action of a parent and/or pediatrician. Unlike other lens wearers, the very small child has meager opinion about the visual benefits of the lenses.

Points of great importance for the dispenser to observe are that the lenses are not unnecessarily large. The increased weight may be uncomfortable upon the child's nose and also allow the eyewear to creep down the patient's face. Keep in mind that much of a child's world is above his eye level. Hence, the child will look over the tops of his ill-fitting lenses when an adult is addressed. Also unless large lenses are carefully decentered, large convex lenses will create prism Base Out. This will only further create an extra load on many pairs of eyes which are often manifesting over convergence.

A child who is crippled is used to sympathy but a cross-eyed child is a special kind of cripple who verges upon being an outcast. If the child reacts to this psychological trauma he may be belligerent or unusually precocious. Before entering into the procedure of spectacle fitting the dispenser should spend a few moments to get acquainted with the child. Showing the pliers and tools in a fitting table drawer may open a conversation. A brief trip into the laboratory may accomplish this purpose. Let the child have a millimeter rule in his hands. When the rule is used to make measurements the child will likely cooperate better.

Do not force a small child to sit in a fitting table chair. Let him move around on foot. Restrain him as little as possible when trying on frames for size. Try to set up as pleasant an event as possible so the child will be conditioned to willingly accept his eyewear and to wear it as directed.

Very young children should be fitted with an All-American® headband to hold the frame in proper position. Resistance to this device is usually broken down when the child is told that skiers, automobile racers, and many Olympic athletes wear headbands to keep their glasses on. Riding-bow temples are satisfactory a little later. Skull-fitting temples are the least desirable. All parents should be admonished to bring their children in frequently for the realignment of their children's eyewear. Undisciplined hands are bound to twist and bend eyeframes. This offer is bound to strengthen both customer and doctor relations. T. Keith Lyle, M.D., in his classical book *Squint* gives ill-adjusted eyewear as the second cause among sensory obstacles to the normal development of binocular vision. Thus a dispensing optician has a serious charge in his contribution toward the promotion of good fitting.

When bifocals are ordered, Executive lenses should be preferred because they cover the entire lower field. Set the segments no lower than the middle of the pupils with the head in primary position. Let an error in placement always be on the side of too high.

In 1959 Roy Marks, then president of Shuron Optical Company, wished to improve their line of children's frames. He engaged M.L. Moss, Ph.D., Professor of Anatomy at Columbia College of Physicians and Surgeons to measure the development of children's noses beginning at age three. The sample of patients (154) obtained from the Clinics of the College of Physicians and Surgeons determined several things, some of them not previously investigated.

1. The vertical angle showed slight or no change in the age range 3 to 18.
2. The transverse angle regularly lessens from a mean of 28.2° at 3 to 5 to 23.0° at 16 to 18.
3. At the same time the depth of the nasal bridge increases from a mean of 14.2 mm at 3 to 5 to 19.2 mm at 16 to 18.

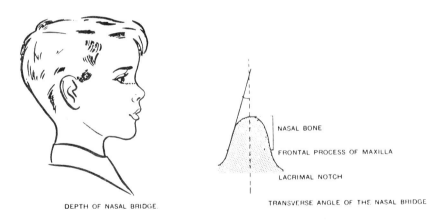

DEPTH OF NASAL BRIDGE

NASAL BONE

FRONTAL PROCESS OF MAXILLA

LACRIMAL NOTCH

TRANSVERSE ANGLE OF THE NASAL BRIDGE

Figure 126. Children's nasal bone research.

Conclusions:

A. Differences related to sex are trivial. Boys' and girls' noses in the designated area show no material difference in shape or growth until near puberty.

B. Greater attention should be paid to the transverse angulation of the pads of children's frames.

C. Increased surface area of the pad is essential.

These findings are corroborated by Fleck et al.* as shown in Figure 126. The pressure upon the nasal surface when the angle at the base of the transverse angle is flat (a $= 90°$) is one G or 100%. As the sides of the nose become more nearly parallel, the thrust upon the pads increases from angle a $= 90°$ (one G or 100%) to 19 G at $3°$ (nearly vertical) with almost 6 G at a common 10% angle.

In their description of their new line of children's frames to the professions and the trade, Shuron presented some significant thoughts:

1. Children are not miniature adults.
2. Until this time no *real* child's frame line had been available.
3. Authoritative data provided the base for frames for a developing nose.
4. The increase in the transverse angle with no change in the vertical angle showed the way for frame designers to make their plans.
5. Pedioptic® frames are guaranteed against all breakage in normal use for one year from purchase.

Upon rare occasions a dispenser has a dramatic experience that confirms the importance of his occupation. Few incidents compete with the event of a cross-eyed child's eyes becoming immediately straight when a pair of plus lenses are fitted and the stress on the accommodative-convergence reflex is balanced!

"COSMETIC" FITTING OF EYEWEAR

Since 1940 when Better Vision Institute enlisted Eddie Senz of Paramount Pictures and Lilly Dache to professionally provide advice and establish guidelines on the matter of the cosmetic (or makeup) effect of eyewear, there has been a constant stream of professionals and others who were self-proclaimed experts writing,

---

*Fleck, H., Heynig, J., and Mütze, K.: *Die Parxis der Brillenanpassung.* Leipzig, VEB Fachbuchverlag, 1960.

lecturing, and demonstrating how to select and fit an eyeframe that would improve the wearer's appearance. The Westmore brothers (of motion picture makeup fame) had a chapter on eyewear in their *Beauty Book*. Perc Westmore had practically researched the subject by having a case full of frames from which he fitted and finally selected the size, shape, and color of eyeframes (his word) for ladies who came to his salon for consultation.

Tura® eyeframes with a very limited number of eye shapes changed the emphasis of frames by accents on the brow line and endpiece. This eyeframe maker introduced anodized aluminum. By this plating process, many attractive pastel colors were made available. Because of the limited elasticity of aluminum, these frames did not hold their adjustment very well for some head shapes. These frames (and Monroe Levoy who developed them) should receive unrelenting gratitude from the entire trade and professions. These frames were a precursor to the establishment of eyewear as fashionable and an accepted accessory. From this new attitude toward eyewear emerged the era of more frequent eyecare and more elaborate eyewear.

Following closely upon this innovation, teenagers developed a fad of wearing old style metal frames with small oval-shaped lenses. They were named "granny glasses." The fad exploded into the "in" thing. Everywhere young ladies wore tinted lenses down their noses (like granny) or up in their hair—they had to be worn! Before the small stock of these old frames was exhausted, the metal eyeframe makers quickly introduced many new styles of octagonal, round, and other shapes in gradually increasing sizes for both men and women. The rush for metal frames brought a number of new frame makers into the field, many of whom had scant experience in eyeframe making.

After many years of emphasis upon carefully fitted bridges (as many as 75 sizes), new lens sizes and shapes were featured while two or three bridge sizes were expected to fit all noses from Grecian to Oriental.

With the new diversity in styles, eyewear purchasers were for the first time developing definite tastes. The historical optical store with the frames in the cabinet drawers quickly became passé. The new order of things demanded display cases and many frames in sight. Purchases were made from the frame "in hand" like ready-to-wear clothing. The days of using and replenishing frames from a large inventory were gone.

Even the larger dispensing firms who have historically carried a large reserve stock of every eyeframe have been forced to follow the methods of ready-to-wear dress and clothing stores. Manufacturers are now using nine months as the style life of a modern frame. When this is compared with previous style lives of up to ten years, even the most sophisticated inventory control finds increasing quantities of obsolete eyeframes in the modern market. As with ready-to-wear, the eyeframe shown to the customer is sent to the laboratory for use. Except for a very few "bread and butter" items, dispensers plan no reserve eyeframe stock.

Jacques' Fifth and Sixth "ages" of spectacle wearers include after-cataract and subnormal vision problems which are discussed separately. Among these Senior Citizens are a large number of doctors' patients who have comparatively clear and well-functioning eyes which require bifocals and trifocals. Taste for eyeframe styling of this group returns to more conservative designs for the most part.

One should not misjudge the preferences of this group. Many of them are prosperous. The reason for which some mature ladies may avoid new eyeframes is not financial. It is often that the eyeframe in use is *comfortable*. Hence, as much emphasis should be placed upon comfort as a more modern style. It behooves the dispenser to deliver a *comfortable* new eyeframe.

Double Gradient Story

In about 1958, Perc Westmore drew the attention of dispensing opticians to the cosmetic advantage of moderate sized plastic eyeframes for middle-aged women. The bottom rim of their eyeframes coincided with the lower orbital margin and obscured the creases or fullness of the lower lids of many of these ladies. The large lens sizes of "fashion" eyewear nullify this cosmetic advantage. A possible remedy is a double gradient lens in which the lower tinted zone is high enough to cover the unsightly area and is not dense enough to interfere with the usefulness of the bifocal segment.

The presentation of this notion requires tact and the density of the tint should be arrived at by demonstration and discussion. The use of antireflection coating is questionable for these instances. Success with this concept has great customer relationship advantages.

These customers (and they are customers, because by this time they have had several prescription changes in their lifetimes) are frequently discriminating about a comfortably fitted frame. Among them are a few lonesome people who tend to use the occasion of a realignment of eyewear as a social event to lighten the monotony of the daily routine. An experienced optician learns to recognize them. He knows that he should not attempt any radical changes in the adjustment. His duty is to carefully check the straightness of the frame and possibly tighten the temples slightly. This work must not be done hurriedly. A running conversation on some comfortable subject is a good part of the service and a cordial invitation to heed their After care Appointment Card is indispensable. Among these customers are some who, through their families and friends, are business builders. They are customers with whom good public relations are especially important. It is wise to recommend that they come in during the early part of the day when their "eyes are fresh" (and also before the usual midday traffic congestion).

INITIAL ROUTINE

This approach is not necessary for the customer who has had a prescription filled before. In this instance there is only one thought that should be conveyed: "We are so glad to have you return to us for your new glasses." There is nothing that pleases an old client more, nor is more deserved, than an expression of gratitude. This would be covered by, "We try very hard to do good work and take good care of doctors' patients who come to us and it is so nice when we see them come in again." The dispenser who follows another who previously took care of the patient should quickly make some complimentary remark to the effect that although he did not have the pleasure of caring for the patient before, he will make every effort to do as well as Mr. _____.

Equally important are the questions and remarks that are taboo.

An expression of surprise or dismay at a strong or complicated prescription, reference to the poor state of the patient's eyes, or direct questions in the same direction are UNFORGIVABLE. Let the patient tell his own story about defective vision and so forth. If he is not disposed to discuss the subject, the whole matter should be ignored. Simply stated, an ophthalmic dispenser's First Commandment is: *An optician shall never comment upon or express an opinion pertaining to a patient's vision or eye health.* Many patients ask leading questions about doctors, diseases, treatments, and surgery. A number of these people are sincere but confused about the educational background and requirements of an optician; the confusion about ophthalmologist, oculist, eye physician, optometrist, and optician is far from cleared up. One must be patient as he replies to all such questions: "I do not have a doctor's education (or education to examine eyes) and can say nothing of value to you on a subject in which I have no training." Naturally it could be offensive to express this thought so tersely. It should be tempered to suit the occasion, but the spirit of the thought must not be varied. One way to say the same thing is to say, "You are in the hands of one of the best trained doctors in this area. He can and will tell you what you want to know about your eyes. My business is glasses and if there is anything I can tell you or do for you with glasses, I am anxious to help. I feel sure that when you discuss this matter with your doctor he will give the information that you want. Then if there is anything we can do to make you more comfortable, do return. Surely all of us working together can make you happy." Occasionally this story will not quite fit. The patient may have said that the doctor has given an unsatisfactory answer and he wants to get other advice. As a last resort, there is only one thing to say, "Your doctor referred you to us and you can readily appreciate the ethics of the situation. We cannot refer you to another doctor."

Your comments upon the old eyewear worn by the doctor's patient may lead to much discord. Be generous about the poorest kind of fitting, by saying something to the following effect: "That is probably not the way I would have fitted you, but we all have different opinions how things should be done. I am going to try very hard to make you happy with your new eyewear."

Nothing is to be gained by the use of an optician's technical language or vocabulary in conversation with a patient. It has been said that when a person uses words that you do not understand, he is doing either of two things—deliberately avoiding a direct answer or "talking down" to you. To do either is impolite. Mostly the optician uses his own vocabulary because it is natural and specific to him. Sometimes an optician's enthusiasm about some fine point in fitting, or a new lens or frame design, starts a lengthy discussion that cannot be expressed easily in other than our own vocabulary. Avoid such situations!

There is probably no patient who is quite so disconcerting as the one who lays down a new prescription and says something like this: "I see he has added a quarter to the spheres in both eyes and changed the axis in my left cylinder. By the way, what do you charge for these in Orthogon?" A flood of questions runs through the optician's mind: "Is he a doctor, and should I recognize him?" "Is he an optician to whom I should quote a professional courtesy?" or "Is he a layman with some superficial knowledge?" A direct question such as "Are you an eye physician?" will usually clear the fog, but even then, the optician will feel constrained because he knows he must not say or do anything that may be at variance with the previous preceptor and thereby provoke a technical discussion that interferes with the work in hand.

An optician should go out of his way to develop a vocabulary for use with laymen. Let it be something like this: for bridge, *nose-piece;* for endpiece, *hinge;* for temple, *bow;* for segment, *reading part;* for pupillary distance, *distance between eye centers.* He should learn to generalize and make simple statements that the *patient can repeat.* "Lens manufacturers' distributing facilities now make it possible to promptly supply you with the highest quality and most advanced lens styles nowadays." Isn't that better than saying that "CR39 and Aspheric Lenticulars are in stock?" or "We do toughen your lenses to increase impact resistance. It won't make them completely breakproof, but they will be a whole lot safer and pass FDA standards." This is one way to refer to case-hardening or chem-tempering. Most manufacturers write advertising that is too complicated for the patient to hear only once and be able to repeat well enough to tell what has been used to take care of his eyes. It is wise to tell the story somewhat like this: "The lenses we now supply are like a fine camera lens; whether you look through the center, as you do when driving, or down at the edge, as you do in reading, the focus is always precisely the same." Reference to "marginal aberration," "skew rays," "oblique astigmatism" is gibberish to most persons. Since these phrases mean nothing to a layman, they arouse no mental pictures and likewise create no interest. Everyone known that there is more than one quality of camera lenses and that the expensive ones are used by professionals because for some reason they are better. It is logical for the patient to think of wearing the best lenses in front of his eyes. There is nothing wrong about calling the lenses by their trade names, but the important thing is to create the proper mental picture, so the customer can talk about his eyewear.

As far as the prescription itself is concerned, *do not venture a thing!* There are several typical questions: "Does by new prescription show that my eyes are better (or worse)?" "Which one of my eyes is better according to this prescription?" "The doctor said my eyes are the same but these figures are all different, why?" In every instance possible, ask the patient, "What did your doctor say?" If he says that he did not ask, tell him to find out from his doctor. When simpler remarks finally fail, compare the prescription to a prescription for medicine and say that you, like a pharmacist, know the general type of condition for which such a prescription is written, but neither the pharmacist nor you would know precisely what the prescription implies in an individual case. Then remember last of all the strength or lens thickness story—how that many persons with very strong lenses see better than average through them and how others can not be improved with either strong or weak lenses. The power of a spectacle lens does not tell the condition of eye health.

As soon as the dispenser feels that he is *en rapport* with the patient he may begin the work of filling the prescription. A recent survey revealed that the most consistent complaint about ophthalmic services was not price or end results. The most frequent remark was that patients felt as if they had been rushed through the transaction.

Despite the widely separated needs of individual patients, for the optician the undertaking sheds many of its complications if an underlying routine is followed. The proper answers to three simple questions provide the care and attention the patient desires:

1. What are this patient's problems?
2. What are *all* the possible methods and ways by which I can care for such a case?
3. What is the best way in *this* case?

Procedure at the dispensing table involves personal relationship between optician and patient. The simple expedient of inducing the patient to talk about himself and his eyes or his doctor will promptly assist in establishing *rapport*. A small establishment in a small community staffed with opticians who have lived in the area for years has no problem. All of the customers are acquaintances or friends. However, when the community grows and new and unacquainted dispensers are added to the staff, attention must be given to the opening remarks in order to prepare the proper atmosphere for the transaction.

What Is Your Vocation?

A dependable opening is the question, "What is your vocation?" This question is essential when serving a presbyope and frequently provides significant information for the care of younger customers when extended to avocation. It can salvage underwater and ski glass service from sport shops!

Watch the customer's expression as you ask the question. Occasionally there will be a change of facial expression that suggests, "Why do you ask?" Follow up quickly with *all customers,* "You may be curious why I asked that question, but if I know how you use your eyes most of the time, I can be of more help to you in the selection and fitting of your new lenses and eyeframe."

Learn to routinely ask the question of all customers, even children. When the child hesitates (as you can expect), say, "I am going to put down *student.*" You have accomplished what you wish to achieve with adults. You wish to get some notion of how and where he uses his eyes. Further, it often provides a subject of conversation, particularly if you direct your questions to let him talk about his activity. Even the side-effects of this important routine are incalculable. Think what it means when caring for a customer who is not pleased with your service. Some time ago, "Supt. of Schools" helped a whole lot when a reply was composed to placate this irritated customer. A move was made that caused him to be an enthusiastic customer.

Study the dialogues that follow until you can easily use them from memory. This is really the modern approach to outstanding dispensing.

For the person who answers, "Retired," ask "What is your principal hobby or activity?" For all of the well-known employments—such as schoolteachers, machinists, electricians, bakers, and so forth—reach for the copy of Clarke Holmes' *Occupational Guide* and turn to the appropriate pages. Say, "Do these pictures suggest things that happen in your day?" The reply should open a rewarding conversation. All specialized vocations would bring the same remark, "I'm not familiar with your activity, but I have a book that may help us." Open *Occupatonal Guide* to his activity and ask, "Do these pictures suggest your vocation?"

For the presbyopic customer, pull out the lens demonstrator tray and say, "Because we all use our eyes so differently on the job, it takes a large number of lens designs to meet our needs."

For a homemaker, open *Occupational Guide* to page 52 and comment, "We seldom realize the versatility required of the eye of a homemaker." Pointing to the pictures is a sure means of opening a conversation which leads to the choice of preferred multifocal.

For people with desk jobs who have a weak prescription and may therefore frequently remove their glasses, about the only recommendation will be to choose a plastic frame.

Tell how FDA requires all glass lenses to be tempered to increase impact resistance, also, how they are tested by dropping a $5/8$ inch ball bearing on them from a height of 50 inches. Further, tempered lenses are warranted for breakage from any cause for one year (two years by some dispensers). Recommend CR39 hard-resin lenses for reduced weight and safety.

If the conversation concerning multifocals has lead to a large segment, show a 28 mm flat-top and tell how the dividing line can be set higher. Then draw to his attention how the lower field will be blurred at his feet. Show a small segment and talk about how it gives freedom in walking but has a smaller reading area.

With every case take an extra moment to show some special trifocal and double segment lenses. If you are a multifocal wearer, show your double D lenses and remark how they fit your special needs, also how you must also have a pair of regular flat-top lenses or something similar for street and social wear.

What is Accomplished With This Procedure

1. By sincere discussion of the customer's activities find if he has any special lens needs.

2. Demonstrate the advantages and limitations of the several lens forms.

3. Bring additional information to doctor's attention (particularly about intermediate distance fields with reading additions of + 1.75 or more) when the conversation with the customer discloses this information was not given to doctor.

4. Assist the customer in the selection of lens types based upon his visual needs rather than "something some friend wears" or some lens form into which you have a developed habit of fitting.

Attitudes or Impressions to be Avoided

1. You must not convey a thought that you are trying to "sell" something the customer does not need.

2. You must be careful to not confuse the customer by showing too many lens forms. Gradually eliminate the styles shown until you reduce to not more than two types (usually a large and a small, or high and low) to meet all needs.

3. You must not accept any lens orders that you are not sure the customer thoroughly understands how they fulfill his needs.

Preparation for Procedure

1. Study pages 3, 4, and 5 in Holmes' book, *Occupational Guide*.

2. Reread this section on ophthalmic dispensing.

3. Carefully read and reread sections on several different voca-

tions to learn how to make use of Holmes' subject matter as well as his pictures.

4. Practice on the procedure as outlined.

When ℞ order forms are printed again place a small box near the name in which to write the vocation.

First Bifocals

When a prescription with a reading addition of + 0.75 to + 1.50 is presented, you should ask, "Are these your first bifocals?" When the answer is most likely "Yes," ask, "Does the thought of the appearance of them bother you?" Observe the customer's words and actions carefully at this point. If he seems to not be disturbed at the thought, use the standard presentation.

On the other hand, if the customer seems tormented with the prospect of having to wear bifocals, as you present the tray of multifocal demonstrators reach for the Younger, Varilux, or Ultravue. Describe and demonstrate the advantages of a progressive power lens. Demonstrate how it is totally invisible when worn. Remark that it is a very difficult lens to manufacture, hence costs somewhat more than many other lens types. Let the customer's desire to conceal his bifocals lead the transaction.

FITTING PROCEDURE

One well-known optician had a rule in his establishment that a dispenser must silently read new prescriptions entirely through two times before taking his eyes off the paper. This man had observed through the years that prescriptions hurriedly read are often misread. He believed, and possibly quite rightly, that a hurried glance at a prescription is sometimes mistaken by the patient as a disparaging attitude toward the prescription or the doctor's efforts. Be that as it may, the pause gives the dispenser time to ponder the prescription.

As previously stated, a large percentage of all lens prescriptions are for not more than a total of 2 Diopters. Lenses within these limits have no unusual physical characteristics. The fact that large numbers of prescriptions are not complicated can lull an optician into a false sense of security. In the fifteen seconds re-

quired to read and reread a prescription, there is time to visualize
the lenses for contour, weight, and thickness. With practice, the
lens powers can be mentally reduced to their spherical equivalents. The patient's probable visual ineffectiveness without the
lenses can be estimated. To this point, the prescription has disclosed whether the lenses will have ordinary or unusual proportions, and by their ~~~~ uggest the patient's dependence upon
the le~   nd visual efficiency. Reduction of an
                         to spherical equivalents is a good
                         change in lens effect and prepare the
                         is great.
                         ns and measurements to be made
                         nterfere with a discussion in which
                         hy he is getting glasses and when
                         m. Sometimes such a conversation
                         ests that the patient has not de-
                         ould have to the doctor. On occa-
                         lieves complications for all con-
                         t the optician may proceed with
                         vertices of the *fitting triangle*
                         nose, and the tops of the ears)
s   centers for near may be meas-
u

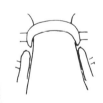

ape analysis.

Un   investigation and report
upon   or, skeletal structure, muscles,
and ne   ... the areas contacted by eyewear is found in
Die Praxis der Brillenanpassung written by Heinrich Fleck, Jutta
Heynig, and Karl Mütze and published in Leipzig in 1960. It is
regrettable that it has not been translated because it contains a

fund of mechanical analysis about frame fitting. Maybe I am somewhat biased because they have copied a good number of my illustrations in the first edition of this book. As could be expected, the colored pictures of young ladies wearing the then current frame styles appear dated.

Their comments only emphasize the importance of surveying the understructure of the bone of the nose before attempting to select an eyeframe. Palpation of the area of the bridge with the thumb and forefinger is the only means by which the shape of the bone can be surveyed. Many times the flesh on the nose appears quite symmetrical, but palpation discloses that the nose has surely been broken in childhood and apparently a splint was not applied. Now all of the slope of the nasal bone is on one side while the other is approximately vertical. Hence one pad will carry the whole weight while the other is ineffective. As shown in Figure 127, the crest of some nasal bones is much wider than the sides, again a pad problem is presented. (As an aside, these are the noses upon which *pince nez* stayed on safety during a windstorm.) Often the solution is a saddle-type bridge with pads. In this way the weight at the nose can be distributed over a larger area. A wraparound rimless or frame bridge can also be plier-fit to the shape of the crest of the nose and the rocking-pads adjusted to share the weight.

Palpation may seem an unnecessary and time-wasting effort until the information provided prevents a disgruntled customer and a "do-over." Make the procedure routine! The fact that the customer is already wearing glasses should not deter you from palpating the nose. The odds are large that your predecessor did not survey the fitting area when he selected a frame. With additional information you may be able to satisfy the customer and explain how you have accomplished your purpose. Individual care is rewarding.

The ideal nose is one that has a regular slope of from 15° to 25° from the vertical and about the same amount of angle transverse toward the front. The variations would be too numerous to mention. The optician's concern is at what point a pair of pads will come to rest. There are some Oriental and Ethiopian noses that seem to have no spot to suggest a seating place for a pair of pads. Such noses cannot support glasses either comfortably or well. The frame must be virtually pulled up on the nose and held in place by the temples. The sway-back rather than arch of a retroussé or turned-up nose often has no resting place for a pair of pads and a saddle or unfit type of bridge is the only satisfactory approach in plastic frames. In extreme cases these bridges must not only be set below center, they must be set behind the plane of the lenses in order to let the lenses clear the lashes. This type of nose presents a difficult problem in rimless glasses. Both blanked and bent bridges are forward of the lens plane in all regular styles and few of them can be readjusted to any great amount. An old-style wide cylinder saddle bridge is often the best solution.

A properly shaped nasal bone with what seems to be healthy covering is a very large contribution to a good fitting. However, the two other legs of this three-legged stool (the *fitting triangle*) are also important. So far as the alignment of the lenses is concerned, the presence of a notch between the external ear and head is all that is necessary. Greater significance is found in those instances when the tops of the ears, and with them the mastoid processes, are considerably above or below the pad position on the nose. When the ears are unusually high, the imaginary triangle slopes to the front and the spectacles even tend to hang on the temples when the head is in primary position. Low ears cause the converse, that is, a slope from the pad position on the nose or nasal apex to the apices at the ears. Temple pressure is in the direction of *back* and *down* and if the septum is not shaped to give a good resting-place for the pads, the glasses will slide down the nose at the least deviation from an accurate adjustment and temple tension.

To continue the evaluation, an optician must rise to get an unobstructed view of the space behind the patient's ears.

Only from a standing position can a dispenser see the positions of the bends of the temples at the tops of the ears and note whether they are equally spaced from the skin surface. The patient may be asked to turn his head and thus present one ear at a time to the optician, but the vertex distances cannot be compared from this position. The shape of the external ear does not seem to suggest the shape of the crotch that may be found behind it. It is imperative that the optician get an unobstructed view of these areas. The important points in this observation are the shape of the skull behind and below the top of the ear and the shape of the notch between the back of the ear and the head. In these areas the tips of the temples are contoured to make the *lock* that holds the pair of glasses securely in front of the eyes. At this time the dispenser visualizes the inclination of the triangle and, with the weight of the glasses as described by the prescription in mind, decides on the preferred type of temple and whether there appears to be any special fitting problem.

Now a measuring device is useful. It is not new but it reduces "fitting table time" at delivery and helps to promote customer satisfaction. It is a pair of calipers to measure the breadth of the skull over the ears. These are made in England by Archer® or in Australia by Martin Wells.

At the zylo bench the temples are set by filing at the joint or bending to open to about 5 mm less than the caliper measurement. This assures that the first time the new eyewear is placed on the customer's head it will feel comfortable. The dispenser will not be confronted with laboratory work to spread or narrow the temple alignment, thus tying up a fitting table, delaying a customer, and stopping his regular work to do laboratory procedures.

Again, this is zylo work that should be ordered by the dispenser (temple spread 145 mm, angle 10°) and executed before the customer comes in for his eyewear. Failure to follow this procedure may lead to necessary work for a precise fitting being overlooked to "save time" or hurriedly and possibly not as well done by a dispenser under the tension as it could have been done by a laboratory technician.

This sort of approach is used in England to the point that frame working and fitting equipment are far removed from the fitting table. Frames are practically fitted to start. One operator says that multiplying the number of fitting tables by eight equals all of the productive hours in a store. Any obstacle or unnecessary work done to delay progress at the table interferes with business income.

Temple Types

There are three temple types to be considered from the aspects of both utility and anatomy: paddle, skull, and riding-bow. Straight (or paddle) temples are especially desirable for reading glasses because the glasses can be put on and taken off with ease. For the same reason they are attractive to women who may have their hairdress over the ears. These temples hold the glasses in position with a direct pressure against the sides of the head if the sides are reasonably parallel. A very long head may require such very long straight temples to accomplish a good fitting that the design is impracticable. A spatula-type temple, that is, a temple that turns slightly down behind the ear top toward the mastoid process, changes the direction of the line of force and because of the shape of most heads the holding bend of the temple tip is much closer to the ear top and the temple can be much shorter. There are many variations of this temple style, called "club" "ambassador," "knobby," "spoon," et cetera, in which the designer has widened or otherwise altered the tip of this shorter temple to improve its holding power. A point of no small concern is the width of the notch at the ear top. When a patient's ear lies close to his head, the bulk of the temple at that point must be considered. Wire core temples are usually somewhat thinner than solid plastic temples but even these may need some handwork with a file for some individuals. Pressure against the upper part (helix) of the outer ear is very uncomfortable for most patients. Some temple designs are thinned down considerably at this point to forestall this difficulty.

The temple style called "skull" in most manufacturers' catalogues is usually much lighter weight than the straight or spatula design. It is intended to be bent abruptly slightly behind the crotch at the top of the ear and then to be fitted pretty much to the shape of the crotch between the head and outer ear. It is intended to extend slightly beyond the bulge of the mastoid process. The point where this temple makes the greatest pressure against the head becomes the pole of the line of force, with the top of the ear serving as the fulcrum. The undersurfaces of the tips of some skull temples have been serrated to increase the friction and retard the temples from "crawling up."

Again you are admonished to carefully estimate the necessary temple length to accomplish a good fitting. Many imported frames have only one length available. Avoid using those designs which are not backed up by a selection of temple lengths by the importer. Let your competitor use them and have his customers constantly push their frames back up into place.

After these observations and consideration with reference to the bridge and temple design of the frame, the interocular distance should be carefully measured with full attention to the monocular differences (see Fig. 105) .

Frame Selection

With the prescription carefully read and analyzed, the measurements and observations of the patient's face completed, a dispenser is prepared to discuss the patient's ocular needs. A layman remarks, "When I get new glasses, I want them like his." The interpretation of that sentence is that he wishes to have a *frame* like the one he has seen. In all likelihood, he has given no thought to the lens style. An ophthalmic dispenser who directs his first question toward the desired type of frame often gains much useful information. "Let me show you some of the latest frame styles." To some customers, "Let's look at some of the new frames that are fun to wear." Most people are willing to look, but the customer who feels he is satisfied with what he is wearing and does not wish to have a new one will usually say something to the effect of "I'd like to use this one. It is all right, is is not?" The dispenser has been asked for professional advice. He should now remove the frame and carefully check the bearings and look for worn parts. The bridge width, lens size, and temple length must also be considered. If the frame is badly worn, it should be remarked that although it is satisfactory now, the material is becoming brittle and likely will not last as long as the new prescription. In the event that an important improvement can be made in the fitting by a frame change, there should be no hesitation to demonstrate the difference, but the decision should rest with the customer. Occasionally the old frame may be unsatisfactory to the point of interfering with the fitting. In this case, the dispenser should explain that he will be censured by the doctor if the glasses do not perform as they should. The patient should be shown, if possible, what the trouble is by demonstrating what is to be accomplished with the correct size in frame. In some instances the use of the glasses made to the new prescription will suggest a new type of frame. For example, the old glasses are reading glasses in a zylo frame and the new prescription is for bifocals which, because they may be worn constantly, may suggest a dressier, lighter weight eyeframe. Assuming there is doctor's permission, one may suggest that the old glasses be retained as spares. If the lenses are not badly scratched, they may be dyed or surface-coated to be used for outdoor wear. The increased addition in the new prescription forces the patient to hold his reading matter much closer to his eyes than with his old prescription. This may be disconcerting to him in some of his activities at an intermediate distance such as music, card-playing, ironing, or gardening. Then, too, each increase in addition reduces the depth of focus for the wearer. The first pair of bifocals with approximately $+1.00D.$ added to the distance prescription has tremendous versatility. The wearer still has sufficient accommodative amplitude to see everything in his intermediate field, 67 to 100 cm (25 to 40 inches), through the distance part of his lenses. In the reading segment he can see up to 20 or 25 cm (8 or 10 inches) from his eyes if necessary and can use the reading part out to almost 1 meter (40 inches), the focal distance of the reading addition. Each successive increase in the addition for near-point reduces this latitude until finally at $+3.00D.$ addition, vision is very poor as little as 2 or 3 inches on either side of 33 cm (13 inches), the focus of the addition.

Although it seems logical that the old glasses with a weaker addition could always provide comfort for the patient, there are exceptions. The old prescription may be so poorly fitted that it is uncomfortable to the patient and he does not wish to wear it at all. Again, the eyes may have changed enough that the doctor has said that it will be harmful for the old glasses to be worn. If either of these situations obtains, it will not take long to find them out. When the doctor does not wish for the old lenses to be worn, he will have told his patient and this will be promptly remarked.

Because you have taken the interocular distance and observed the fitting areas on the nose and behind the ears after you have studied the prescription, you will understand any limitations that may exist with reference to the type of frame that can be best fitted. In the event the patient expresses a desire for a frame type that is not well suited or cannot be worn successfully, it is your duty to *demonstrate,* not tell, why you take exception to the choice. Occasionally the exception is not too marked and may be a matter of opinion. In such instances, yield gracefully and fit the glasses as desired. It may be only such a matter as a wish for straight temples by a person who does not have a good head shape for them and that you would expect the glasses to tend to slide down the wearer's nose. It is wise to make a notation on the order that the subject has been discussed. If doctor or patient is later dissatisfied with the fitting it is good to have a record that exception has been taken.

When a frame is desired by the patient that will actually interfere with the performance of the lenses—that is, hold them too far from the eyes, let them slide down and drop the centers and reading portions or let the lenses severely touch the lashes—let the wearer know that the doctor will take exception to the fitting because it is interfering with the proper performance of the prescription. If the customer does not yield, have a consultation with another dispenser, if possible. This procedure, if tactfully presented, does impress the doctor's patient that it is not a personal or biased opinion and that a sincere attempt is being made to solve the problem. Begin by saying something to the effect that you do not wish to leave anything undone to please, while at the same time discharging your responsibility both to the doctor and to him. Leave the table and briefly discuss the fitting with another dispenser. After introducing him to the customer, step aside while he looks over the problem. This is an occasion when an optician's vocabulary is used while you converse about the case in front of the patient. It is usually best not to arrive at a decision in the presence of the patient. Walk away from the table together, then return with the new plan. In that way it is not obvious who made the decision and no one has "lost face."

If, after the demonstration and consultation, the patient insists upon the impossible and you are thoroughly informed and know that no one else can do more than you can, it is best to let the patient leave without undertaking to fill the prescription. Be sure of your ground in this instance and carefully tell the patient why you cannot accomplish his wishes. Do not be dogmatic nor allow yourself to become irritated. Say that you would like to make the glasses, but that you do not dare risk complications with the doctor by making up unsatisfactory glasses that compromise his prescription. If you have been correct in your premises, frequently the patient will return after discussing the matter with his family, other opticians, or his doctor.

An optician should never impose his opinion with reference to color, weight, or material of the frame, or the shape of the lenses as long as the function of the prescription is not involved. Avoid projecting a preference before the patient has made some kind of sign or comment to lead you. This part of the fitting (that is, the style of the glasses) is almost completely a psychological affair. This is the point where the work of a dispensing optician begins to differ from a pharmacist. A medical prescription can be filled in only one way and is the same for all people. The same lens prescription may be given to a large number of persons, but when their individual needs and tastes have been satisfied, the glasses will be utterly different. Patient participation in the transaction produces the difference.

The regular G.I. spectacles supplied to the Armed Forces bore a similar approach to a pharmacist's handling of a medical prescription. Properly adjusted servicemen's glasses accomplish what the doctor has prescribed from the physiological and physical aspects. The frames were sturdy and not in bad taste, but they were *all alike*. The complaints about the glasses were mostly centered on the impersonal appearance and style. This comment could be considered unique in face of the fact the customers were wearing uniforms.

Experience teaches that taste is a very personal thing. What is very pleasing to one person or in one place may be totally undesirable to another or elsewhere. During World War II, an extremely masculine Naval Aviation Officer from Argentina was in California. He was having a prescription filled before leaving for home. When he was shown a pink (flesh-colored) zylonite frame, he remarked that he couldn't wear that feminine color in his country. He chose a light blue frame, which he considered a manly color. Who can say that he is right or wrong about such a matter?

In the end, the patient and his eyes will be best served if he can be supplied as nearly as possible with what he wishes to have as far as spectacle design is concerned. If he feels that the glasses are outstanding or contribute to his personal appearance, he will likely wear them as much as his doctor has prescribed. His interest in them will help sustain him in the first few days while he is undergoing the usual newness of a prescription change. If the end result is something that he feels is unsightly and that his optician or doctor has more or less forced upon him, the whole affair works out badly for doctor, optician, and patient.

So long as the holder for the prescription lenses keeps them properly and comfortably placed before the eyes, its purpose is served. It is an optician's duty to agreeably show many, if not all, styles of the type of frame desired by the patient. From a wide selection, the patient can be more sure of his choice.

Selling methods for eyeframes have changed drastically with the introduction of so-called "modern styling." Some type of a wall display became necessary. Some of these displays are so inartistically designed that they add very little more to the walls of the store than the shoe boxes of the old time shoe store.

It may be interesting to review the origin of the new approach. Optometrists complained to Jack Copeland, of Bausch & Lomb, Chicago, that it took as long for a patient to select a frame as it did to conduct an examination. He had a furniture designer make some wall cases for eyeframes and told the optometrists to let their patients take their time making a selection while he proceeded with another eye examination. Thus, the length of appointment times were reduced.

Some dispensers who had a strong attachment to previous procedures referred to the new approach as an optical "cafeteria" without any professional guidance. The elapse of time and new frame designs caused them to reconsider. The previous large selection of bridge sizes were reduced to two or three. This made it less likely that the customer would select an improper bridge size. A price tag on the inside of a temple virtually obliterated price discussion. Dispensers have found that customers who are waiting to be served have virtually selected a new frame before coming to the fitting table. Thus the discourse on whether a new frame is desired is answered. In that same activity which ladies name "shopping," handling frames in the display occupies them until they can be waited upon.

The old style store is gradually disappearing. A good variety of eyeframes conveniently displayed simplifies fitting table procedures. A dispenser's expertise in styling is displayed when the customer wishes help in deciding between two or three frames. This is the time when the introduction of another somewhat similar but more daring design may quickly conclude the choice. For those dispensers who have not had the advantage of a course in art and composition in school, Rudolph Arnheim's *Art and Visual Perception* (University of California Press) is outstanding as a source for information on the cosmetic styling of eyewear. It should be read cover to cover.

Unless the doctor's patient has made his/her independent selection of the eyeframe, it is very important that lower and higher priced eyeframes be shown. If the transaction becomes one with the finality of a purchase in pharmacy, there is the possibility of great liability. The patient is vulnerable to anyone who may ask him what he paid for his glasses. There are always persons who seem to know how to get bargains that only they know about. If, to further complicate the situation, the prescription change has been large or it is the first pair of bifocals or trifocals that require some adaptation and if dissatisfaction about frame selection is added, the patient may become a liability to both the optician and the doctor.

There is a procedure that reduces to a minimum all these complications. It *must* be followed if an optician is not to risk poor public relations. Simply show everyone at least one other frame or lens style that costs less than the one he is about to purchase. Do not force it or the patient may become offended or confused. Show it and if the difference is something that is easily seen, demonstrate or explain the difference. If the patient actually changes to the less expensive frame, it is what he should have. In most instances he will continue with his first choice, but he will no longer be vulnerable to the person who talks about lower-priced glasses. He has seen them and knows why his glasses cost more. Doctors are never pleased when the story the patient tells them sounds as if the optician were dogmatic about the design of the glasses; the doctors are surely not pleased when the report smacks of "high pressure."

A dispensing optician should never forget that the vast majority of patients are direct references from doctors, and if the transaction causes his patient to feel that he has been mistreated, the doctor has "lost face." It is so easy to provide doctor protection for a patient who complains about price. Always show a range of prices and the doctor will be able to ask safely, "Weren't you shown less expensive glasses?"

There is an old story that J.P. Morgan, the financier, said, "All persons have two reasons for everything—the one they give and the real one." Doubtless many of the patients who return for re-adjustment or to the doctor with unexplainable complaints are dissatisfied with the physical appearance of their glasses. They are often hoping that by some means the doctor or optician can be induced to make a change that will present an opportunity for a liberal policy of exchange; makeover, directed by management following Marshall Field's attitude, has been found to enhance public relations. Let prescribers and your laboratory know your attitude. The occasional customer who strains fairness is tremendously offset by those whose finished eyewear is unpleasant or has been criticized by other family members. In those instances, the altered appearance and the means by which it happened provides a wonderfully complimentary "word of mouth" advertising event.

Although the optician must not lead the choice, it is incumbent upon him to make tactful suggestions or give advice that avoid disfiguring or uncomfortable glasses. Children *must* be supplied CR39 lenses and preferably plastic eyeframes. Most metal eyeframes are too easily bent. This is the technical ability upon which the doctor depends and is one of the reasons that causes him to refer his patients. Experience teaches an optician how to approach the situation and keep the patient from deciding upon unsatisfactory design.

Spectacles are usually much easier to design when rimless mountings or metal frames are fitted. In these styles there can be a wide range in the choice of lens shapes and other details. The contours of the lenses and bridges of these glasses are reasonably independent. Plastic frames on the other hand demand an entirely different approach. The shape of the nasal end of a lens in a plastic frame has a direct bearing upon the fitting and adjustment of the glasses. The weight of plastic spectacles is greater than that of rimless or metal framed glasses. It is essential therefore that the contact area on the nose be as large as possible. The shapes of nasal bones at the point where spectacles rest can be classified into three types (Fig. 128) :

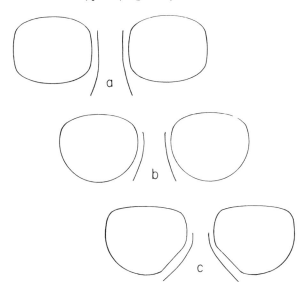

Figure 128. Lens shapes required to properly distribute weight on different nose shapes.

1. The nose with nearly parallel sides. A square oval lens shape produces a contour in the area of the pad that produces a good fitting surface (Fig. 128*a*).

2. An average slope against which an average difference pear

shape such as P3 provides a good contact surface (Fig. 128*b*).

3. The nose that flares out rapidly and requires a narrower DBL (distance between lenses) with a flattened area in the lower nasal quadrant (soulé) like the perimetric lens shape (Fig. 128*c*). Some plastic frame makers attempt to design their frames to have a more or less universal fit. It is a common practice among them to shape the pad and surrounding area with a convex surface. In this way the bearing or contact surface tends to be concentrated in one spot unless the underlying bony structure is concave.

At least one pattern book is available in which more than 1600 lens shapes are classified by shapes and proportions. Makeup (cosmetic) principles are discussed and a procedure to make such shape modifications as described above is presented in it.*

Routine palpation of the contact area on the sides of the nose discloses the actual shape of the nasal bone and indicates the required shape of frame and pad. Not only the basic shape, but the "difference" and size of the lens must be considered. The contour of the area at the end and slightly below the geometric center of a pear (P) shape changes rapidly as the difference in length and breadth is altered. The y-axis tangent through the geometric center of a P3 pattern is decidedly more nearly vertical than the tangent to the same point of a P6 when the difference between the dimensions is 6 mm. As a lens increases in size, the ratio between length and breadth for the same shape decreases and thus again the contour is altered. For example, when the size of the lens is 36 $\times$ 30 mm, the ratio of the dimensions is as 12 is to 10 or 1.20 : 1. A larger lens, say 52 $\times$ 46 mm, edged to the same pattern, is a ratio of 1.13 : 1. In the first case, the length of the lens is 20 percent or $^1/_5$ greater than the width. A difference of 6 mm in the larger lens reduces the ratio to only 13 percent and therefore it more nearly assumes the characteristics of a round lens. A standard pear shape (P3) frame can run the gamut from a poor to a proper fitting by changes in lens size. It must be kept in mind that irrespective of the size or shape of a lens in a plastic frame, the

---

*Stimson, R.L.: *A Pattern Book and Cosmetic Fitting*. Los Angeles, Superior Optical Company, 1966.

contour of the lens area in contact with the nose should not vary materially from the contour established by the shape of the side of the nose.

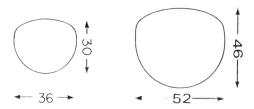

Figure 129. Ratio of dimensions for different lens shapes.

Adequate glazed fitting models are necessary at the fitting tables to accomplish consistently satisfactory work. Many poorly fitted glasses are directly chargeable to an inadequate set of fitting frames. In fact the best practice is to place the final frame on the patient to acquaint him with its appearance and to give the dispenser the opportunity to confirm his decision. Lack of well-selected frames breeds either of two troubles. If the fitter is conservative, he tends to concentrate on a single shape and size for all patients. A large number of compromises with fitting principles occur in a "production line" approach. Competent ophthalmic dispensing is nothing if it is not an individualized consideration of each patient and his particular prescription and frame fitting. At the other extreme, when a dispenser tries to use his imagination too freely and conjectures how other shapes and sizes may fit while he uses a different model on the patient's face, a great deal of patient dissatisfaction and "make-overs" are assured. Facing the wide variety of frame styles and lens shapes, this is certainly an erroneous approach to fitting. From the patient's side it is difficult for him to visualize the end result of an item with which he has so little experience. It is a common experience for most persons to have had some kind of a disappointment with reference to tailored clothing, and the purchase of clothing is a more frequent experience for everyone. Because of the patient's lack of familiarity with the subject, it is not remarkable that it is difficult for an optician to create, with words alone, the precise mental picture of the appearance of a pair of glasses. Paradoxically, the most highly skilled dispensers work from the most diversified sets of fitting models. Some experts wish actually to prefit the particular frame for the patient before the lenses are put in it. Therefore one is not safe to imagine he is becoming expert when he attempts to take shortcuts and guess at his measurements. Clarke Monroe, a master craftsman, regularly glazed a modified frame with coquille lenses to demonstrate to his customer the effect of his designing.

Many of the innovations in plastic frame design have originated in zylonite frame factories which have little or no connection with the lens manufacturers or prescription laboratories. As we shall see, some of the designs that have been widely accepted have presented many problems for dispensers and optical laboratories. The majority of the unusual designs have been made for women whose features are smaller and whose interocular distances are narrower than those of men. As is shown (Fig. 130), in this typical lens shape, the upper temporal quadrant draws the mechanical center out and up. A large number of the lenses for such frames must be decentered rather large amounts. This adds to the requirements of the lens size necessary to fill the prescription. The blank size of the single vision lenses only a few years ago was 48 mm diameter and was considered adequate. Uncut single vision lenses are now 65 mm and still there is insufficient area to account for the extended corner or corners of the asymmetric lens shape.

The present trend to large and larger lens sizes means larger

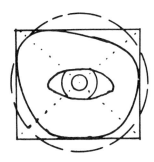

Figure 130.   Minimum blank size to accommodate asymmetric lens shape.

material and prescription prices. The dispenser who does not know in advance the size of lens blank required (68, 71, or 75 mm) takes an unnecessary loss.

Minimum Blank Size Determination

A simple method of blank size determination has been developed. A dispenser is obligated to use it before quoting a price to a customer. It alerts the dispenser to the possible delay in obtaining materials to execute the order. The information about blank size must be found at the fitting table. Everyone is aware of the poor public relations with the customer arising from an improperly priced order.

Let us also review the points at which the error may be noted: (1) uninformed stock clerk may put too large or too small lens blank on the order; (2) materials inspector may find the error; (3) surface grinding layout may detect the error; (4) finishing layout may stop the order with small blanks; (5) edging will see an incomplete lens, *but in no instance is an unnecessarily large (and costly) blank ordinarily challenged.*

Were it not for the incoherence, I should like for this section to be at the front of the volume. Once established, use of this procedure will pay for this book in a few days and earn a further return from then on.

The foundation of the determination is the Equivalent Diameter (ED) of the lens shape at the size ordered. Figure 130 shows how much larger than the Boxed Dimensions a round blank must be to produce the lens. In Figure 131 the radius and diameter of this round blank are demonstrated. It shows that, if a compass were set at the center of the Box and the compass opened to the distance of the greatest dimension of the lens and used to draw a circle with this radius, it would demonstrate the size of the round blank required for that particular size. If the compass is closed to touch the box at the ends of the "A" measurement, the long corner will protrude out of the smaller circle. This protrusion is a constant increase for any lens size of this shape. (See the difference between the ED and A dimensions in the specifications given for the pattern of any eyeframe.) This protrusion has been named Equivalent Diameter Extra (EDX) and *is as important*

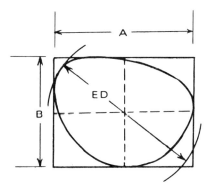

Figure 131. Equivalent diameter of an asymmetric lens shape.

as the A or B dimensions.

The EDX should be shown on the temple tag of the frame so that it will be convenient for the dispenser to calculate the Minimum Blank Size (MBS). As an alternate, some firms have file cards for each frame style; less convenient, the dispenser may refer to this card to find the EDX. Frequently the specification chart may show a fractional difference, such as:

A	B	ED
52	45	55.3

Complete the ED to 56 or EDX 4. This provides a safety factor for rough edges on blanks.

EXAMPLE:

Interocular Distance	62/59
Lens length	54
+ DBL	18
= Lens centers	72
— Interocular Distance	62
+ Total Decentration	10

℞ order form:

"A" Length	Total Decentration	EDX	MBS
54	+ 10	+ 4	= 68

Hence the Minimum Blank Size is 68 mm.

For a single vision lens, the decentration can be reduced by grinding prism in the direction of the horizontal meridian. The precise amount of prism we put in lenses which are 58 mm blanks is 54 ("A") + 4 (EDX) = 58 mm or 62 mm for safety, but a bifocal would be a 71 mm blank which in the 1977 lens catalogue is an oversize blank.

The order form above tells the stock clerk the blank size required. At each point in production, the question of the required blank size is answered.

When this information is found at the fitting table and the customer resists an extra charge, a smaller frame can be selected in order to use the regular size blank.

Summary of Advantages of MBS Method

1. It shows when an oversize blank must be used.
2. Since it is established at the fitting table, it assures correct pricing.
3. It gives the dispenser notice of possible delays due to non-stock lens blanks at the time of the order.
4. It instructs the Stock Clerk the precise blank size.
5. It answers the questions of laboratory technicians.

Minimum Bifocal Blank Size

The centers of the reading portions of multifocals are the reference points. Hence the MBS as found above cannot be reduced by grinding prism in the distance portion. Round segment blanks can be rotated to place a round segment in the proper position. Flat top segments are generously decentered to assist when the optical center must be decentered from the mechanical center of the blank.

THE EDX FOR SOME LENS PATTERNS

American Optical Co.		Victory Optical Mfg. Co.	
Liner	3	Bentley	5
Teddy Bear	3	S643	3
Rowdy	3	S579	4
School Girl	3	7115	2

Universal Optical Mfg. Co.
Ladybrow   5
Charmbrown   4
Stateman   4
Newport   3

Transworld Optical Co.
Cutie   4
Chi Chi   3
Flounce   0
Commander   4
Sweetie   2
Classic   1

Marine Optical Co.
Tech   2
Marauder   5
Host   2
Jr. Miss   0
Indeed   3

May Mfg. Co.
Half Eye   2

Spencer   4
Signature   1
Surrey   2
Trafalgar Square   7
Sports Car   2
Go See   4

Artcraft Optical Co.
Leading Lady   5
Beauty Lite   4
#299 Rectangular 3
#294 Octagon   1

Liberty Optical Mfg. Co.
Libby   5
Spokesman   4
Par Nine   3
Miss Jones   3
Wanderlust   2
Understudy   2
Redhead   3
Take Charge   2

LENS PATTERNS

It seems incredible that the number of lens patterns (formers) has increased from a handful to the point of almost 7,000 in my firm's laboratory. What was once a small detail has now become a prodigous task. Leon Totten, past president of BVI, designed a pattern rack for us that will hold 17,000 patterns. This problem is not exclusively a large laboratory problem. If the patterns for only the ten most popular eyeframes each year since Harlequin were retained, there would be 3,000; and they must be retained, because some zylo frames last a very long time. Since the advent of metal frames, which have an interminable life and require precise lens shape and size, retention of patterns for these frames is essential. Figure 132 shows the size and detail of Totten's rack. It is something that a good "do-it-yourself" man can build. Totten's detail drawings for the job are obtainable from me at no charge. By its design, it can be easily altered in size to meet the needs of a laboratory of any capacity.

A pattern maker is a great help for any laboratory but at the end of making a special pattern, an important decision must be made. It is what to do with the pattern. Not appreciating what will develop, these patterns may be placed on a "special pattern" rack. As the years go by, the retrieval of one of these patterns becomes a time-consuming and often unfruitful search. There is a relief by sending the pattern out with the job and letting the pattern rest in the customer's record file envelope in the store. By this method, the pattern is ready for a lens replacement or a new pair of lenses to the frame at any time in the future.

The boards of Totten's pattern racks are identified by letters A,B,C. . . The rows of patterns on the boards are identified by letters A,B,C. . . The nails for the patterns on each row are identified by numerals, which for the size of the board used is twelve on each side; that is, 1 to 12 on one side and 13 to 24 on the other. Hence the identification of the location of any pattern would be, for example: AB 12; CM 24; FF 19; or KA 4. This information must be available to the dispensers so that this identification is written on the order. If the temple tag on the eyeframe is long enough, the number should appear on it. By this means, there is no interruption of the free flow of the order in the laboratory. This method avoids the selection of the wrong pattern (and as the number of patterns increases, some designs are so nearly the shape of others that they are almost indistinguishable.)

When the edger has used the pattern, it is dropped in a small bin which is identified by the first letter of the pattern number. Thus the pattern can be handily located if it is needed before it is returned to the pattern board. When several patterns accumulate in the bin, they are easily placed on the single board where they belong.

FRAME CATALOGUE NUMBERS

It is most important to give serious consideration to the identification of frames and lenses. Use of manufacturer's names for frames and their colors leads eventually into an impenetrable maze. A frame price book will become ponderous in a short time and, because of frequent price changes, can easily become undependable and costly (underpricing).

The solution for this problem was found more than twenty-five years ago. It is to replace written names with numbers. Start with it and avoid many heartaches. Change to it if you have started with frame names and color names. The number notation is simple. The first numeral identifies the source. This is followed by a letter which identifies the category of the frame, which is followed by the item sequence of purchases from an individual source.

Starting at the first of each year, the item number for each first frame purchased from each manufacturer is number 1 followed by a dash and the last digit of the year. For example: 20F1-8 for 1978. This procedure keeps the catalogue numbers small and at the same time records the number of styles purchased from each manufacturer. The date identification measures the obsolescence of each style. It is easy to distinguish two-year-old frames which

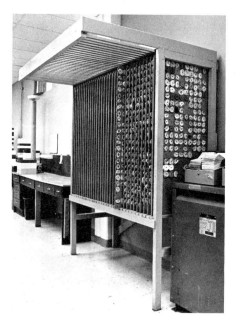

Figure 132A. Totten lens pattern rack.

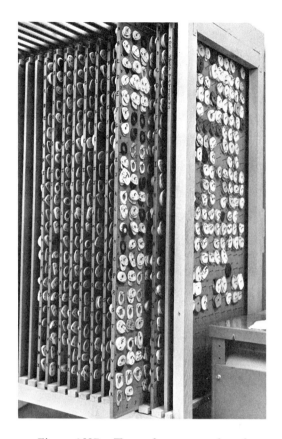

Figure 132B.   Totten lens pattern board.

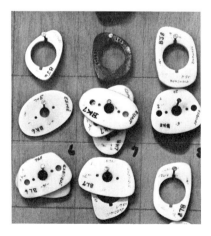

Figure 132C.   Detail of pattern rack.

are to be closed out even if an incentive is necessary. The number is valuable to your accountants at tax time to properly evaluate your inventory and, when necessary, to "write off" outdated items.

8 D 2/7		GB50 (MF 9)		+5	C	5
CATALOG NUMBER		PATTERN		EDX	SHAPE	DiFF
EYE	BRIDGE	COLORS		MISC. INFO		
56	19	10 medium shell (11)		Front: 30.85		
59	19	41 brown fade (10)		F/O:		
- - - -	- - - - - - - - - - - - -	91 grey fade (20)		41 brown fade		
	Bridges measure 17					
					7/20/77	
TEMPLE LENGTHS		LENS	REG.	IND.	PROF.	TEMPLES
140- 145 MM		+1	.85		.85	.00
TEMPLE TYPES		DATE				
skull		7/20/77				
				GEOFFREY BREENE # 50		

Figure 133. Lens information card.

The catalogue number is on the first line of the frame information card (see Fig. 133) for the style. Use of the Rolodex information card file by dispensers prevents orders for bridge sizes, lens sizes, temple lengths, or colors which are not available. The card also gives the pattern number and EDX for the lens shape. The prices of frame parts are on the card. The colors of frame materials are also coded. Manufacturers' names are avoided. Let us say the color code for the above frame is 12. All of this information plus the sales price can be written on a standard price tag for the right temple of the frame: 1F1-7 12 $28.50. This procedure disposes of a frame price list. The maker and category identification simplify the inventory form for year's end. Price increases can be made by placing a piece of a tag over the old price.

Frame Source Numbers

The original list should be your principal suppliers in alphabetical order, spacing them at the fifth digit. Then, as there are additions or changes, there is space for new names, still in alphabetical order. The example below illustrates:

05   Adensco
10   American Optical Co.
15   Art-Craft
20   Artoptic International
25   Avant-Garde Optics, Inc.
30   Bausch & Lomb
35   Christian Dior
40   Flairspecs, Inc.
45   Hudson Optical Corporation
50   Liberty Optical Mfg. Co., Inc.
55   Marine Optical Inc.
60   Martin-Copeland Co.
65   May Optical Co.
70   Menrad
75   Optyl Corporation
80   Rodenstock USA, Inc.
85   Shuron-Textron

Frame Categories

The frame category list could be as follows:

A   Rimless
B   Men's plain zyl
C   Men's ornamented zyl
D   Children's zyl
E   Children's metal
F   Ladies' plain zyl
G   Ladies' ornamented zyl
H   Men's outdoor
J   Ladies' outdoor
K   All metal frames
M   Men's zyl combination
W   Ladies' zyl combination

Frame Color Code System

The color list could be as follows:

1   Crystal, Clear

2 Flesh (Not Pink)
3 Black
   30 Blackwood
4 Brown
   40 Brownwood
   41 Brownsmoke
   45 Brown Satin
5 Bronze
   50 Seal Briar
   51 Dusty (Light Brownsmoke)
   55 Bronze Satin
6 Cordovan
   60 Redwood
7 Blue
   70 Bluewood
   71 Bluesmoke
   75 Blue Satin
8 Slate
9 Grey
   90 Greywood
   91 Greysmoke
   92 Gunmetal
   95 Grey Satin
10 Demi Amber
11 Demi Blonde
12 Smoke Amber
13 Gold (Yellow Gold-Filled)
   135 Gold Satin
14 Silver (White Gold-Filled)
   145 Silver Satin
15 Pink (Not Flesh)
   155 Pink Satin
16 Red
   161 Crystal Red
   165 Red Satin
17 Yellow
18 White
   185 White Satin

19 Orchid
  195 Orchid Satin
20 Green
  21 Crystal Green
  22 Olive
  23 Green Satin

Dispenser Information

An easily read price on the frame, like prices on clothes, is advantageous when a customer is selecting a frame from a display. A half length tag is put on the left temple with dispenser's information. The EDX and PATTERN NUMBER (3 —— LB18) makes it possible for the dispenser to know the size of the lens blank required and thus the price of the lenses. The second set of letters and digits facilitates the laboratory order.

This is an example:

8	= Made by Victory Optical Mfg. Co.
M	= Man's Metal-Zylo Eyeframe.
4-8	= "Atlas," the 4th Victory item stocked in 1978.
4-8P	= Panel Temples.
$\overline{\text{8M4-8P}}$	is the sum and tells the story.

The eyeframe inventory list is subdivided by the different categories of eyeframe. Under each, the eyeframes are listed in the numerical order of manufacturers. Knowing the kind of eyeframe and who made it, one can quickly turn to the group of all such frames available.

The number of the frame is very advantageous to the dispenser. He copies the number from the temple tag on the order form in little space, and he is very specific. Frame numbers are very convenient in telephone conversations. They also assist in arranging merchandise in the stock department. Bin cards and stock order cards are much simpler with numbers rather than names.

LENS CATALOGUE NUMBERS

Equally important is the identification of lenses by catalogue numbers. Like the numbering of frames, this simplifies data processing for sales analysis and inventory control. Although these analyses may be some time in the future for a new business, the records are in line when the time arrives.

Four elements describe almost any lens, with an additional element to describe lens treatment or processing of the finished lens.

Material and Category

The first number indicates lens material and category.

4 Plastic
6 Industrial 3 mm
8 Cataract
9 High Index (Zeiss Hilite)
X Balance

Lens Type

The numeral before the letter is descriptive of the lens power or powers of the lens.

0 Plano
1 Single Vision
2 Bifocal
3 Trifocal
Σ Masterpiece Single Vision
90 Frosted Lens
91 Chevasse Lens
92 Pin Hole Lens
93 Occluder Lens

Color

The letter indicates the lens material and its color or tint. This is the base of the code.

A   Clear
B   Green #1
C   Green #2
D   Green #3
E   Green #4
F   Cosmetan
G15 B & L Grey
G/2 G15 Lt.

H	Photochromic
K	Kalichrome (Noviol)
M	Miscellaneous
S	TruColor
S/2	Lt. Shade
T	Therminon
U	Uniform Density
X	Pink #1
Y	Pink #2
Z	Pink #3

Multifocal Design and Width

The numbers following the color code indicate the multifocal design. In a two digit number, the first number indicates the type of multifocal, e.g. 1 = seamless; 2 = flat top; 4 = round; 5 = one piece; and 8 = cataract. The second digit describes the width or other detail of the type.

1	Executive
2	Curved Top (Ful-Vue)
3	Panoptik
5	Varilux II
6	Ultravue
10	Younger
13	Kryptok
14	RedeRite

Flat Top

20	20 mm
22	22 mm
25	25 mm
28	28 mm
20/35	35 mm
20/40	40 mm

Round

40	20 mm
42	22 mm
40/16	16 mm

One piece

50	Ultex A (38/19)
51	Ultex AL (38/24)
52	Ultex B (22)
54	Ultex Lge. Field
56	Univis B
57	Univis R

Cataract

80	Flat Top 20
82	Flat Top 22
83	Flat Top Lent.
84	AO Lent. "E"
85	Panoptik Lent.
86	Aolite Asph. Lent.
87	PanAspheric B & L
88	Hyperaspheric
89	Welsh Aspheric

Special Treatment

The letters and digits that follow describe special treatment to the edged lens.

E1	Equatint #1
E2	Equatint #2
E3	Equatone #3
E4	Equatone #4
G	Gradient Density (Top)
GG	Gradient Density (Double)
AA	Fashion Colors for Plastic
S	Super Coat (Antireflection)

Dispenser Information

These are some examples of the use of the catalogue numbers:

1A = Single Vision, clear glass

2D3 = Bifocal, Green Tint #3 (Rayban) Panoptik Regular.

3A25/6 = Trifocal, clear glass, Flat Top 25 wide, 6 mm intermediate.

2X25 = Bifocal, Pink Tint #1, Flat Top 25 wide.

2A22/2A22 = Double D Bifocal, clear, 22 wide.

A more complex example:

8   = Cataract
2   = Bifocal
A   = Clear Glass
85   = Panoptic Lenticular
S   = Surface Coat

82A85S

Thus, 82A85S is the catalog number for Supercoated Panoptik Cataract Lenticular Bifocal Clear Glass (6 digits and letters replace 54 letters!).

It is obvious that any means by which an optician can reduce the above essay when he is busy with a customer at the fitting table has merit. Some of the side effects are that the color and

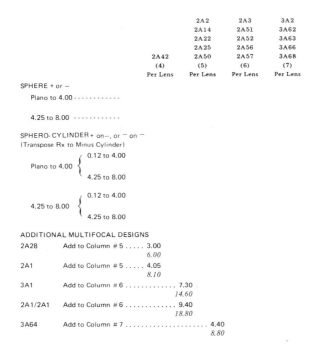

SUPER-TUFF (CASE HARDENED)
MULTIFOCALS

		2A2	2A3	3A2
		2A14	2A51	3A62
		2A22	2A52	3A63
		2A25	2A56	3A66
	2A42	2A50	2A57	3A68
	(4)	(5)	(6)	(7)
	Per Lens	Per Lens	Per Lens	Per Lens

SPHERE + or −

Plano to 4.00 · · · · · · · · · · · ·

4.25 to 8.00 · · · · · · · · · · · ·

SPHERO- CYLINDER + on−, or − on −
(Transpose Rx to Minus Cylinder)

Plano to 4.00 { 0.12 to 4.00 / 4.25 to 8.00

4.25 to 8.00 { 0.12 to 4.00 / 4.25 to 8.00

ADDITIONAL MULTIFOCAL DESIGNS

2A28   Add to Column # 5 . . . . . 3.00
                                    6.00
2A1   Add to Column # 5 . . . . . 4.05
                                    8.10
3A1   Add to Column # 6 . . . . 7.30
                                    14.60
2A1/2A1   Add to Column # 6 . . . . 9.40
                                    18.80
3A64   Add to Column # 7 . . . . 4.40
                                    8.80

Pair price in italics

Figure 134. Lens price list page.

kind of glass, segment diameter, and lens processing are all written in one place on the order. Thus the errors of omission in writing, processing, and inspecting the order are at minimum. The codes can be typed on one $8\frac{1}{2} \times 11$ paper and copies conveniently placed at points of vantage to familiarize the laboratory and stock department staffs. Copies will also be advantageous in the stores after the first printing of the new lens price list. It is surprising to note the rapidity with which the staff learns the numbers. This is explainable because the vast majority of lenses are grouped in a few designs.

Because lens color and segment diameter are a part of the catalogue number, there is no reason to have places on the ℞ order or customer record for these specifications. One user of catalogue numbers remarked that many dollars had been saved on "remakes" when lens color was no longer omitted from the laboratory order.

When a tray of Multifocal Demonstrator Lenses is prepared for the fitting tables, the catalogue numbers can be easily imprinted on the plastic handles of the demonstrators.

Special Lenses, Processes, Etcetera

If the right and left lenses differ, write a separate catalog number for each lens.

Example: $\dfrac{42A22 \quad \text{(Flat top, clear 22 segment)}}{90 \quad \text{(Frosted glass)}}$

Balance—For a balance lens, prefix the entire catalog number with X.

Example: X1X (Balance Lens Single Vision Pink Tint #1)

Prism—Place a $\triangle$ sign after the catalogue number.

Example: 2A50$^{\triangle}$ (Bifocal Clear Ultex A with Prism)

Trifocal—If the intermediate segment width is other than standard, write the depth of the intermediate segment followed by a slash (/) mark before the number indicating the style of lens.

Example 3A 8/25 (Trifocal Clear 8 mm Intermediate Flat Top)

LENS SHAPE ALTERATIONS

Most of what follows is totally inapplicable to large lens size "fashion" frames; however, the principles described are still of value in the fitting of lightweight, moderate-sized plastic eye-frames.

Oftentimes the fitting of a plastic eyeframe can be materially improved by reshaping the nasal side of the lens. This alteration is done by flattening the lens at the point where the pad contacts the nose. This modification is called *soulé*. The laboratory must have very specific instructions, if this work is to be done properly. A highly satisfactory method is to draw an outline of the shape of the lens, show how much of the periphery is to be affected and the amount of lens to be removed. There are frequent instances when it is unsafe to have the work done before the frame is partially fitted, then the optician can do or direct the work with more accuracy. Round lens oxfords can often be fitted very satis-factorily by this method when they are unsatisfactory otherwise. Adjust the oxford as usual, then mark with an ink-stick the center of the point of contact. Flatten a distance of 15 or 20 mm on the edge of the lens with the center slightly below the contact point. In this way compensation is made for the rotation of the axis of the lenses because of the slightly reduced DBL.

Many of the asymmetric shapes of the Debutante® family can-not be safely modified to any great degree. Occasionally a change in lens size will help. In rare instances, the lens shape can be rotated to accomplish the purpose without destroying the cosmetic effect of the frame. A slight increase or decrease of the brow angle often improves the appearance and fitting in an individual case. There are times when the shape of a slightly different style can be put in the frame. A glazed sample should be prepared for this last undertaking. The alteration may accomplish the fitting but be highly unsatisfactory for the wearer.

After the contour of the slope has been established, the remain-ing consideration is the bevel of the nose. Again palpation with the finger tips will have indicated the necessary contour for the pad. This final part of the fitting is usually done at the time the glasses are delivered. There are extreme cases, though, that should be considered at the time the order is placed. A flattened nose of the Oriental type may require a pair of pads to be reset more nearly parallel with the lens plane. To accomplish a good surface contact for the pads on some straight-sided noses, the pads must be removed and reset at approximately 90° to the lens plane. It is frequently advantageous to have this work done in advance so that the cemented surfaces are dry and will readily permit working with a file.

Some reference has been made by manufacturers to the effect that raised endpieces have on the adjustment of the glasses. From the point of view of the *fitting triangle*, the position of the end pieces has no effect on the position of the lenses. Whether the endpieces are high or low, the apices of the *fitting triangle* are still the ear tops and nose. In common with many other designs, Ful-Vue temples are not in the straight line from ear top to nose but the stress or tension required in fitting is seldom great enough to produce torque.

The position of the endpiece has moved up through the years. At one time practically all lenses were oval. Although the holes on the nasal side of the eyeglass and occasionally a saddle bridge mounting were drilled as much as 3 mm above center, the endpieces were regularly fitted on the 180° line of the lens. As the pear (or drop) shape appeared, some endpieces were set 2 to 4 mm above the midline. Radical change awaited the advent of the Ful-Vue design. In it the endpiece was set 30° above the old position. New lens shapes were developed for the mountings.

The high endpiece is an improvement in the appearance of the vast majority of cases. An elevation of about 15° above the datum line (the midline of the "B" dimension), called Low-Bow, is more satisfactory on some faces than the regular 30° Ful-Vue (or Hibo®). When the ears are lower than average, the temples slope down to the ear tops and either accentuate the length of the face or make the low ears more noticeable. Lower endpieces are definitely indicated for these faces.

In geometry, the Golden section (or Divine Proportion) is that if a line segment is divided into segments such that one is the mean proportion between the whole line and the other, the line segment is said to be divided in extreme and mean ratio. This proportion is about the same as two is to three. It has been presented to us in many of the art forms of the past and present. The beautiful contour of a Grecian vase is an example of the Divine Proportion. Many of the present lens designs are closely related to it. A large number of dispensers prefer the Low-Bow endpiece position because it reflects this proportion in what they call "balance."

Much has been written on the styling of glasses—that is, the proper style of bridge for nose, lens shape for face, etcetera. There are a few simple observations that seem to be true. (a) In much the same way that a plaid coat accents shortness and stripes accent height, a high arch bridge seems to elongate some noses, while a low wraparound bridge that crosses the nose only slightly above the datum line does not have that effect. (b) Rounded lens shapes ordinarily look best on angular faces and, conversely, rectangular or straight-side lenses fit well on round faces. (c) If the contour of the top of the lens follows the general curve of the eyebrow, it will be inconspicuous. A greater arc causes a "raised eyebrow" expression while a flatter line tends to look severe. (d) The outside end of the lens should be in conformation with the line of the side of the head. Then no new line is set up when the wearer's face is viewed "full-face." (e) The width of the lens must leave some clearance from the cheek at the bottom. Lenses that are too close "steam up" easily. Lack of ventilation behind the lenses makes the eyes uncomfortable. Lenses that are made too wide have to be adjusted away from the cheeks and this interferes with the best lens position. (f) The cosmetic effect of the

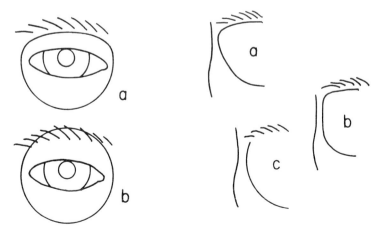

Figure 135. Cosmetic effects of lens shapes.

shape of the lower temporal area of the lens creates an illusion with reference to the cheekbone. A squared effect seems to raise the cheekbone and accent it. A rounded curve or slope away from the face has the opposite effect.

Now any optician who becomes dogmatic and tries to dictate lens shape, etcetera, will find that at some time, no matter what opinion he may project, he will be in direct variance with some of the spectacle-wearing public's taste or as least its wide acceptance.

In the recent rebellion against all things that suggest conformity, eyeframes were grotesquely shaped and sized and glasses (outdoor and regular prescription) were deliberately worn at half mast on the nose. The dispenser who cannot respond to the times is badly out of touch with a large percentage of his customers.

Stylists declare an arched shape above the eyebrows provokes a startled look. Probably it does, but most everyone wore round lenses one day. During World War I, it was a military convenience to standardize on 40 mm round lenses. They could be delivered to the hospitals as edged lenses and rotated in the metal frames to the prescribed axis. In this way, each spherocylindrical lens could fill many prescriptions. When the war was over, the public accepted the new round shape for all kinds of glasses. It was several years before doctors were able to discourage the use of round lenses. They had the bad habit of loosening in the frame and rotating to other than the prescribed axis.

The end to the fad was helped by the advertising of the metal mounting manufacturers. Someone conceived the idea of Colonial (octagonal) shaped lenses. This shape could hardly be put in a plastic frame and was difficult to fit to a metal frame. The eight-sided shape was new and different for rimless glasses. It soon appeared on long, oval, and round faces and the public enjoyed the glasses. For several years there were many new lens shapes designed, and practically all showed the octagonal influence. The advent of Ful-Vue frames soon after 1930 brought the lens shapes back toward pear-shaped (P3) lenses. The Ful-Vue idea was produced in a rimless endpiece and rimless lenses followed suit. Opticians talked about lenses following the shape of the orbit and rimless lens shapes were developed with different arcs at the top to follow the brow-line. Attention was soon paid to the slope of the side of the nose. A lens shape called "perimetric," first de-scribed by Thorington in 1897,* was revived. The top of the lens was slightly flatter than the conventional pear shape and the nasal side of the lens had a "nasal cut" (soulé) of a little more than a millimeter. The shape was a prompt success because it did fit the orbit of many faces.

Then about the time a rut was forming in public taste and fitting habits, a startlingly new frame was presented. Its trade name was Harlequin. The lens shape was about that of the aper-ture of a domino mask. The long axis of the lens was tilted up severely at the temporal end and the endpiece of the frame was as high as the end of the eyebrow (Fig. 136). The frame violated most of the fitting rules in use at the time. The brow-line was intersected by the top of the lens, the lower temporal field was much smaller, bifocal segments were small in the long oval lens. Opticians were in dismay. Some of them almost refused to fit the frame and the majority were doubtful about both the acceptance and utility of the frame.

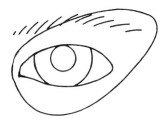

Figure 136. Harlequin shape intersects the eyebrow diagonally.

A new word, "upsweep," came into the style vocabulary of women. Hair was being dressed on the top of the head again and the upsweep of the lines of Harlequin took the fancy of many women. It was a bit too extreme for some, so there was soon a wide choice of variations. Frame makers engaged fashion design-ers for their factories to keep abreast of women's styles. All this activity had a marked effect on the acceptance of glasses as a part of a woman's ensemble. Pictures in style magazines began to show

---

*Thorington, J.: *Methods of Refraction*. Philadelphia, Blakiston, 1947, pp. 381-382.

women wearing or carrying glasses. A few women's stores in the larger cities added fancy sunglass and spectacle frames to their lines.

Thus it is seen that taste in spectacles, like taste in anything else, is a very personal thing. In that it is a perception of excellence, it does not need to be logical or scientific. It might be said that a doctor's work is to arrive at a proper prescription and the dispenser's work is to translate the prescription into lenses that will perform as the doctor intended, but the appearance of the glasses, so long as it does not interfere with function, is in the hands of the wearer of the glasses. It is an optician's duty to have a thorough understanding of conventional fitting principles, but he must not attempt to force his personal opinion.

By demonstration, a customer's decision can usually be swayed from an inadequate combination. The less a layman is expected to visualize what an optician is attempting to describe, the less disappointment and misunderstanding can come into the transaction at the final adjustment. No optician's stock is complete without a few pairs of plano coquille (glazing) lenses. It is an unnecessary expense and time-consuming gesture to make up a "mocked-up" sample for ordinary orders, but there is nothing quite so satisfactory to both optician and patient as a model that shows precisely how a specially designed pair of glasses will look. It takes little time and effort to cut and mount a pair of plain lenses to the special size or shape the customer has described. If the effect is wrong, little has been lost and nothing is quite so convincing to the customer of a sincere effort to please. How much easier it is to offer to make up the idea than to argue why it is wrong and try to create an interest in something else. On occasion a dispenser has had a good idea given to him when he has kept his mind open by use of this approach. The expense of the lenses, the delay in finished work, and the extra visit in the store are more than repaid. The exacting patient appreciates that his special request or desire is receiving special attention. By this procedure, the optician avoids the loss of materials or prestige from a pair of glasses that must be made over because of disappointment caused by a layman's poor judgment or an optician's description which was misunderstood.

After the frame type and lens shape and size have been decided, the concluding decision is the style and length of the temples. Some frames are designed for only one type of temple, so length is the remaining measurement. In other instances, the intended use of the glasses determines the preference. Outdoor glasses for adults or glasses for children are frequently fitted with riding-bow temples for the sake of security. Many rimless or metal-framed glasses for constant wear are also chosen with riding-bow temples because a lighter adjustment of the glasses can be accomplished with some head shapes. Skull temples are indicated for all casual glasses. They are almost a necessity with some styles of women's hairdress. Persons with crippled hands or arms usually favor skull temples because they can be handled with one hand.

With the frame decided upon, the optician's attention again returns to the lens. Corrected curve "best form" lenses are used for all carefully filled prescriptions today. The posterior curves of the low powers of all of these lenses (which approximate Tscherning's ellipse) average point −6.50D. Therefore the glazing lenses in the sample show the approximate plane of the posterior lens surface. Corrected curve lenses have usually been designed for a separation of 13.75 mm from the corneal surface, but a slight reduction in this calculated distance does not materially affect the formula. The lenses are corrected for a 30° angle from center. With the lens closer to the eye, the same rotational angle does not intercept as large an area of the lens. It is accepted practice to fit the lenses so that the lashes barely clear the lens surface. There are many advantages in having the lenses close to the eyes, one of the most important of which is the fact that the lens size subtends a larger angle of the visual field. This is particularly important with reference to bifocal segments. A prominent nose, overhanging brows, or deep set eyes may preclude the possibility of fitting the lenses as closely as is desirable. Within limits an optician should, whenever possible, sacrifice the cosmetic effect of large lenses and manage the shape in such a way as to get the lenses closer to the eyes when strong lenses are fitted to this type of face.

A more common experience is the patient with a flat nose, prominent eyes, and long lashes. Rocking pads can often be adjusted to lift the lenses away from the face, and occasionally a slight amount of reconstruction by building up fixed pads on plastic frames will solve the problem. Deepening the base curve is occasionally attempted and *should be avoided*.

Increased concave curve on the back surfaces of lenses to increase clearance for lashes accomplishes much less than it appears. Even with a lens as long as 48 mm, the difference in the depth of curve between —6.00D. and —9.00D. is only 1.8 mm (Fig. 137). The cost of this gain is usually all out of proportion to the patient. The extra work in making the lenses on a special base increases the selling price of the lenses considerably. The bulging curves of the lenses are sometimes unsightly and only accentuate proptosed eyes. The lenses are difficult to retain in a frame unless the shape is nearly round. The most recent recalculations for marginally corrected lenses have tended toward flatter rather than deeper curves. All together it is much more satisfactory to use a little more imagination or ingenuity in the choice or fitting of the frame than it is to attempt to accomplish so much of the fitting by alteration of the profile of the lenses. The magnifying effect of increased curvature of the front surface of the lens should not be overlooked (see page 113).

The position of the optical centers, both vertical and horizontal, can become a part of a wearer's visual habit. Myopic eyes seem to be slightly more sensitive to changes than those of the hyperope. It is important, therefore, always to know the location of the centers of the old lenses when a new pair is being ordered. If the

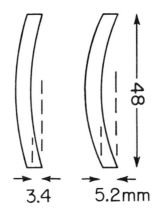

3.4   5.2mm

Figure 137. Small difference in depth on base curve increase.

old lenses were made in your own laboratory, the old records should suffice. It is worthwhile to routinely locate the centers of patients' old lenses in the lensometer. It is an absolute necessity when only one lens is being replaced. Some opticians decenter both lenses up large amounts to avoid using oversize lenses. If they are found to be unusually high or low, the subject should be discussed with the patient and possibly even with the doctor. The pantoscopic angle difference between the new and old eyeframe is another significant factor.

Saddle bridges should be avoided for babies and small children. The weight of the glasses on the bridge of an undeveloped nose can deform it seriously and permanently. Children's frames are now made to distribute the weight of the glasses over the widest possible area. A dispenser should encourage mothers to return frequently for him to observe and, as the occasion demands, alter the fitting of the contact area of the bridge as the nose begins to take shape during normal growth.

Occasionally after middle life, a skin condition may develop on the side of the nose in or near the point of contact of a pad. The simplest relief is a saddle bridge with a very shallow crest fitted to the top of the bridge of the nose. A 5 mm cylinder bridge made of solid gold is the best type in metal. The lenses should be made of CR39 hard-resin for lightness and the lens size should be minimum. Plastic saddle bridge frames are often useful for patients with nasal lesions. At the present time no manufacturer offers these frames from stock, but they can be had on special order. Only four or five bridge sizes are needed to care for these cases. In any event, many of these bridges will have to be individualized and rebuilt.

Frequently the tissue of the nose is badly deranged after injury and specific areas become especially sensitive. In some instances, the crest of the nose is more tolerant of pressure than the sides. A saddle bridge, rebuilt if necessary, often solves these problems.

EYEFRAME REQUIREMENTS

From time to time efforts have been made to interest the spectacle-wearing public in having more than one pair of glasses. Efforts have been made to classify eyeframes for certain social or other purposes, without much avail. The American public seems to express its independence in such matters. Rimless glasses are seen on the golf-course and colored lenses in a plastic frame are seen with formal clothes.

However, there is a minimum to spectacle requirements that will stand up against most arguments. The only resistance the wearer may have is that the optician cannot give him a better reason for having the glasses than the patient's excuse for spending the same money on something that he believes will give him greater enjoyment out of buying and having.

Even the wearer of low power prescription lenses is a candidate for a lightweight eyeframe with clear lenses for indoor use and a pair of photochromic or tinted lenses in a plastic frame for outdoors. If the prescription is for near use only, the doctor may wish his patient to have plano lenses in his sunglasses. The moderate power single vision prescription should be duplicated, for safety against loss or breakage, and different types of frames will prove to be restful. One pair could be designed for social wear. Outdoor glasses to prescription are indicated as above.

Presbyopes, especially women, who have weak plus or minus distance prescriptions are a special group. Many of them will not regularly wear glasses, and therefore the many kinds of casual glasses should be discussed with them. They may not wish to have their distance prescriptions made in clear glass, but will enjoy a dark tint for sports and outdoors. Very small segment bifocals should be discussed. Reading glasses for home should be plastic or plastic and metal with skull or straight temples. A small glove lorgnette in plastic or metal to wear on a cord or chain is a "must" for these women. As an alternate many styles of Spec-grips® are available with metal chains or braided cords. Otherwise shopping and marketing are a bore if reading glasses must be put on and taken off at each change of fixation distance. Non-folding oxfords or plastic straight-temple frames should be suggested to men in this group. More than one pair is not extravagance. These individuals continually leave their glasses behind.

Confirmed spectacle wearers who have become presbyopic are quite different again. To start, they should have a pair of clear bifocals with moderate size segments for ordinary use, a pair of very large segment bifocals for reading (or a pair of reading glasses for convenience and to serve as "spares" for breakage) , and a pair of dark-tinted lenses with small reading segments for daytime automobile driving and outdoors. Any special vocation may require special consideration, such as double segments. Later, the moderate segment clear lenses should be trifocal lenses after the total reading addition becomes as much as +2.00D.

REVIEW

1. What is an optician's First Commandment? Why is it so important?

2. What are some of the disadvantages that may arise from the use of technical language in conversation with a patient?

3. State three questions that a dispenser should ask himself before he proceeds with a fitting.

4. Explain fully why it is necessary to palpate the nasal bone in the area between the eyes.

5. Discuss the advantages of a catalogue numbering system for lenses. For frames.

6. Explain the Minimum Blank Size routine.

7. When should straight temples be avoided?

8. What is the important difference in the effect of lens shapes upon fitting when rimless and plastic frames are used?

9. Discuss the reason for attaching the pad to the guard arm above center.

ADDITIONAL REFERENCES

1. Marks, Roy: *An Investigation of the Anatomical Changes in the Shape of Children's Noses.* Rochester, Shuron, 1959.
2. Arnheim, Rudolph: *Art and Visual Perception.* Berkeley, U of Cal Pr, 1954.
3. Westmore, P.: *The Westmore Beauty Book.* Chicago, Korshak, 1956.

Chapter 10

SINGLE VISION PRESCRIPTION ANALYSIS

◆◆◆◆◆◆◆◆◆◆◆◆◆◆◆◆◆◆◆◆◆◆◆◆ ◆◆◆◆◆◆◆◆◆◆◆◆◆◆◆◆◆◆◆◆◆◆◆◆

The subject of "getting used to glasses" is important to an ophthalmic dispenser and some of the rudiments of the scientific
principles involved should be surveyed. As discussed in Chapter
4, the optical image on the retina is not sensed or interpreted at
the point of stimulation. It is projected as an object in space in
front of the eye. The ramifications and complications of this subject have attracted the attention of physiologists and psychologists
for many years.* That we are born with the faculty of localizing
objects in space is proved by the ability of a newborn baby to fixate
a bright object. Kant (1787) contended that this innate function
was unchangeable, but Nagel, Helmholtz, and others have followed
Locke (1690), who considered the appreciation of space to be
acquired by experience. Recent research seems to indicate that
an adult's perception is a combination of intuition and trial and
error.

In early life, vagueness or imperfection may be partly due to
poor coordination. However, it is apparent that a high degree of
discrimination is dependent upon the sensitivity of the retina at
the point where the image is formed. Because of an undeveloped

---

*Helmholtz, H. von: *Physiological Optics,* Vol. III, Menasha, Banta, 1924 p,p.
1-36.

Duke-Elder, Sir W.S.: *Text-Book of Ophthalmology.* St. Louis, Mosby, 1934,
pp. 1048-1058.

Emsley, H.H.: *Visual Optics.* London, Hatton, 1946, pp. 329-340, 493-505.

Southall, J.P.C.: *Introduction to Physiological Optics.* London, Oxford U Pr,
1937, pp. 221-231.

Parsons, Sir J.H.: *An Introduction to the Theory of Perception.* Cambridge,
Mass, Cambridge U Pr, 1927, pp. 152-160.

Gesell, A., Ilg, F.L., and Bullis, G.E.: *Vision, Its Development in Infant and
Child.* New York, Hoeber, 1949, pp. 155-161.

Prince, J.H.: *Visual Development.* Edinburgh, E. & S. Livingstone, 1947, pp.
8-21.

macula, visual acuity is quite low for the first year of life. The widely separated nerve-endings in the extreme periphery of the retina cannot produce the high degree of visual acuity of the retina in the region surrounding the macula (Fig. 138). The sharpness of the retinal image contributes to the accuracy of the projection. The aberrations of the optical system of the eye cause some degeneration of the image in the margin of the retina.

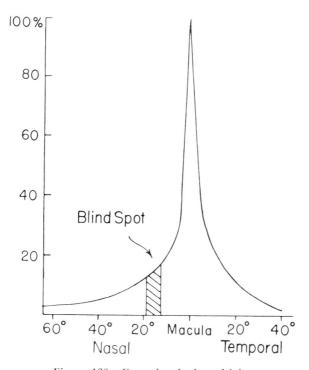

Figure 138. Central retinal sensitivity.

Figure 138 portrays the retinal sensitivity of the right eye. Since the optical nerve enters the eye from the nasal side, the blind spot is shown at 15° to 19° on the nasal side. The projected visual field is a reversed image of the retinal surface, the blind spot (Mariotte's) is on the nasal side of the retina and projected in the temporal field.

Ametropia, which affects the quality of the image over the

whole retina, affects perception of objects in space. Thus, the uncorrected hyperope learns to associate the additional amount of accommodation with all distances, the myope's acuity diminishes beyond his far point and becomes progressively worse toward infinity. The astigmatic patient associates some degree of meridianal distortion with all things in space. Pulfrich (1922) has also demonstrated that a difference of about 12 percent in the illumination of the two retinal images is enough to disturb spatial perception.

Contemplation of this subject as a problem in geometric optics for monocular vision is reduced to insignificance when the complexities of binocular vision are considered. The individual visual fields are limited by the brows, nose, and cheeks. The fields superimpose (Fig. 139a) when the eyes are in primary position to provide an area about 60° on either side of the fixation line *(z-axis)* in the horizontal meridian and about 70° up and 75° down where all objects are imaged in both eyes.

On either side in the horizontal meridian for another 30° to 35°, objects are seen by only one eye. When the maculae of the two eyes are fixed upon a single object, the retinal images of the two eyes are mentally interpreted as one object. For a short distance in all directions surrounding the maculae, corresponding areas and even corresponding points of the retinas are stimulated by the object space surrounding the fixation point **M** in Figure 140. It

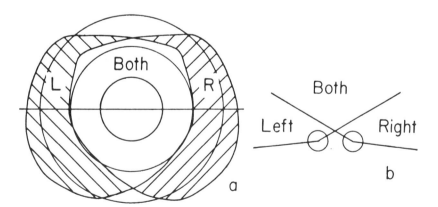

Figure 139. Area of binocular vision.

is apparent, however, that an object at point **Q** makes different angles at the nodal points of the right and left eyes and corresponding points of the two retinas are not stimulated. When point **Q** is not too far removed from the fixation point, the object is seen double (physiologic diplopia), because the two images Q'_R and Q'_L are different distances from the images of point **M**.

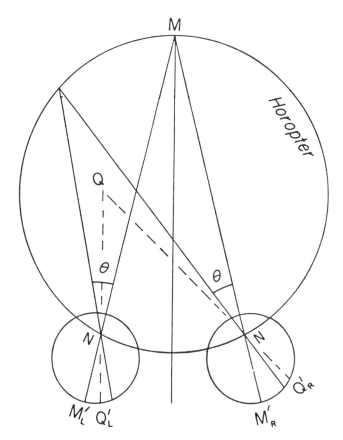

Figure 140. Horopter (projection of retinal correspondence).

By several means the location of the projection of corresponding points of the retina in the object space have been located. The first investigator, Aguillon (1613), named this surface the *horopter.** Study of the performance of the two eyes from a geometrical point of view led to the statement that two eyes looking at a single star had parallel visual axes. Hence all other stars would make identical angles with the visual axes and the images would fall upon corresponding retinal points. Perception of these identical images as single images is known as fusion. Subsequent research by Hering, Hillibrand, and most recently Ames, Glidden, Ogle and others at Dartmouth Eye Institute has established several facts:

1. Fixation at shorter distances than the sky causes the *horopter* to curve toward the viewer on both sides.
2. The location and contour of the surface is different for every pair of eyes.
3. Discrimination pertaining to spatial projection varies greatly with different individuals.
4. Environmental changes that alter this perception affect some patients severely.
5. The period of readaptation after a change varies from immediacy to a matter of months.

The fourth and fifth observations occasionally involve an ophthalmic dispenser. Now and then a first prescription, or a radical change, produces dizziness or nausea at the adjusting table and temporary unsteadiness when the patient attempts to stand or walk. In most instances the necessary adjustment is promptly made and compensation is complete in a day or so. Sometimes the patient will return even after several days with a complaint that the sidewalk runs uphill or downhill or that everything is tipped at an angle.

---

*Ogle, K.N.: *Binocular Vision*. Philadelphia, Saunders, 1950, p. 14ff.

Techerning, M.: *Physiological Optics*. Philadelphia, Keystone Press, 1904, pp. 304-312

Stevens, G.T.: *The Motor Apparatus of the Eyes*. Philadelphia, Davis, Co., 1906, pp. 177-194.

Southall, J.P.C.: *Introduction to Physiological Optics*. London, Oxford U Pr, 1937, pp. 221-231.

Luneburg, R.K.: *Mathematical Analysis of Binocular Vision*. Princeton, Princeton U Pr, 1947, pp. 61-73.

Waters, E.H.: *Ophthalmic Mechanics*. Ann Arbor, Edwards Bros, 1947, pp. 61-64.

Study shows that the possible changes that have taken place through the environmental change of even a very weak prescription are tremendous. The relationship between accommodation and convergence is altered by the lenses. Convex lenses relieve (inhibit) accommodative effort; but since the same amount of convergence is still required for all points, the ratio between the functions is changed. Concave lenses clear up visual acuity at distance and enforce a greater accommodative effort at near. Unless the prescriptions for the two eyes are identical, the images at corresponding points are equally clear for the first time. Practically all spectacle lenses change the retinal image size to some degree and in most instances dissimilar prescriptions produce unequal magnification. The rapid absorption of the new conditions by the vast majority of all lens wearers is a compliment to the physiological and psychological adaptability of these individuals.

Referring to the prism experiments recommended in Chapter 3, these alterations to accommodation-convergence association are easily understood.

1. *Hyperopia:*
    R + 1.00
    L. + 1.00

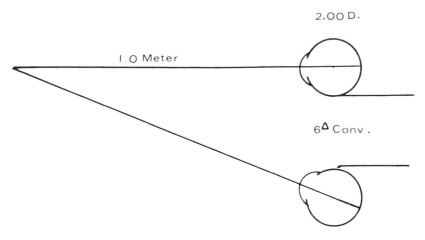

Figure 141. Rearrangement of hyperope's accommodation and convergence with lens correction.

To see at one meter without glasses this pair of eyes accommodated +2.00D. (+1.00D. to overcome the hyperopia and +1.00D. for the fixation distance).

With +1.00D. lenses, now only +1.00D. of accommodation is required but the same amount of convergence (about 15ᐃ) is required. Formerly when they viewed at distance +1.00D. accommodation was associated with *no* convergence.

The prism Base Out in the experiment demonstrated (converging more than the habitual amount) this patient's new stress is upon *Positive Fusion Convergence.*

2. *Myopia:*
   R. − 2.50
   L. − 2.50

As would be expected, with concave lenses conditions are reversed.

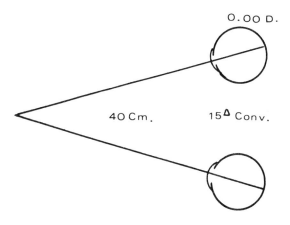

Figure 142. Rearrangement of myope's accommodation and convergence with lens correction.

At infinity all objects are blurred without lenses, but at 40 cm, the focus of − 2.50D. spheres vision has always been keen without any accommodative effort. But these eyes have associated 15ᐃ convergence with no accommodation.

With the prescription lenses, vision is now clear at distance without accommodation and also *no* convergence can be tolerated.

At 40 cm 2.50D. accommodation is now required but no more convergence than was formerly used at this distance. The restraint was to not to converge more because accommodation was now activated. The burden is now upon *Negative Fusion Convergence* to restrain the associated convergence.

The prism Base In experiment described on page 31 was a demonstration of using less than the habitual amount of convergence with a certain amount of accommodation. Remember the "drawn" feeling when very much prism Base In was placed before your eyes?

3. Astigmatism:
This problem of adaptation is not so easily explained because, as you remember, there are five different possibilities where the rays were directed for hyperopic, mixed, and myopic astigmatism. Further, the axis could be at an oblique angle which would twist or distort vertical and horizontal lines. Relief from the acceptance of these twisted images required considerable adaptation.

A useful device to acquaint the reluctant and occasionally irritated patient with his new glasses is to have him take them home and not wear them until the following morning. Tell him to put his glasses beside his bed and immediately upon awakening in the morning put them on—before he gets out of bed. Tell him to keep them on and that if he must remove them, to keep his eyes closed; if the glasses become intolerable he may take them off and leave them off for the remainder of the day. Instruct him to repeat the process every morning for a week, then come in and report. In practically all instances, the adaptation will be complete. This presents a first step in aftercare and therefore *must* be followed with personal contact by telephone. However, those who do come back a week later do have something wrong. Occasionally some kind of change in the prescription or lens form is required; even a change of the style of frame has been known to help! It is a good practice to have a reminder to phone those patients who do not come in after about two weeks. It signifies interest in their comfort and occasionally repairs relations when the customer thinks that no further help is intended.

In the foregoing discussion it was assumed that the eyes continued to stand in the primary position. Identical prescription lenses before the eyes produce symmetric and tolerable prism effect from decentration as the eyes verge in any direction. Along with the spatial perception adjustments for the power and shape of the lenses, the patient quickly learns to accept the displacement in the extra axial portions of the prescription lenses and finally he is totally unaware of it. This adaptation includes very strong lenses such as those required after cataract surgery. This adjustment to a new visual space tends to refute lengthy discussions about symmetric prism effects of lenses at all distances from the lens axis. Despite the large amount of prism that appears in a geometric construction of his lenses, he learns to rectify the displacement in much the same way the image in the rear vision mirror of an automobile is interpreted. The mirror reports that an automobile is coming down out of the clouds for a head-on collision, but experience, not vision, tells the driver to pull over toward the side of the road to let the car pass him from the rear.

When the prescription lenses are not identical, a new effect is producted at all extra-axial points. Dissimilar amounts of prism are generated by decentration. This effect is directly related to the difference in the powers of the two lenses and the distance and direction the intercepts of the z-axes of the eyes have moved from the optical centers of the lenses. When the refractive error of the two eyes is not equal, the condition is called *anisometropia*. In clinical refraction procedure, the term is usually reserved for those cases where the prescriptions are markedly different. From the aspect of spectacle fitting, there are likely many prescriptions with rather small differences that produce optical effects like those with large differences in lens power. Careful customer records for bifocal patients must have a line to show the optical difference in lenses and, when corrective measures are instituted, whether dissimilar segments or slab-off are needed and how much. Whether the induced imbalance is significant for an individual case will be disclosed in the eye examination because it is a function of the patient's (a) monocular visual acuity, (b) muscle balance, (c) tendency for suppression, and (d) general nervous condition.

Aside from prism generated by the vergences in which the eyes turn equal angles in the same direction, there is also the function of convergence when the z-axes turn toward one another and intersect at the fixation point. At the lens plane, the axes intersect the lenses about 2.0 mm to the nasal side of the optical centers for infinity when the eyes converge at the reading distance. This amount of decentration is rather insignificant in the majority of lens prescriptions. However, when Prentice's rule is applied to the power of cataract lenses, $+10.00D. \times 0.3$ cm equals $3^{\triangle}$ Base Out, which if it is not overcome by additional convergence effort means that objects are separated about 12 mm at a reading distance of 40 cm (16 inches).

It is common practice to consider the lens power in a single meridian and calculate the prism effect through that direction for the required amounts. For some purposes the method is satisfactory but as the prescriptions for the two eyes vary, many important effects can be easily overlooked if the effects of the lenses at all extra-axial points are not investigated.

BOEDER'S ISOBARS

In 1939 Paul Boeder, Ph.D., used illustrations in his book *Analysis of Prism Effect in Bifocal Lenses* which graphically show the distance at which units of prism are generated by decentration. The shapes of these isobars are circles for spheres, parallel lines for cylinders, ellipses for generic $(+ \smile + \text{ or} - \frown -)$ spherocylinders and hyperbolas for contrageneric $(- \smile + \text{ or} + \frown -)$ lenses. It is regrettable that all these shapes cannot all be drawn with simple tools because they demonstrate lens effects so dramatically. The illustrations to follow are scaled to 50 mm round lenses. The wedges represent the direction of the bases of the prism induced by decentration.

EXAMPLE:

O.D. $+ 1.25$ D.

O.S. $+ 0.50$ D.

What is the optical difference of these lenses?

O.D.		O.S		O.D.
$+1.25$	$-$	$(+0.50)$	$=$	$+0.75$

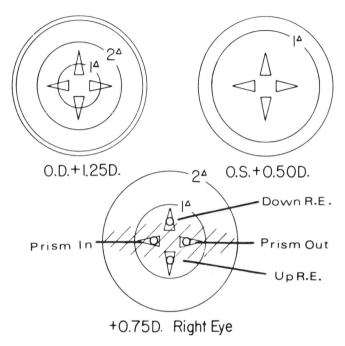

O.D.+1.25D.   2ᐃ   O.S.+0.50D.

+0.75D. Right Eye

Figure 143. Zone of comfort with dissimilar lenses.

It is always necessary to keep in mind which lens is the minuend (the lens from which the other is subtracted) in order to know the direction of the base of the prism. The prism effect at extra-axial points for this patient is similar to a prescription of +0.75D. before the right eye and plano before the left. Since the difference, or remainder, is a plus sphere, the prism base is always toward the lens center. When the eyes turn away from primary position, these are the effects:

Both eyes Right   15 mm, +0.75 × 1.5 = 1.12ᐃ Base In
Both eyes Down   8 mm, +0.75 × 0.8 = 0.6ᐃ Base Up Right Eye
Both eyes Left   10 mm, +0.75 × 1.0 = 0.75ᐃ Base Out
Both eyes Up   12 mm, +0.75 × 1.2 = 0.9ᐃ Base Down Right Eye

If the individual's tolerance of induced prism is found to be 0.5ᐃ in the vertical meridian and 2.0ᐃ Base In or Out across the horizontal meridian, the zone of comfortable binocular vision with this pair of lenses is confined within the shaded area shown in the lower diagram of Figure 143. When the fixation lines intersect the lenses inside of this area, the asymmetric prescription is tolerable.

There are no complications in finding the differences between spheres, plane cylinders, and even spherocylinders when the cylinder axes are coincident or at right angles to one another (Fig. 144).

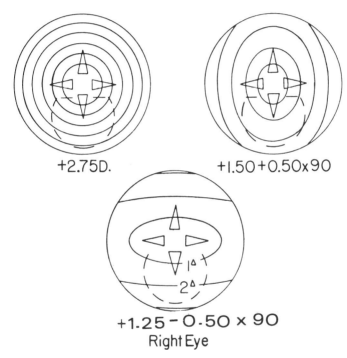

+2.75D.   +1.50+0.50x90

+1.25 − 0.50 × 90
Right Eye

Figure 144. Extra-axial prism in anisometropia.

EXAMPLES

1. ℞:
   O.D. +275
   O.S. +1.50 + 050 ×90
   Subtracting   D.D. +275
                  O.S. − 1.50 −050 × 90
                  ─────────────────────
                  +1.25 − 050 × 90

Notice that the isobars of the left lens are vertical ellipses. It follows that these isobars have the same position whether the lens is expressed with plus or minus cylinders. It is interesting to note that the diagram representing the optical difference is horizontal ellipses which can be transposed to $+0.75 + 0.50 \times 180$ still with horizontal elipses. On occasion it may be difficult to decide which lens is the minuend (stronger). When the power or sign of the cylinders seems to obscure the difference in lens strength, reduce the two lenses to their spherical equivalents.

2. ℞:

     O.D. $-1.00 + 3.50 \times 60$
     O.S. $+2.50 + 1.00 \times 150$

$$-1.00 + \frac{+\ 3.50}{2} = +0.75D., \text{ the spherical equivalent}$$

$$+2.50 + \frac{+1.00}{2} = +3.00D., \text{ the spherical equivalent}$$

Therefore, the right lens is subtracted from the left (that is, change the signs of the powers and add). Since the axes of the cylinders are at right angles the right lens is transposed to

     O.D. $+\ 2.50 - 3.50 \times 150$

in order to bring the axes in agreement.

         O.S. $+2.50 \ +1.00 \times 150$
    (−) O.D. $+2.50 - 3.50 \times 150$

When the signs of the weaker lens have been changed to subtract, the powers are:

         O.S. $+2.50 \ +1.00 \times 150$
    (+) O.D. $-2.50 \ +3.50 \times 150$
             ——————————
             $+4.50 \times 150$ (O.S.)

The difference between the lenses in this prescription is the effect of a strong cylinder with the axis near the horizontal meridian. From Table IV it is seen that $150°$ ($30°$ from 180) $= 25\%$. Hence, $0.25 \times +4.50 = +1.12D.$ is the lens curve in the horizontal meridian. In the vertical meridian $30°$ from $90° = 60°$ or $75°\%$. It follows that $.75 \times 4.50 + +3.37D.$ is active. If the limits of prism tolerance of the previous case are applied in this instance, the '"zone of binocular comfort" is limited to the axial area in Figure 145.

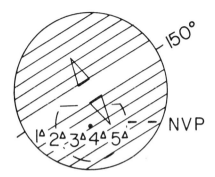

Figure 145. Zone of comfort in anisometropia.

Each 3 mm of vergence of the eyes in the vertical meridian creates $1^\triangle$ in the opposite direction before the right eye. The average reading position of 8 mm below center means about $3^\triangle$ Base Up before the right eye which is insuperable. The results as experienced in the prism experiment are vertical diplopia, usually followed by suppression of vision of one eye. The prism effect is reversed about center and is especially distressing in the upper temporal and lower nasal areas. The reversing stresses against fusion convergence should cause a never-ending problem for these eyes in any area except the paracentral zone of the lenses. Some possible assistance for the bifocal reading segment area would be $4^\triangle$ slab-off on the left lens ideally at axis 150.

3. When the cylinder axes of the two lenses are crossed obliquely, the calculation of the difference is a bit more tedious, but all the more important. Frequently rather innocuous looking prescriptions induce prism effects in the area of the bifocal segments which may preclude binocular reading comfort. Conversely, many lens prescriptions that seem rather formidable are shown to be quite tolerable when analyzed. The vector method described in "Combining Obliquely Crossed Cylinders" in Chapter 5 serves handily for this problem.

The rules to combine obliquely *crossed cylinders* are supplemented by the *power difference* rules for these lenses:

a. Reduce the prescriptions to spherical equivalents to determine the minuend (stronger lens) .

b. Change the signs of the weaker lens and add the lenses.
c. Combine crossed cylinders.
   (1) Transpose the cylinders to plus values.
   (2) Choose the largest usable unit and plot the cylinder (A) with the axis closer to zero (180°) on metric polar coordinate paper.
   (3) Double the difference between the cylinder axes and add this amount to the axis of the first (A) cylinder. Plot the other cylinder power (B) in this meridian.
   (4) From the ends of the lines **A** and **B,** draw the lines to complete a parallelogram. Use a compass for accuracy.
   (5) The diagonal of the parallelogram is the power of the resultant cylinder (**C**).
   (6) Find the midline between the axis of the diagonal and the axis of cylinder **A.** This is the axis of **C,** the new cylinder.
   (7) Some spherical power is induced when oblique cylinders are combined. The amount is half the difference between the resultant cylinder and the sum of the original cylinders or

$$\text{The induced sphere} = \frac{(A + B) - C}{2}$$

For example
    O.D. $+ 1.75 + 1.50 \times 60$
    O.S. $+ 1.00 + 2.00 \times 85$
The spherical equivalents are

$$+1.75 + \frac{+1.50}{2} = +2.50$$

$$+1.00 + \frac{+2.00}{2} = +2.00$$

Hence, left lens power is subtracted from the right.
    To substract, change the signs of the left lens and add
        $+1.75 +1.50 \times 60$
        $-1.00 -2.00 \times 85$

$$+0.75 \begin{cases} +1.50 \times 60 \\ -2.00 \times 85 \end{cases}$$

To combine these crossed-cylinders
(a) Transpose to cylinders with the same sign

$$+ 1.50 \times 60$$
$$- 2.00 + 2.00 \times 175$$

(b) $175 - 60 = 115°$ $115 \times 2 = 230°$

The diagonal of the parallelogram is 1.55D.

The midpoint of the side of the parallelogram between the diagonal and the axis of cylinder A is 19°.

The induced sphere is:

$$\frac{A + B - C}{2} = \frac{+2.00 + 1.50 - 1.55}{2} = \frac{195}{2} = +0.98$$

The total sphere is:

$$+0.75$$
$$-2.00$$
$$+0.98$$
$$\overline{-0.27}$$

The combination is $-0.27 + 1.55 \times 19$

With the axis 20° from 180° (horizontal) the vertical curvature of the cylinder is $88° \times 1.55 = 1.35$D. The total vertical effect is $-0.27 + 1.37 = 1.10$D. Hence at the N.V.P. 8 mm below center $= 0.8^{\triangle}$ Base Up Right Eye.

Since the vertical power of this optical difference is substantially $+1.25$D $(+1.55 - 0.27)$ the vertical limits of the "zone of comfort" are about $\pm$ 5 mm from the optical axis. As was shown, pantoscopically inclined lenses have the optical axes (lens centers) in the vertical meridian 4 to 6 mm below the primary position. Hence, the wearer of this prescription can be provided with comparatively comfortable vision for the ordinary use of eyes. Only vertical vergences will require the head to be turned up or down to retain comfortable binocular vision.

Finding Lens and Prism Powers by Lensometer

The lensometer can also be used to make a rapid estimation of this difference in power. Choose from stock an uncut lens of the power of the minuend. Choose a lens of the power of the weaker lens with *opposite signs*. In this way the power of the weaker lens is being subtracted to find the optical difference. Lay out both lenses for the prescribed axes. Carefully stack the weaker lens on top of the minuend and place both lenses in the lensometer with centers and horizontal lines in proper position. A spot of balsam secures them. Find the power of the combined lenses. This will agree very closely with the plotted or calculated result. A small but inconsequential error in lens power is induced because the weaker lens is slightly removed from the nose of the lensometer.

When the lens is plotted by zones, one can instantly appreciate the prism effect. Figure 146 is plotted as a 50 mm round lens. For example, if the eyes turn an angle of 45° to the right (to the edge of a 50 mm lens) in the horizontal meridian, only 0.47 prism Base In is generated. When the eyes turn to the left, the prism is Base Out. However, when the eyes are raised or lowered, prism is generated more rapidly. One Prism Diopter is generated for each 4.8 mm. The prism is Base Down Right Eye when it looks up and Base Up when it looks down. As you have already learned, the ability to overcome prism in the vertical meridian is very limited.

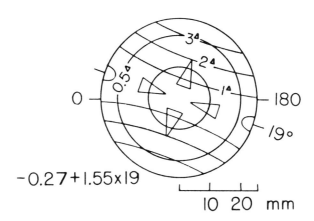

Figure 146. Extra-axial prism of resultant contrageneric (− ⊃ +) lens.

LENS PLACEMENT

Probably the first attempt to produce individualized lenses was to place the optical centers of the lenses at the centers of the pupils. Helmholtz* was the first to describe and give the terminals of the

*Helmholtz, H. von: *Physiological Optics*, Vol. I. Menosha, Banta, 1924, pp. 350-358, 392.

line to accurately set the centers of the lenses. This line has been named the Helmholtz base line. It connects the centers of rotation of the two eyes, and its length is established when the P.D. is measured. However, this axis is only one of the three dimensions of a prescription lens. These dimensions are: (1) the horizontal axis, the 180° meridian or x-axis, (2) the vertical axis, the 90° meridian or y-axis and (3) the optical axis which perpendicularly intersects the x, y plane in Figure 147 and projects through the center of rotation of the eye, the z-axis.

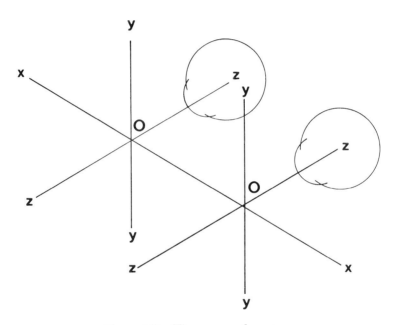

Figure 147. The *x*-, *y*-, and z-axes

The construction in Figure 147 is valid only when the lenses are set precisely vertical and when the eyes are in primary position with fixation at infinity. If the lenses are tipped forward at the top (pantoscopic angle), the axis of rotation is not the x-axis as illustrated in Figure 148. It moves back to the terminals of the Helmholtz base line at the centers of rotation of the eyes.

If the lenses are rotated to reduce one vertex distance while the vertex distance before the other eye increases, the rotation is

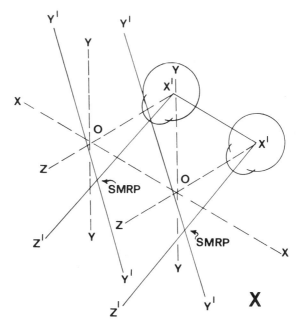

Figure 148. Tilted on x-axis.

not on the y-axes in Figure 149. The new rotation axis is at or very near the center of the bridge. Both lens axes are forced to the right or left of the centers of rotation.

Tilting the eyewear so that one lens is lower than the other is not a rotation upon the z-axes, as shown in Figure 150. The lenses rotate upon the midpoint of the line between the point of contact of the pads of the bridge. This point is on or very near the axis of the cyclopean center which is the projection of the binoculus. Thus, the common intersection points of the individual lenses are in disarray. This situation has received small, if any, attention in our literature. Disregard of any of these axes causes the prescription lens to deviate from the power described by the prescriber.

Long ago, lens makers knew little more about aberration than that an angled or a tilted lens created an astigmatic image, hence books on spectacle fitting concentrated on this one factor for many years.

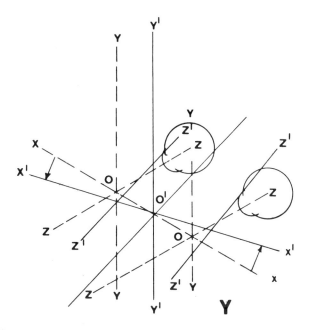

Figure 149. Turned on y-axis.

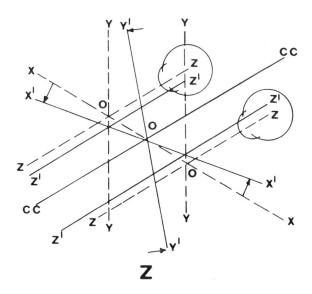

Figure 150. Turned on z-axis.

322   *Ophthalmic Dispensing*

In 1890, C.H. Brown, M.D., started a series of articles which were later published in a book entitled *Optician's Manual** in 1896. He made reference, probably the first, to the practice of tipping the bottom edge of lenses toward the cheek.

> Pantoscopic glasses, so-called, have the upper part of the rims flattened in order to permit the wearer of reading glasses to see over them in looking at distant objects; the lenses are also set, as a rule, obliquely to the direction of the side pieces, but perpendicular to the visual axis in reading.

Thus, he had given the optical justification for the placement of the plane of the lenses at an angle to the face plane.

At the time this was written (1896), the astigmatism of a titled lens was the only central aberration published. Calculated for a thin lens, the mathematics involved was simple. It is interesting to note that practically all writers since Doctor Brown have limited their discussion of improper lens placement to this one aberration. Despite the fact that point-focal lenses were described and designed within the next ten to twenty years, and oblique (marginal) aberrations of lenses were carefully described, the correct position of the lens center in the vertical meridian was totally neglected. True, this phase of lens designing involves lens thickness and lens curves (profile) which intails third order mathematics. Unfortunately, scientists, such as Tscherning, Ostwald, Wallaston, Gullstrand, and von Rohr, described their work in langauge that only those who were competent in advanced mathematics could apprehend. It would seem that practically all subsequent writers did not, or could not, make the effort to simplify and clarify the importance of lens axis, thickness, surface curvatures (profile or Base Curve) and vertex distance. At the risk of becoming laborious, I have listed a sample of the discussion of tilted lenses (induced axial aberration) as each author has repeated no more than what has been said before by previous writers.

In 1907, Taylor† said,

---

*Brown, C.H.: *The Optician's Manual*. Philadelphia, Keystone, 1896, p. 105.

†Taylor, H.L.: *The Manipulation and Fitting of Ophthalmic Frames*. Birmingham, H & H Taylor, 1907, p. 82.

Percival, A.S.: *The Prescribing of Spectacles*. Bristol, John Wright & Sons, 1910, p. 131.

. . . the centers of the lenses . . . 3 mm or so lower than the visual axis . . . in addition, provision must be made for tilting the lenses, so that their plane shall be perpendicular to the visual axis in this position of the eyes, and this is effected by angling the joint downward upon the eyewires, the sides being 10°, 20°, or more out of the perpendicular with the lenses.

In 1910, Percival[†] gave a detailed description of the aberration induced by lenses that have their axes tilted 10° to 35° from the visual axis, to become temporary spherocylindrical lenses after cataract surgery, but made no mention of inclining lenses to correct the tilted lens effect in eccentric (reading) angles. In 1916, Pixley* said, ". . . and the lenses tilted back a little at the bottom, so that the line of vision will be at right angles to the plane of the lenses when reading. . . ." Sir Duke-Elder,[†] in 1928, added little to what had been said before. In the same year, Olsho's[‡] book reporting research since 1920 made a great stride in establishing a line of communication between ophthalmologist and optician by his proposal of a "base line" which used the outer canthi as its end-points. Despite this huge improvement over previous suggestions for the determination of the *"x" axis* of the lens space before the eyes, it was not complete. It did not discuss the vertical position of the center.

Four years later, E.T. Hartinger* agreed with Doctor Olsho, but took exception to the vertical height of the base line.

With all due respect to the doctor for his theory, which is a decided

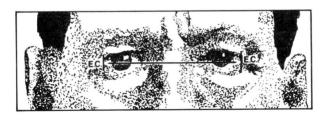

Figure 151. Line joining outer canthi.

*Pixley, C.H.: *An Optical Primer*. Chicago, F.A. Hardy, 1916, p. 171.

†Duke-Elder, Sir Stewart: *The Practice of Refraction*. Longdon, J & A Churchill, 1928, pp. 263 and 281.

‡Olsho, S.L.: *The Coordination of Refraction with Spectacle and Eyeglass Fitting*. Philadelphia, Pelham Pub, 1928, pp. 3-7.

improvement upon thoughtless fitting, I do not think it is low enough. Where it is possible, fit glasses 2 or 3 mm below a line from one canthus to the other.

Thus, he demonstrated that he had misunderstood Doctor Olsho's intention. The doctor was describing a line or axis and not a definite position (vertically) of it.

In 1964, Epting and Morgret[†] wrote,

> When a lens is tilted, its spherical power is changed and cylinder is induced. The relationship between the amount of tilt and these changed powers is stated in Martin's formulae for tilt.

In 1968, Bennett[‡] wrote a new edition of Emsley and Swaine's *Ophthalmic Lenses* and in it he made a most admirable and complete discussion of optical centers and lens tilt, concluding with the comment that the subject had been sadly neglected.

Drew,[§] in 1970, presented the most extensive story about vertical centering to offset aberrations but, in his usual lighthearted manner, did not emphasize the importance of his presentation.

Dowaliby,[‖] 1972, discussed the effect of lenses tilted on the optical axis and gave several examples, but made no mention of means to dispose of the objectionable result in prescription lenses.

It remained for Fry and Ellerbrock[¶] to develop and set forth the *inexorable* relationship between the angle of lens plane and position of the vertical lens center. They demonstrated how the lens axis should ideally remain congruent with the visual axis in all directions of the eye rotation. Except for contact lenses, which are adherent to the eye, this is not possible. But, when the individual pantoscopic angle has been determined, the lens plane

---

*Hartinger, E.T.: *The Opticians Dispensing Manual*. New York, E.T. Hartinger, 1932, p. 42.

†Epting, J.B. & Morgret, Jr., F.C.: *Ophthalmic Mechanics and Dispensing*. Philadelphia, Chilton, 1964, pp. 114, 206, 269.

‡Bennett, A.G.: *Ophthalmic Lenses*. London, Hatton Press, 1968, pp. 166-168.

§Drew, Ralph: *Professional Ophthalmic Dispensing*. Chicago, Prof Press, 1970, pp. 210-212.

‖Dowaliby, Margaret: *Practical Aspects of Ophthalmic Optics*. Chicago, Prof. Press, 1972, pp. 171-175.

¶Fry, G.A. and Ellerbrock, V.J.: Placement of optical centers in single vision lenses. *Optometric Weekly, 32*:933-936, September 25, 1941.

should be parallel to it. Hence, the optical centers of the lenses are regularly slightly below the visual axis in primary position, because the lens plane is slightly inclined away from the brow line. This geometric approach to the matter concludes and defines the required angle of the lens tilt.

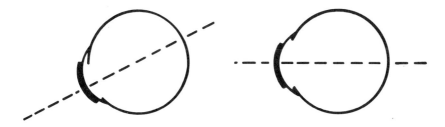

Contact lenses

Figure 152. Contact lens axis is constant.

When a lens is tilted from a vertical position, the lens center must be lowered the distance **OA** which is the tangent of angle θ. This is also the angle at **C**, the center of rotation of the eye. If the distance of the vertex of the prescription lens is 27 mm from the center of rotation **C**, the distance **OA** the lens is lowered is:

$$\mathbf{OA} = \mathbf{AC} \tan \theta$$

EXAMPLE: at 2° tilt

$$\mathbf{OA} = 27 \tan 2° \ (.0349) = .9423$$
$$= \text{approximately 1 mm}$$

From this equation, a table can be set up.

TABLE XIV
CENTER DROP WITH PANTOSCOPE ANGLE

Pantoscopic Angle	Drop Optical Center
2°	1.0 mm
4°	1.9
6°	2.8
8°	3.8
10°	4.8
12°	5.7

Because the angles are small, the ratio of approximately 2:1 is consistent. Therefore, the center of the lens is lowered 1 mm for each 2° increase in pantoscopic angle. Despite their otherwise thorough paper, they slighted the clinical application of their observations.

In 1963, Davis* wrote an extensive discussion of pantosopic angle and vertical lens center placement. He does not give the means of clinical application. His effort was only to ". . . point out and illustrate better relationships and to indicate factors which must be considered. . .".

Recently, Sasieni† spent considerable space in the section on frames explaining the position of lens centers in inclined lens planes, but he failed to pick up the subject again in the lens section of his comprehensive book and apply the information to the individual fitting.

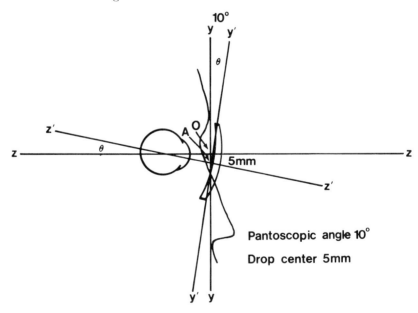

Figure 153. Center position of tilted lens.

*Davis, John K.: *Optical, Cosmetic and Mechanical Properties of Ophthalmic Lenses.* Southbridge, Mass., American Optical Co, 1963, pp. 31-34.

†Sasieni, L.S.: *Principles and Practice of Optical Dispensing and Fitting,* 3rd Ed. London, Butterworths, 1975, pp. 155-156.

Major Reference Point (MRP)

Major Reference Point, first used by Fry and Ellerbrock, is defined in the ANSI-Z80.1‡ glossary as "That point on an uncut lens which satisfies all of the specified distance prescription requirements and which is marked MRP.

1. For a prescription lens which is not decentered, this point is congruent (identical) with the optical center (z-axis. of the lens.
2. For a decentered lens, this point is placed at the appropriate decentered position to meet the specifications of the laboratory order.
3. For a planocylinder, this point has no dimension in the meridian of the cylinder axis; however, it has a specific position in the other principal meridian.
4. For a planoprism, this point is assigned the position of the geometric center of the prescription lens shape.
5. For a spherocylinder with prism, this point is that position where the precise amount of prism and prism base direction are specified.

In many places in this text the word *center* or *x-axis* is used instead of MRP. In each, the text implies a centered (not decentered) lens.

Once Fry and Ellerbrock's reasoning has been absorbed, it becomes very clear that, since Brown's first reference to lens tilt in 1896 until 1941, no other writer has clarified the required position of the lens center in the vertical meridian. Fry and Ellerbrock established the optical principle most capably but, like previous writers, paid scant heed to how these data would be clinically applied. Like all other half-told tales, this phase of prescription lens fitting has been largely a subject of controversial opinions. Actually, their work is based upon physiological optics but, until their paper, most of the criteria had been based upon anatomy, such as "lines perpendicular to the sides of the head," "real horizontal line," "high eye," "brow line," etc.

Let us first explore the fact that each person has an individual

---

‡American National Standards Institute: *Z80 Lens Standards.*

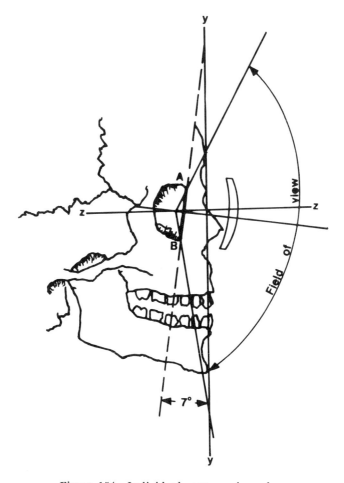

Figure 154. Individual pantoscopic angle.

pantoscopic angle. This angle is established by the shape of the skull (as described by Olsho) in the area of the orbit and shows the bony landmarks of the vertical limits of the field of view, namely, the upper rim of the orbit A and the corresponding point on the lower rim B. Thus, an overhanging brow would limit the upper visual field or a full cheek bone would have similar effect on the extent of the lower visual area. When the line of sight is at the midpoint of AB, the visual fields are practically symmetric in the vertical meridian. Investigations in the past have shown the habitual position of the eye is very near that position most of the time. Although we may momentarily move our eyes away from this position, such as to read, the head will soon be inclined forward and the eyes return nearer to the midpoint position. Bifocals demand that the eyes remain depressed for nearpoint vision. It has been maintained that this alteration of habit sometimes contributes to the task of learning to wear bifocals.

When the plane of the lens and spectacle rim are parallel to the line AB and the lens center is at the point of the lens plane which projects the lens axis through the center of rotation of the eye, the lens is at some inclination to vertical when the face plane is vertical. This inclination or angle is the individual's pantoscopic angle. From this it follows that the optical centers of prescription lenses must be some distance below the pupil center when the eye is in primary position. The distance is a function of the pantoscopic angle. Fortunately, the position of the eyeframe bridge on the nose and the shape of many lenses combine to set the center of the lens pattern below the pupil center in primary position.

Thus far, I have presented this subject in its classical form. The geometrical optics involved and the physiological limits determined by the shape of the orbital area are consistent, but the means of the clinical application of these data has not been discussed.

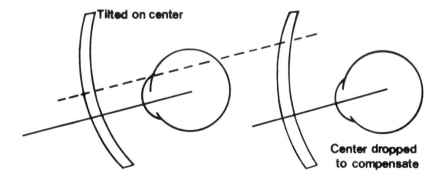

Figure 155. Center dropped to compensate.

Historic Frame Fitting

Let us trace the individualization or custom fitting of eyeframes. At the beginning of the twentieth century, practically all spectacles had saddle bridges and easily adjustable endpieces. The approximate bridge size was selected from a sample set. When the completed eyewear was presented for delivery, a few deft bends with appropriate pliers rolled the bridge crest forward or backward as well as raised or lowered the bridge, and finally perfected the crest angle to lay flat on the nose. Small twists of the endpieces altered the temple angles to tip the bottoms of the lenses toward the cheeks. Hence, the completed spectacles were customized at the fitting table, often by the man who had produced the glasses. Even the distance between lens centers to match the P.D. was easily adjusted. Bifocal segments were ordered 3 mm down and $1\frac{1}{2}$ mm in for everyone and the proper individual position was established by plierwork on the bridge. In all truth, the glasses were fitted (or customized) at the fitting table. These circumstances demanded few specifications, aside from lens power, at the time the order was taken. However, eyeglasses required more attention in order writing. Little could be done at delivery time to make basic changes of these mountings.

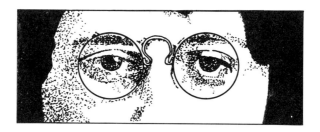

Figure 156. Centered eyeglasses.

After 1920, when imitation shell (zylonite) frames grew in popularity, the former *laissez faire* was diminished. But still, there were 48 bridge dimensions from which to choose. Little bridge modification could be made on these frames at delivery time. In about 1920, gold pads were attached to the sides of the crests of metal saddle bridges to take the weight of the glasses.

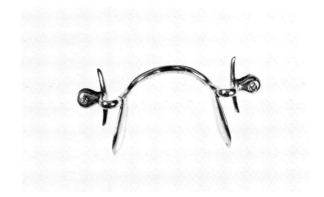

Figure 157. First pad bridge.

This change required more careful bridge selection. The design could not be used for flattened noses. Shortly, adjustable pads, which were attached to the bridge (now called center) independent of the crest or shank, became popular. Many designs followed which were arched to simulate hoop spring eyeglasses.

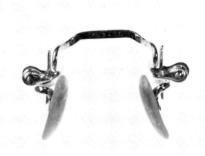

Figure 158. Rocking pad bridge.

The endpiece joints were vertical, hence, the temples opened perpendicular to the lens plane. Thus, the endpiece had to be twisted to angle the temples downward and cause the lenses to tip away from the brows and toward the cheeks. Concurrently, a zylo rimmed frame and a metal rimmed frame with zylo covers on the rims became very popular. Both had saddle bridges and were as adjustable as ever. Rimless mountings returned to popularity, mostly fitted with variations of octagonal shaped lenses. From the aspect of individualizing the eyewear, it became principally the selection of lens shapes.

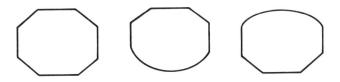

Figure 159. Variations of octagonal shape.

The first important variation from saddle bridges came in the form of keyhole bridges. These were bridges that rested on the sides of the nose and were ordinarily made in only three widths for adults. Small frames for children were made with two or three narrower widths. Temples could still be easily angled to account for low or high ears or instances when one ear was higher than the other. The width of the bridge established the point of contact

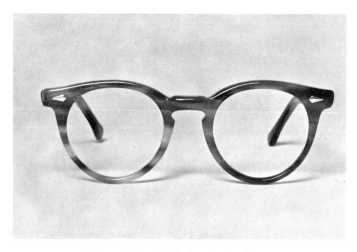

Figure 160. Keyhole zylonite frame.

(high or low) on the nose. Ethiopian and Oriental noses did not wear these bridges well because of the limited adjustability of the nose pads.

Shortly after 1930, there was an abrupt change to a pear-shaped lens shape in a metal frame with the temples 15 or 30 degrees above center (Ful-Vue).

These frames gave a foretaste of what was to follow. The temple angle could not be altered because the endpiece was too short to grip with pliers. The frame was followed by Ful-Vue rimless mountings which were most difficult to adjust. The next mounting, with the endpiece attached to the bridge by a bar which lay behind the top of the lens (Numont), revived all of the fitting conveniences of old-time mountings. The endpiece could be freely twisted or turned.

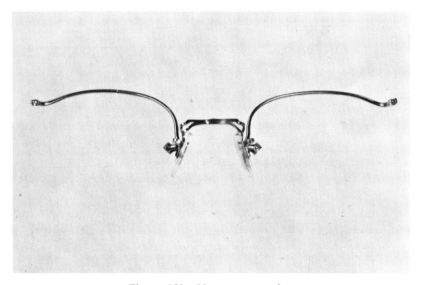

Figure 161. Numont mounting.

Then came a myriad of lens shapes in lightweight plastic frames. They had mitered endpieces which still provided the opportunity for moderate temple angle changes. Then, the manufacturers learned that a butt joint temple was generally accepted. Since this design is decidedly easier to manufacture, it soon virtually re-placed mitered ends. The butt joint is scarcely adjustable be-cause removal of stock to make a neat fitting on an altered inclina-tion causes the temple to open wider than desired.

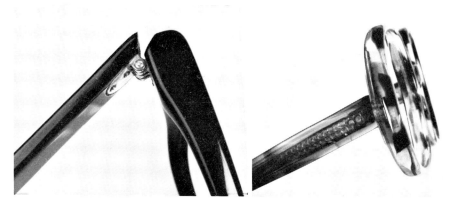

Figure 162. Mitre (left) and butt (right) joints.

Next followed an interval in which cosmeticians and motion picture make-up artists entered the scene. Their efforts were to set up rules by which lens shapes could be selected which would give the illusion of altering face shapes toward the desired classic oval shape. The Westmore Brothers, Hollywood's famous motion picture make-up family, devoted an extensively illustrated chapter on this subject in their *Beauty Book*.

About 1960, teenagers took over the notion of making eyewear conspicuous rather than a secondary item. The practice of cos-metic lens design and the makeup artists precepts were forgotten, first, for young prescription lens wearers and, finally, for grade school children to grandparents.

This abrupt change in eyewear designing precipitated unending problems with reference to lens centering and additional lens weight. Fortunately, Pittsburg Plate Glass Co. alleviated this latter crisis by the introduction of CR39, a plastic lens material. The matter of center locating and "wrap around" lenses still remain.

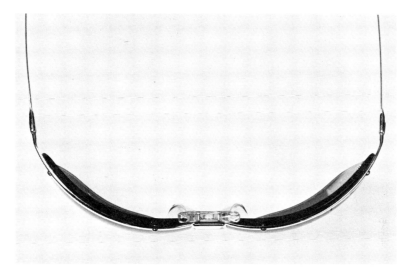

Figure 163. Wrap-around rotation on y-axes.

Along with increased lens size and a shallow unadjustable saddle bridge, which was reduced to two and occasionally three sizes, these frames had butt temple joints with buried, rather than riveted hinges. Such zylo frames have little, if any, adjustability. This impass virtually precludes traditional individualization of zylo frames at delivery time.

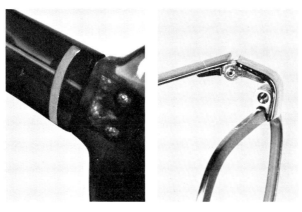

Figure 164. Unadjustable zylo hinge.

Metal frames have also kept abreast of these limiting design changes. The conventional hinge and temple have been replaced by streamlined joint, which is ten or more millimeters behind the lens plane. Few dispensers have tools to grasp the front of the frame to permit twisting of the front part of the joint to alter the temple angle. Thus, the inclination of the lens plane is virtually fixed by the manufacturer. Rimless mountings are the only remaining lens holders which can be altered with conventional pliers (including the Numont pliers). Hence, the traditional approach to frame fitting at delivery has essentially disappeared.

In the late 1950s and early in his professional career, R.C. Welsh, M.D., Ophthalmologist, Miami, Florida, received a number of referrals for cataract surgery from optometrists in his area. He returned the patients to them, after surgery, for their new lenses. Repeatedly, the patients returned with sadly defacing eyewear, which had large, thick, decentered lenses that did not produce as good visual acuity as he had obtained at his refraction. He became obsessed with a desire to find the means to provide acceptable lenses that truly expressed his prescription. He observed that when a strong plus lens was ground to knife edge, it was round if the prescription were a sphere and that it was oval if a spherocylinder. He also noted that the lower nasal side of an assymetric lens shape was very thick because it was closer to the optical center of the lens than the "long corner" on the upper temporal side of

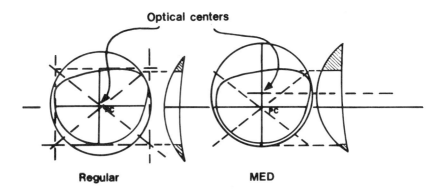

Figure 165.   Regular and M.E.D. lens cutting compared.

the lens which remained very thin. Thus, a lens with knife edge at the "long corner" would have the thickness of 4 to 7 mm decentration on the lower nasal side.

Totally disregarding undesirable optical effects in order to improve the cosmetic effect, he decentered the lens to the bottom of the knife edge uncut lens and obliterated the in-out thickness difference. He named this Minimum Equivalent Diameter (M.E.D.). Now, the only thick edge of the lens was at the top because of the decentration up. This decentration varies from 5 to 9 mm according to the lens shape. There is also a horizontal decentration of 0.5 to 2.0 mm out depending upon the lens shape. Compensation for this latter factor requires a smaller lens size or reduced DBL to accommodate the Interocular Distance (P.D.).

As we have learned, the vertical decentration up reduces the associated pantoscopic angle toward zero and can raise the multifocal segment above the desired position. To ignore the pantoscopic angle change can induce a tilted lens effect that prevents the lens from performing as its vertex power in any direction.

From Doctor Welsh's point of view, there was another gain. The uncut lens could be made slightly smaller with a corresponding slight reduction in center thickness.

Dispensometer®

Returning to our original problem, there is a need for an instrument that is attachable to the selected frame which (1) provides the means to find the individual pantoscopic angle and (2) provides the location of the datum line for the lens as fitted in the selected frame. From this, the precise vertical position of the optical center is determined; (3) from the datum line, the position of the top edge of a bifocal segment is precisely determined; (4) the temple angle of the frame is measured.

Such an instrument has been developed. It provides the specifications of:

1. Pantoscopic angle
2. Vertical position of lens center
3. Top edge of multifocal segment

When the laboratory adjusts the frame to the specifications on the laboratory order which are obtained by the Dispensometer, frame alterations at delivery time are reduced to minimum.

Hence, the new order of the day is to first determine the individual pantoscopic angle, then find if the frame under consideration provides, or closely approximates, that angle before the selection is confirmed.   It can be contended that such precision is unwarranted because the effect of lens tilt is not great when the power of the distance prescription is small.   Such laxity would dismiss corrected lenses, accurate measurement of P.D., the appropriate separation of lens centers, and equal vertex distance.   Much of the laxity in this area of dispensing is chargeable to the fact that a measuring device has not been available to provide the necessary information for the dispenser.   Errors, because of precise information in this phase of lens fitting, are a major contribution to the disparity of lens function in the correction of aphakia and are also a cause of "these lenses are not as comfortable as this other pair."   Relatively unadjustable eyeframes have forced the use of a means of stipulating complete specifications for the eyewear on the laboratory order if high quality dispensing is to be accomplished.   At last, individualized eyewear *must* be specified at the time the order is written.   This predicament has been overshadowed by the enthusiastic acceptance of "modern" fashion frame styles.   These conditions force a totally new approach to precise dispensing.   The days of plier and file work at delivery time have virtually disappeared.   The eyewear must be designed and specified at the time the order is accepted because few alterations *can* be made after the lenses are fitted to the frame.

Use of the Dispensometer

The Dispensometer is essentially an aluminum parallelogram to which an inclinometer with protractor are fitted on the end, to indicate the vertical and horizontal meridians.

The eyeframe, which the customer has tentatively selected, is now placed in the instrument to find if the temples tilt the frame at, or very near, the wearer's true pantoscopic angle.   Assuming that the frame meets these conditions, or the temple joints can be angled to properly angle the frame, it is now viewed from the front.   First, the temples of the frame should be adjusted to bring the horizontal (datum) line symmetric with the pupils. The patient should now be directed to look straight forward (primary position) so the position of the lens pattern center (datum line) can be measured on the vertical scale. Usually, the center line will be below the pupil center, but recent fashion lens shapes, which extend above the brow line, may have center lines at or above the pupil center. When the location of the datum line has been found, reference to the inclinometer will indicate the inclination of the lenses. By the terms of Fry and Ellerbrock's formula, the lens center will be placed 1 mm below the pupil center for each 2° of pantoscopic angle. Thus, it is apparent that the lens center will frequently be decentered up from the pattern center.

Hitherto, without proper instrumentation to make this measurement, the position of lens centers in the vertical meridian have been discussed in the literature but virtually nothing has been done to put the information into clinical use. Thus, until now, few lenses have been properly rotated on their x-axes, nor have the lens centers been in the proper position for the lens axes to be congruent with the visual axes. For the proper placement of multifocal segments, reference is again made to the horizontal (datum) line on the plastic bar and the vertical scale is read at the point below the line, usually in the area of the lower lid, where the top edge of the segment should be placed. For comparison, a previously satisfactory pair of bifocals can be used to establish the exact position. Thus, the segment position is found without calculations and it is the number of millimeters below the pattern center (datum line). If there has been vertical decentration of the lens center, the distance of the point to the optical center of the lens will be less or more than the segment dimension. Do not let this be confusing.

One measurement is an optical specification and the other is a relationship between the location of the geometric center of the particular lens pattern before the eye and the location of a borderline of lens powers. One dimension is related to the lens power and performance of the whole lens and the other is related to the use of a particular area of the lens.

Record of the temple angle should be made on the customer's file card for duplication or future adjustment of the frame. It should be noted that another frame resting differently on the nose with a different lens shape and the joint set at a different position could present a quite different specification.

Univertex

The symmetry of vertex distance of lenses is controlled by the angles of spread (or flair) of the temple joints. No means has been previously provided for the dispenser to specify the angle (or angles) he desired which was based upon measurement. Now, a tool has been devised for the purpose.

The schematic frame has no nose pads. It is provided with two cups which rest upon the upper eyelids like the Distometer, thus setting the two lenses equidistant from the eyes. The joints of the frame are spring-loaded to cause a small pressure on the temples at the ear tops. Protractors are attached to the front to indicate the individual angles of spread (or flair).

Since a large number of skulls are slightly asymmetric, these angles are frequently slightly different. If this detail is specified, no fitting table time will be consumed to balance the vertex distance of the lenses.

Hence, if the interocular distance has been precisely measured and the lenses are in perfect planar position on both the x- and y-axes, the lens axes will project symmetrically and parallel to intersect both of the centers of rotation. The mechanical adjustment of the frame has been done in the laboratory, as it should, and individualized eyewear has been provided to the wearer from specifications.

The temples of this schematic frame are slidably adjustable for length. The scale on the temple refers to mm length to the bend. The bend of the temple is intended to be sharp enough to set the bend somewhat behind the crotch at the ear top. This type of temple adjustment can be specified and will leave only the end of the temple to be altered.

At this point, two of the axes of the three-dimensional lenses and eyewear have received our attention:

1. Rotation on the x-axis was discussed and established in the measurements and positioning of the pantoscopic angles of the lenses.

2. Rotation on the z-axis was fixed by the congruence of the base line of the eyes and the 180° line (datum line) on the Dispensometer.
3. Rotation on the y-axis was fixed when the vertex distance of the lenses was set.

Only one point has not been discussed. It must be correct (or corrected) before any of the specifications of the eyewear are valid. The bridge of the eyeframe must not be twisted. This error would counter-rotate the lenses on the x-axis and the lens axes could not simultaneously intersect the centers of rotation.

Visual sighting down on the eyewear or from the end of the eyewear reveals this imperfection.

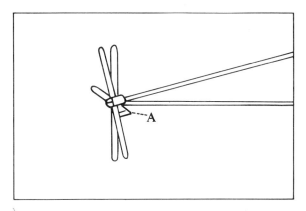

Figure 166. "Propeller" twist of lens planes.

The Measuring Cards of long ago had two slots in them about 10 mm wide and each about 45 mm long. The finished eyewear was placed in these slots at the final inspection and the bridge was bent to let both ends of each lens rest against one edge of the slot. This inspection proved that the lenses and frame were all in a straight line. This inspection could also be made by using the edge of a mm rule placed perpendicular to the lenses. This inspection was valid at the time when lenses were comparatively small, 42 or 44 mm long with practically no decentration. But, present-day oversize lenses and much decentration force a new approach. As can be seen in Figure 167, the temporal end of each lens is much behind the nasal end. Since this asymmetry varies with the dioptric curve of the back surface of the lens and the decentration, another approach must be made to assure the straightness (absence of y-axis rotation) of the eyewear.

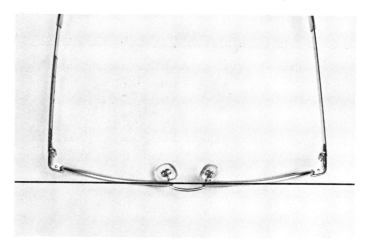

Figure 167. Inspecting straightness of x-axis.

Find the distance of the lens center from the nasal edge, then, at an equal distance on the temporal side, place a small, contrasting colored, ink dot on the top rim of the frame. These reference points and the nasal ends of the lenses should describe a straight line. When this has been accomplished, the optical axes of the lenses will be parallel and should simultaneously intersect the centers of rotation. Disregard the extended portion. It will be in the right direction.

This discussion of inspection is not done to relieve the laboratory of its work. It is only presented to suggest the means of checking the work received from the laboratory.

EXTRA-AXIAL COMPENSATION

Ellerbrock* has made a lengthy study of the correction of aniso-

*Ellerbrock, V.J.: *Some Effects Induced by Anisometropic Corrections.* Columbus, Ohio St U Pr, 1941.

Ellerbrock, V.J. and Fry, G.A.: Effects induced by anisometropic corrections.

metropia at Ohio State University School of Optometry. In one report on forty-seven cases that were largely optometry students he drew the following conclusions. (It must be remembered that the subjects were prepresbyopic and were not forced to use extra-axial areas in the use of the reading portions of bifocals.)

1. No symptoms without compensated lenses, none indicated, none fitted 17%
2. Symptoms without compensated lenses, more comfortable with them 61%
3. No improvement with compensated lenses 22%

From these conclusions he recommends that prism compensation or bicentric grinding for single vision lenses should not be used indiscriminately. His experience shows that about three-quarters of those who have had symptoms of headache, asthenopia, and/or diplopia are improved by compensation. He also raises the question of aniseikonia and special center positions for special vocations.

If a patient who has a prescription for anisometropia is wearing glasses, it is wise to mark the optical centers of the lenses in the lensometer and to check these positions with the Dispensometer as worn by the patient. Isometric (identical) prescriptions seldom present a problem in moderate powers whether the old lenses were set higher or lower than the new fitting. On occasion, however, a poorly made pair of glasses with an asymmetric prescription may induce a vertical prism of considerable strength. The prescribing doctor may be pleased to discuss your observation and consider the effect of the lenses on his refraction findings.

For Example: Old lenses, ℞ O.D. +2.00
                             O.S. +1.00
                    For reading only.

Optical centers are 2 mm above the fixation line z-axis for primary position. Visual axes intersect lenses 8 mm below primary position when normally depressed for reading. The difference in the lenses is +1.00 before the right eye. The optical

*Am J Optom, 19:*444-459, 1942.

Ellerbrock, V.J.: Further study of effects induced by anisometropic corrections. *Am J Optom, 25:*430-437, Sept. 1948.

centers are 10 mm (2 + 8 mm) above the reading position. Therefore, $1^\triangle$ Base Up before the right eye is induced when the eyes are depressed for reading.

There is little difficulty when a pair of lenses is used for only one fixation distance. When the center of the above prescription are placed at the proper distance below center, the decentration and prism effect disappear in the reading field. The correction lenses for anisometropia to be used for general purposes often present a greater problem. Bicentric grinding precludes the possibility of the axes of the two separate areas from violating the extension of the wearer's z-axes.

There are two other solutions. When the locations of the optical centers for distance vision and reading position have been found, the lenses can be centered at a compromise point between the locations. The centers of the pair of lenses described above might be placed midpoint between distance and near fixation, which is 4 mm below the intersection of the axes for primary position. When the eyes are in the primary position, $0.4^\triangle$ Base Down before the right eye is induced, and when the eyes are depressed to the reading position, the prism effect is reversed to $0.4^\triangle$ Base Up because the center of the right lens is above the z-axis. If the patient fatigues in either of these positions, he may tip his head back slightly for distant vision or drop his head a little farther for reading and use the optical axes of the lenses for either fixation distance.

A greater difference in the lenses before the two eyes may require prescription lenses with two centers (bicentric), in which the prism effect is neutralized at some extra-axial point. It may be that E.D. Tillyer was the first to use slab-off to create a bicentric lens. It is certain that he converted a bicentric bifocal to a monocentric lens by slab-off on the segment side of an Ultex bifocal. The appropriate amount of prism (according to the addition) was ground off the curve of the distance portion with the dividing line tangent to the segment to offset the "jump" of the 19 mm radius segment. The lens was marketed under the name of Tillyer Monocentric Bifocal. The short life of this lens design may suggest the possible unimportance of "jump" to the average bifocal wearer.

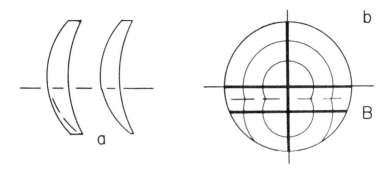

Figure 168. Slab-off surface to create bicentric lens.

In Figure 168*a*, the lower part of the front surface of the weaker plus or stronger minus lens is ground off (using the same dioptric curve on the anterior surface) to generate prism Base Up in the lens to balance with the companion lens at the predetermined point. The patient learns to use this pair of single vision lenses much like a bifocal wearer. He finds a point on either side of the dividing line at which the prism effect disappears and thus he may have comfortable binocular vision for both distance and near.

The accuracy of the prism neutralization is checked on the lensometer. Dot the uncompensated lens at the extra-axial point at which the lenses are to be balanced. Place the lens in the lensometer with this dot on the axis of the instrument. Note the amount of prism generated. Slide the compensated lens into position with the corresponding point on the instrument axis. The target will be in the same position as the other lens if the prisms are equal.

A novel method of measuring the amount of prism introduced by the slab-off is shown by Morgan and Peters.* They derive the formula which shows that when a standard lens measure is used to measure the compensated curve on either side of the dividing line and then the center pin of the gauge is placed on the dividing line with the other pins in a line perpendicular to it, the difference in the dioptric curves is the amount of prism in Prism Di-

---

*Morgan, M. and Peters, H.B.: *The Optics of Ophthalmic Lenses.* Berkeley, U of Cal Pr, 1948, p. 45

opters introduced by the bicentric grinding (Fig. 169). The lens measure provides a means of quickly checking either finished lenses from the laboratory or unknown lenses.

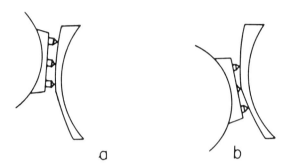

Figure 169. Checking amount of prism generated in slab-off with lens measure.

EXAMPLE

The gauge reads +6.00D. on either section of the lens and reads +7.50 D. when set as shown in Figure 169b.

7.50 − 6.00 = 1.50 = 1.5$^{\triangle}$

Therefore, the prism Base Up effect of the slab-off is 1.5$^{\triangle}$. The utter simplicity of this measurement makes it most useful.

An alternate method to measure single vision bicentric lens prism is to bisect the nose of the lensometer with the dividing line. Adjust the position of the lens carefully until the images of two targets, seen on the reticle, are equally illuminated. The total separation of the center cross-lines as measured on the concentric circles on the reticle is the amount of prism in the compensation.

DISSIMILAR OBJECT DISTANCES

It can be easily demonstrated that when a spectacle lens is placed at the primary focal point of an eye (about 15 mm in front of the cornea), the lens has no effect upon the retinal image size.*   That is to say the retinal image is brought into focus but is not changed in size.   When the lens is brought closer to the eye or moved farther away, some magnification or minification results. The change in image size is approximately 0.1% per diopter per millimeter of change.   It follows that low-power lenses can be moved rather large amounts without much effect on the image size.

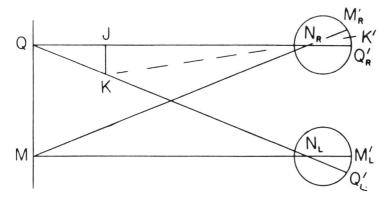

Figure 170.   Effect of dissimilar object distances.

When an eye is used singly, a rather large change in image size may go unnoticed; when objects are clearly seen by both eyes, a remarkably small difference in the images of the individual eyes is readily discerned.   When both eyes are fixed on **M**, images **M'**$_R$ and **M'**$_L$ in Figure 170 fall on the maculae of the two eyes. These images are mentally fused into a single impression which is visually projected and the object is perceived at the point **M**. The object **Q** is also imaged on the two retinas at points **Q'**$_R$ **Q'**$_L$, equal distances to the left of the images of **M**.   Points **M** and **Q**

*Laurance, L.: *Visual Optics. The School of Optics.*   London, 1920, pp. 361-370.

Cowan, A.: *Refraction of the Eye.*   Philadelphia, Lea & Febiger, 1945, pp. 192-198.

Duke-Elder, Sir W.S.: *Textbook of Ophthalmology,* Vol. IV.   St. Louis, Mosby, 1949, pp. 4560-4564.

Linksz, A.: *Physiology of the Eye,* Vol. 1, *Optics.*   New York, Grune & Stratton, 1950, p. 299.

are on the horoptor because the images are falling on *corresponding* points of the two eyes. In other words, if the eyes turn to look at $\mathbf{Q}$, points $\mathbf{M'_R}$ and $\mathbf{M'_L}$ are corresponding distances to the right of fixation. If an object is placed at point $\mathbf{K}$, which is in the same direction as $\mathbf{Q}$, the image of $\mathbf{K}$ falls on the left eye at $\mathbf{Q'_L}$ but the image on the retina of the right eye falls on point $\mathbf{K'}$ between points $\mathbf{Q'_R}$ and $\mathbf{M'_R}$. The position of image point $\mathbf{K'}$ on the retina and its distance $(\mathbf{Q'_R K'})$ is quickly calculated from similar triangles:

$$\frac{\mathbf{Q'_R K'}}{\mathbf{KJ}} = \frac{\mathbf{N'_R Q'_R}}{\mathbf{J\,N_R}}$$

$$\frac{\mathbf{KJ}}{\mathbf{N_L N_R}} = \frac{\mathbf{QJ}}{\mathbf{QN_R}}$$

If the separation between the nodal points $\mathbf{N_L N_R}$ is 60 mm, the distance $\mathbf{N_R Q}$ is 6 meters (20 feet), the object $\mathbf{K}$ is 50 cm in front of $\mathbf{Q}$, and the secondary focal length of the eye $\mathbf{N_R Q'_R}$ is 17 mm, we find by substitution that

$$\mathbf{Q'_R K'} = \frac{\mathbf{N_R Q'_R}}{\mathbf{JN_R}} \times \mathbf{KJ}$$

$$= \frac{\mathbf{N_R Q'_R}}{\mathbf{JN_R}} \times \frac{\mathbf{QJ}}{\mathbf{QN}} \times \mathbf{N_L N_R}$$

$$= \frac{.017}{5.5} \times \frac{.5}{6} \times .060 = \frac{.00051}{33} = .015 \text{ mm}$$

Thus it is seen that the image of point $\mathbf{K}$ is only .015 mm from the corresponding point. It would be considered no particular feat to perceive that an object stands 20 inches from the wall at a 20 foot distance. In fact, the aviator's test for depth-perception requires discrimination more than five times as great.

If the distance $\mathbf{MQ} = 50$ cm

$$\frac{\mathbf{M'_R Q'_R}}{\mathbf{MQ}} = \frac{\mathbf{N_R Q'_R}}{\mathbf{QN_R}}$$

$$\mathbf{M'_R Q'_R} = \frac{.017}{6} \times 0.5 = \frac{0.0085}{6} = 1.42 \text{ mm}$$

When we refer to the disparity $(\mathbf{Q'_R K'} = .015)$ we see that the lack of correspondence is almost precisely 1.0 percent of the distance $\mathbf{Q'_R M'_R}$. Referred to the horoptor, a distance of 5 mm (1% of $\mathbf{MQ}$) at the fixation distance changes the position of the image the same as an object 50 cm in front of the fixation distance. Hence it is apparent that a difference of 1 percent in image sizes may become a significant quantity. The distance **MQ** in Figure 170 is 50 cm and object **K** stands 50 mm in closer to the eyes. The calculations above indicate that since 1 percent in image-size difference is practically identical with the displacement of the image of **K,** the horoptor would tend to rotate 45° as shown in the dotted line **MK.** In actual experience, such exaggerated distortion of objects in the visual space is not produced. Previous experience and the domination of the report of monocular vision (space perception organized by size of objects, shadows, etc.) prevent such radical departure as suggested by geometric optics. Some individuals, however, are sensitive to such disparity and are distressed by what seems to be a rivalry between the intermittent projection of distorted binocular vision and the impression of the visual space when only one eye is active and vision of the other eye is suppressed. Research in aniseikonia (dissimilar ocular images),* as well as the reports of clinical experience, shows that the majority of successfully treated cases are in the zone between 0.5 to 1.5 percent image difference.

Table III (in Chapter 5) shows the magnification of 1.00D. spherical lens with a constant center thickness and a fixed vertex (z) distance when the front surface power is increased. In Table XV the same formulas have been used to show the magnification

TABLE XV
% MAGNIFICATION OF PLANO LENS

Curve Front of Lens	Center Thickness in mm				
	1.0	2.0	3.0	4.0	5.0
Plano	—	—	—	—	—
3.00	.2	.4	.6	.8	1.0
6.00	.4	.8	1.2	1.6	2.0
9.00	.6	1.2	1.8	2.4	3.0
12.00	.8	1.6	2.4	3.2	4.0
15.00	1.0	2.0	3.0	4.0	5.0

*Ames, A., Glidden, G.H., and Ogle, K.N.: Size and shape of ocular images. *Arch Ophthalmol,* 7:576, 1932.

Duke-Elder, Sir W.S.: *Text-Book of Ophthalmology,* Vol. IV. St. Louis, Mosby, 1949, pp. 4451-4465.

of a plano lens.

It was shown in Chapter 5 that the power factor increases magnification by approximately 2% per diopter increase of front surface power. With that information and the foregoing table, the magnification of dissimilar prescriptions can be approximated.

FOR EXAMPLE

O.D. + 3.25D. Sphere

O.S. + 1.75D. Sphere

magnification factor from power

+3.25 × 2 = 6.5%

+1.75 × 2 = 3.5%

If the right lens has +3.00D. front curve, 2 mm center thickness

1.065 × 1.004 = 1.069 = 7%

The total magnification of the left lens must be increased from 3.5 to 7 percent if the image sizes are to match

7 ÷ 3.5 = 2%

Reference to the table shows that the left lens must be ground with a front curve of

+6.00D., 5 mm center thickness

+7.50D., 4 mm center thickness *or*

+9.00D., 3 mm center thickness.

It is immediately apparent that large differences in lens prescriptions will create image-size differences that are too great to be practically corrected by the shapes of the lenses. In practice, most cases of anisometropia that do not involve large corrections for astigmatism are axial ametropia and therefore do not require image-size correction. Whitwell (1922) prepared Table XVI to serve as a guide in the shaping of lenses for asymmetric prescriptions.

Upon investigation, these general rules will be found to follow the formulas previously set forth. In this whole matter, the conservative approach is to have lenses with similar prescriptions made with similar front curves and center thicknesses. Only when, after careful fitting and adjustment, the patient still has difficulties that

TABLE XVI
SPHERICAL LENSES IN ANISOMETROPIA (WHITWELL)*

One Eye	Other Eye	For the Lens	Make Back Surface
Normal	Hyperopic	Plus	Plane
Normal	Myopic	Minus	Strongly minus
Hyperopic	Hyperopic	Stronger plus	Plane
		Weaker plus	Strongly minus
Myopic	Myopic	Stronger minus	Minus
		Weaker minus	Plus
Myopic	Hyperopic	Plus	Plane
		Minus	Strongly minus

*Taken from Whitwell, A.: Best form of spectacle lenses for correction of small amounts of anisometropia. *Trans Opthalmol Soc, 24,* 1922.

the doctor cannot account for otherwise, should attention be focussed on ocular images. It should be remembered that in a large number of the cases in which dissimilar images are the cause of discomfort, the disparity approximates 1 percent. The first experiment can be directed toward an increase of about that amount before the eye with the weaker convex or stronger concave lens.

Among the advantages of marginally corrected lenses is the reduction of unequal magnification in similar lens prescriptions as compared with the effects of the shapes of some toric lenses. For example

	Front Curve	
	Toric	Corrected lens
+3.00 sphere	+9.00	+6.75 to +8.25
+3.00 +0.50	+6.00	+6.75 to +8.25

which for a standard center thickness of about 3.0 mm produces a difference of 0.6% magnification in the old-style lens.

The thickness factor also emphasizes the desirability of dividing prism power between the lenses in order to control center thickness. Reference to a prism chart shows that the center thickness of a lens is increased almost 0.5 mm for each Prism Diopter and the table shows that lens thickness increases magnification very rapidly.

This discussion is intended merely to present the physical effects of prescription lenses and in no way is to be construed as a discussion of or substitution for the examination for aniseikonia or the production of iseikonic spectacles for the correction of the condition. This special phase of refracting procedure can be undertaken only with the special apparatus such as the Ophthalmoeikonometer® developed at Dartmouth Eye Institute and the complementary prescription lenses prepared by American Optical Company.

This consideration of magnification and imagery has been concerned with axial rays only. The discussion to follow will present the necessity of particular (and in many instances radically different) lens forms for each lens prescription if the same dioptric effect is to be produced when the eyes turn from the primary position toward the peripheral areas.

In Chapter 5, reference was made to lenses designed to image parallel rays as nearly as possible on the far-point sphere at all points of vergence. The lens aberration to be overcome is marginal astigmatism. The designing of a series of lenses to provide substantially the same dioptric power in the center to a distance, say 30°, away from the lens center requires almost an interminable amount of data processing ray tracing.* The formulas require that some assumption be made and that they become constants in the calculations of all prescriptions.

The distance to the back-surface of the cornea **A'P** (vertex distance) in Figure 171, distance to center of rotation **A'C**, and thickness of lens **AA'** must be assumed. The angle through which the eye is to turn, **QCA**, is taken as 30°. With this set of condi-

---

*Hardy, A.C. and Perrin, F.II.: *The Principles of Optics.* New York, McGraw, 1932. pp. 99-106, 437.

Fincham, W.H.A.: *Optics.* London, Hatton Press, 1942, pp. 372-376.

Martin, L.C.: *Technical Optics.* New York, Pitman Pub, 1948, pp. 317-325.

Southall, J.P.C.: *Introduction to Physiological Optics.* London, Oxford U Pr, 1937, pp. 96-101.

Emsley, H.H. and Swaine, W.: *Ophthalmic Lenses.* London, Hatton Press, 1946, pp. 237-248.

Morgan, M., and Peters, H.B.: *The Optics of Ophthalmic Lenses.* Berkeley, U of Cal Pr, 1948, pp. 44-50.

Mason, F.I.: *Principles of Optometry.* Berkeley, U of Cal Pr, 1940.

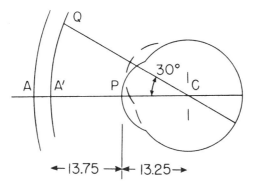

Figure 171. Parameters for best form lens.

tions the "best form" lens can be computed to focus parallel rays on the far-point sphere. When the theory is exercised to the fullest, the forms of the lenses are slightly different when they are designed for near-point fixation.*

Lenses recently designed by American Optical Company called Masterpiece have included as parameters in the calculations intermediate and near-point object distances, also variations in vertex distance. To relieve the variations in cylinder power generated by object distance as well as thickness when the toric curve is on the front surface, this series of lenses has the cylindrical curve on the back surface. Univis Best Form and Shuron® Kurova® lenses also have formulas which are somewhat similar.

In Table XV, the marginally corrected lenses of the larger lens factories are compared. It must be borne in mind that all these series were calculated from the same basic trigonometric formulas which if followed rigidly would require hundreds of base curves.† In practice the bases can be gathered into groups when the limits of tolerance have been established. Usually the fewer the number of bases, the greater the compromise with the theory or the objective. Then, too, the different lens designers have different points

---

*Duke-Elder, Sir W.S.: *The Practice of Refraction.* St. Louis, Mosby, 1949, pp. 294-296.

†Morgan, M. and Peters, H.B.: *The Optics of Ophthalmic Lenses.* Berkeley, U of Cal Pr, 1948, p. 45.

of view, as previously described. It will be noted that despite all these considerations, all precision lenses of the same power are remarkably alike in form. Some of these curves and thicknesses have been altered to meet FDA regulations. When intermediate and near-point object distances are introduced into the calculations, the curves of the whole series are flattened by a diopter or more.

TABLE XVII

COMPARISON OF FRONT CURVES AND THICKNESSES
OF MARGINALLY CORRECTED SPHERICAL LENSES

Power	Optical Masterpiece Bausch & Curve	Thick-ness (mm)	Bausch & Lomb Orthogon Curve	Thick-ness (mm)	Continental Optical Kurova Curve	Thick-ness (mm)	Shuron Optical Widesite Curve	Thick-ness (mm)
+1.00D.	+5.50	2.1	+7.62	2.2	+7.50	2.2	+7.50	2.1
+3.00D.	+7.75	2.8	+10.25	2.9	+9.50	2.9	+8.75	2.9
—1.00D.	+5.50	1.3	+5.62	1.4	+6.50	1.5	+5.50	1.3
—3.00D.	+3.75	0.8	+5.25	0.7	+5.50	0.9	+4.75	0.8

It is now apparent that the choice of lens shapes as suggested by Whitwell for image-size control in cases of anisometropia may be highly unsatisfactory except in a restricted area in the center of the lens. Again the ophthalmic dispenser must weigh the problem and the means of solving it and let judgment reflect all the factors.

Some patients are very sensitive to changes in the form (profile) and thickness of lenses. The discomfort may arise from specular reflections from the lens surfaces (see Chap. 20) or image magnification. Experience shows that hyperopic patients enjoy an increase in the curvature of their convex lenses and many myopes prefer flat lens forms. If an explanation is attempted, the hyperope may be pleased with the slight increase in magnification and the removal of marginal distortion. The increased curvature of the concave lenses produces some image-size reduction and in many cases moves or more sharply focusses the images reflected from the lens surfaces. This second condition is materially alleviated by surface coating, to which reference is made in Chapter

20. Of the two types of refractive errors, myopes seem to observe small differences more keenly.

Much to the surprise of doctors and dispensers, the lower-based Masterpiece series of lenses has been generally accepted by all wearers with negligible complaint that seems traceable to lens profile, producing reduced magnification.

On some occasions when a patient has a shallow bridge and prominent eyes, it is normal to think of deep-curved lenses to provide clearance for the lashes. These are several reasons why the practice should be avoided:

1. It is very difficult to produce a high-quality surface on a very strong convex surface; therefore the lenses are seldom as perfect as they would be on normal curves.
2. The curves of high bases are compensated for thick, strong, convex prescriptions and will therefore be inaccurate for weaker and thinner lenses.
3. Concave lenses must be flatter than average to be marginally corrected. A deep base curve is incorrect.
4. Many lenses with elongated shapes do not fit or hold securely in metal or plastic frames when the curves are deep.
5. The actual gain in vertex depth is much less than it seems. If the curves on a lens 44 mm long are raised 3.00 diopters (that is, from +6.00 Base to +9.00 Base) the increased depth is only 1.5 mm, a distance that can be gained more easily by the adjustment or fitting of the frame.
6. The extra cost to the patient and poor cosmetic effect are last but not least.

REVIEW

1. Why is the retinal spot about 18° nasalward on the horizontal axis (projected 18° temporalward) in the visual field blind? Why is this insensitive spot not observed in regular usage of the eyes?

2. What is the approximate angular width of the field of binocular vision?

3. Describe the horoptor.

4. Discuss the usefulness of Boeder's prism isobars in projecting the comfort of an asymmetric prescription.

5. What is the correct placement of lens center and pantoscopic angle?

6. Why and how much should the lens center be lowered when the lens is angled 10° toward the cheek?

7. Explain the stress placed upon fusion in the peripheral areas of anisometropia correcting lenses.

8. Prepare two anisometropic prescriptions, one a rather small difference and the other larger. Calculate the prism effect at 9 below for each and describe how you would compensate each.

9. Why is the datum line difficult to use as a reference line on plastic frames made in the United States?

10. Above the dividing line of a slab-off, the lens measure reads +6.25D. With the center pin on the dividing line, the lens measure reads +7.75D. How much prism Base Up has been added?

11. ℞ R. +3.75
L. +2.50 + 0.50 + 90

Which lens should have the stronger front curve if an attempt were made to balance the image sizes of the lenses?

Chapter 11

PRESBYOPIC PRESCRIPTION ANALYSIS

◆◆

F inally when the prescription lenses which provide clear vision for distance are no longer suitable for reading because of the onset of presbyopia, patients are forced to make some changes in their habits. Included in this group are those who hitherto have worn no glasses for distant vision and now find it necessary to consider the use of spectacles for near. Equally distasteful to these patients is the fact that the new lenses which make reading a delight also cause an increasing blurriness to all objects much beyond the reading distance. If they would have clear vision, these patients must now learn to put on their reading glasses when accommodation is stimulated for near and as promptly remove them when the gaze returns to distant objects.

When Benjamin Franklin asked his optician to split his distance lenses and reading lenses so that the upper half of his spectacles would be suitable for distance and the lower half for reading, he was making a compromise. He sacrificed half of the area of each of his pairs of glasses so that he could have the effect of wearing two pairs at once. He was less fortunate than many of his neighbors in those days. Their need for a distance prescription was not as great, so they merely looked over the tops of their small reading lenses when they wished to see at a distance. In Franklin's keen judgment, he was willing to dispense with the least used fields of both pairs of glasses in order that his eyes be immediately prepared for all uses. He had individualized the lens prescriptions to his particular needs and convenience.

This individualization of presbyopic prescriptions without doubt is one of the largest and most important activities of an ophthalmic dispenser. To all the considerations described in Chapter 10 that contribute to the judgment of the design of single vision lenses, there must now be added *when* and *how* the eyes are used for near vision. Truly it is not trite to say that multifocal lenses are "fitted to the patient." They must fit into his daily life and activities with minimum adjustment on his part if they are to be a total success.

As pointed out in Chapter 8, presbyopia is a relative term. The condition depends upon the age of the patient, the basic refractive error, his postural habits, and his near-point activities. The date of onset may vary with the individual's state of general health. Some hypertonic persons who can summon a large amount of accommodative power for short periods of time may defer the use of supplementary lenses for several years. At the other extreme some debilitated patients require reading lenses before forty years of age. For these reasons, any attempt to reduce the condition of presbyopia to a mathematical formula is fraught with exceptions. The former infinite accommodative adjustments between the reading point and distance must now be supplemented with and finally almost be replaced by lens power. The advantages and limitations of the near-point addition can be studied from the point of view of the effect of the lenses upon physiological function. One authority* averages the near-point at 28 to 30 cm and states that presbyopia may be said to have set in when the accommodative near-point has receded to 22 cm (4.50D.). The large number of people in England ranging from 5'5" to 5'9" in height, with corresponding shorter arms and closer reading distance, justify Sir Duke-Elder's observation of a somewhat earlier than usual advent of presbyopia. His calculation would agree favorably with the 35 mm and 50 percent reserve as displayed in Table XII.

At age forty-four when the maximum accommodative effort is measured as 4.25D. and the near-point is 24 cm, a prescription for +0.75D. sphere addition is written. The supplemental lens power raises the amplitude to 5.00D. and the near-point becomes 20 cm, but unlike his experience when his accommodation alone accomplished the act, the patient has a far-point through the reading prescription at the focal length of the addition. In this in-

---

*Duke-Elder, Sir W.S.: *The Practice of Refraction.* St. Louis, Mosby, 1949, p. 137.

stance it is 133 cm. Figure 172 shows that with his distance prescription this person can see clearly from infinity to 24 cm and that through his reading prescription he can see clearly from 133 to 20 cm. In the interval between 133 and 24 cm he can see clearly through either his distance or reading prescription.

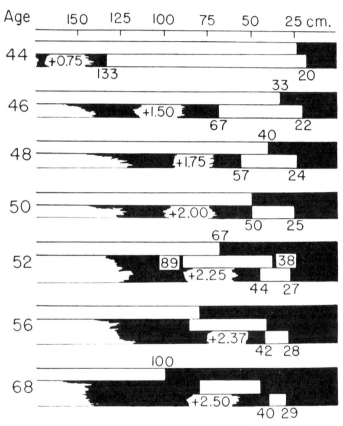

Figure 172. Useful distances of additions.

Characteristic of the first of the three stages of presbyopia, termed *"early presbyopia,"* patients still have sufficient accommodation to permit the clear areas of the distance and near prescriptions to overlap. A few years later when the addition has increased to about +2.00D., the clear areas in Figure 172 and very near the same distance from the eyes. This stage may be termed *"middle presbyopia."* During this period, objects near the far point of the reading addition and the patient's near point (about 50 cm) can be seen clearly through one prescription but not with the other. When the addition has been increased to assist the receding near-point of accommodation, finally the far point of the reading prescription is within the patient's near point. A space now exists in which the eyes cannot see any objects clearly in the interval from about 45 to 80 cm. (Allowance of a depth of field of ±0.25D. is made.) * In this stage of *"advanced presbyopia"* the former continuous accommodation for distance is lost if the eyes must depend upon only two lens powers. It is at this point that, if the patient wishes to (or must) see clearly at all distances, an intermediate prescription is a necessity. Figure 172 shows the effect of an intermediate segment with 50 percent of the reading addition. When the allowance for depth of field is added, it is apparent that the patient can again see clearly at all distances and for many years has overlapping clear areas between the distance and intermediate lenses or the intermediate and reading prescriptions.

A survey of the patient's necessary adjustments will be made. New bifocal wearers can be divided into two groups—those who have been wearing distance or reading glasses and others who have worn no glasses before. The first group already has gone through the adjustment period of "getting used to glasses." These patients have learned to accept the distortion of spatial perception induced by the aberrations, magnification, minification, or size differences of the distance lenses. They have become acquainted with the prism effects of the lenses when the eyes are rotated away from the lens centers. If the prism is more than can be conveniently overcome, they have learned to turn their heads in order to keep their visual axes in the *area of comfortable binocular vision* closer to the lens centers. If the prescriptions for the two eyes were not identical, the additional compensations have been accomplished. Tolerance for the increased chromatic aberration induced by the addition of another lens to the system has been made. Surface reflections which may have been noticed

---

*Davson, H.: *The Physiology of the Eye.* Philadelphia, Blakiston, 1949, pp. 237-239.

at first are now ignored. If the first glasses were for reading only, these patients have learned to accept a blurred image of everything at more than about three feet away. They have learned to vary fixation from distance to reading matter in hand and even walk without the effects of nausea. All this has been accomplished with the single vision lenses and very infrequently indeed has doctor or optician heard much complaint about it.

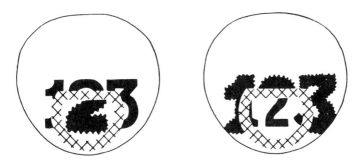

Figure 173. Blur at segment margin.

By the very design of multifocal lenses, the wearer must conform to some new conditions. In any event, in one area of the binocular field, distance vision will be sacrificed at all times. The size and shape of the reading aperture is dependent upon the style of multifocal. Surrounding this porthole is a blurry rim which has been shown to be useless for either distance or near vision (Fig. 173).

If the patient is to become accustomed to the change, the rapidity with which it will be accomplished obviously is affected by the amount his habits must be changed and by his individual adaptability. A careful discussion of the patient's daily activities is necessary. The dispenser can then choose the size, shape, and position of the reading portion of the lenses which will most satisfactorily meet the patient's demands and at the same time not violate his accumulated habits more than necessary.

As pointed out by Percival (see Chap. 5), the actual area of a lens used in the act of ordinary reading is a rectangular spot about 8 × 12 mm. A large number of patients would have a very difficult time with a reading portion that small for several reasons. Although visual efficiency diminishes rapidly (Fig. 130) on either side of the macular area, the blurred segment margin in the indirect field, like a smudged lens, is highly irritating to some persons. They would willingly sacrifice a larger portion of the distance field to have the segment margin set farther away from the fixation axis, hence the acceptance of very wide segments. In any event, the blurred margin or the top of the reading portion is frequently close enough to the primary position to come into the line of fixation occasionally. Until the patient has learned to tilt his head slightly forward and thereby turn the objectionable blur away from distant fixation, there will be some confusion from time to time. Percival's small segment subtends an angle only $19° \times 27°$ or, in terms of a 4 mm pupil diameter, about two pupils high by three pupils wide. For most persons this restriction in the use of lens area after no restraint in a single vision lens would be most unsatisfactory. Further, it requires a certain amount of ocular marksmanship to find the center of a segment of such limited size. When the lateral diameter has been increased about 50 percent to 19 or 20 mm, most patients are satisfied.

One of the most confusing acts for some newly corrected presbyopic patients is the use of stairways. It is frequently necessary to remind them that long ago they have relegated the act of walking up and down stairs to an almost automatic act comparable with eating. A large part of the confusion comes from visual interference with an act that had been largely taken over by the other senses. They must be told to locate the first step by tipping the head to see it clearly, then let the handrail and experience take over the task.

The effect at near-point fixation (Fig. 173) in which only the "window" is clear is a change in the patient's habits that frequently causes the most trouble. Some individuals have a strong habit to change the reading position every few minutes. It is quite instructive to watch a large number of persons reading in a library. Some readers with or without multifocals tend to drop the eyes habitually an angle of about 15° and move the head to look from one text to another. Others squirm about as they look down, then straight forward, or finally, with their heads supported by their hands, actually look above center. Whether these movements are diagnostic of eye fatigue that the new glasses will alleviate, in any event they must be stopped when reading can be done only through the "porthole" in the visual field.

Ellerbrock* has reported a study made on fifty-two pre-presbyopic persons on whom both the habitual tilt of the face-plane and the angle of depression for reading was observed. An ingenious protractor device was used which was set up separated at some distance from the subject and therefore did not interfere with his postural habits. Table XVIII shows the findings. Twenty-eight persons, or 54 percent, depressed their fixation lines (z-axes) 20° to 30°. An equal percentage tilted the face-plane forward by the same amount. In other words, the angle of the reading material is 40° to 60° below the horizon in the majority of cases. The cilia line of the lower lid (the reference line for the top edge of reading segments) is 7 to 9 mm below the center of the pupil when the eye is in primary position. After an average size pupil has traversed the dividing line to the near-vision point, the distance will have increased 10 to 14 mm or 20° to 27° which is not an alteration of habit in the majority of cases. The established habits that can present problems are those in the first and second columns, patients who tilt their heads forward and depress their eyes little or none. It is obvious that they would try to use almost the same area in their lenses for both purposes. Beginning at the time of the writing of the prescription, these patients must be reeducated in their postural habits. Multifocal failures are largely among those who do not respond.

TABLE XVIII

Tilt of Face Plane	*Depression of Fixation Line*			
	0° to 10°	*10° to 20°*	*20° to 30°*	*30° to 40°*
0°–10°				
10°–20°		3	8	1
20°–30°	2	10	14	2
30°–40°		2	4	
40°–50°	1	2		1

*Ellerbrock, V.J.: A clinical evaluation of compensation for vertical prismatic imbalances. *Am J Optom Monograph, 50:*July, 1948.

In the process of the development of the "visual marksmanship" or habit of depressing the eyes the correct angle to engage the reading portions, some patients feel that the chosen reading segments cover too small a portion of the visual field. (If the decision in the selection of multifocals represents careful consideration on the part of the dispenser, a delaying action of readjustments, etcetera, is advisable to give more time for the patient to reform his habits. A supplementary pair of plain reading lenses for some special occupation that requires a larger near-point area frequently can be advised. It is so important to remember that as the area of the reading segment is increased the distance field is disproportionately reduced. When 3 mm is added to the width of the reading segment, the width of the reading field at 40 cm is increased about 50 mm, but the same angle projected to 6 meters (20 feet) covers an area 750 mm in width. Generally, reading segments are larger than needed.

A reasonably dependable rule is "devote the same percentage of area to the segment as the percentage of time the patient devotes to near-point vision." A pair of glasses made for sports or driving need have a segment no more than 16 mm round. At the other extreme is a desk worker whose lenses should have more than half of the area for near-point. It has been offered that larger reading areas for sustained near work allow some head movement behind the lenses and thereby permit the extraocular muscles to have some relief from fatigue of a fixed position. It is obvious that the size and shape of the reading segment limit the ocular movements for near vision. A segment 19 mm wide with pupils 3 mm in diameter and the segment 13 mm from the cornea permits the eye to move about 35° laterally. The vertical movement is voluntarily restricted to a much narrower arc.

Anisometropia! Probably the most overlooked and neglected obstacle to comfortable bifocal binocular vision. The roar of disapproval from conscientious dispensers is deafening!! *We do watch for vertical prism and do compensate for it!*

Yes, the obvious prescriptions are balanced in the lower areas of the lenses in such prescriptions as these:

+3.50 D. Sph.

+2.00 + 1.25 × 90

+2.75 + 0.50 × 180
+0.75 + 1.25 × 90

−1.25 − 1.25 × 180
−1.25 − 2.75 × 180

Such unbalanced prescriptions are too obvious for a conscientious dispenser to miss. The ones overlooked are those with reasonably symmetric sphere and cylinder powers but different cylinder axes which produce crossed-cylinders. For example

+0.75 + 1.25 × 105
+1.25 + 1.00 × 50
= 1.12 vertical at 8 mm = 0.9$^\triangle$

As might be expected this whole subject is controversial. In the literature there is report of patients compensating for as much as 4.0$^\triangle$ to 5.0$^\triangle$ of vertical prism in the reading position. Most patients are not able to overcome that much prism momentarily in a supraduction or infraduction test. At the other extreme is a distinguished firm of dispensing opticians in southern California which has regularly compensated for vertical prism for *all* bifocal prescriptions for thirty-five years. They feel that they have gained gratitude from innumerable patients for increased reading comfort.

The best care for these unfortunate patients will not be regularly attempted until dispensers can quickly and easily estimate the amount of prism at the reading level. Any method that requires graphs and diagrams at the fitting table is foredoomed to failure. If doctor's patient has not previously worn compensated segments or slab-off lenses, there is the matter of explaining the reason for the different styled lenses and an explanation of the additional charge. From the side of public relations these factors thwart prolonged calculations.

By using the table of Vertical Curvature of Cylinders (Table IV), the estimation of vertical lens power and prism power is virtually a mental calculation.

1. Transpose the prescription if necessary to have the same sign on both cylinders.
2. Subtract the sphere powers and jot down the difference.

3. Refer to the chart and find the curvature of the right cylinder under R axis.
4. Find the curvature for the cylinder under the L axis.
5. The maximum vertical prism that seems to be tolerable is 0.75$^\triangle$. Hence all pairs of lenses with 1.00D. (N.V.P. = .8 mm down = $1.00 \times .8 = 0.8^\triangle$) or more vertical power difference should be compensated. Univis R segments will account for small prism compensations and slab-off of flat-top bifocals will be used for 1.5$^\triangle$ or more.

This procedure is an approximation which is more than accurate for the purpose. The following is a slower but more precise method:
1. Find the spherical equivalent of both lenses.
2. Change the signs of the sphere and cylinder of the weaker lens.
3. Add the powers of the lenses.
4. If the cylinder axes are not identical, the difference will be a sphere with crossed-cylinders.
5. Transpose one lens, if necessary, to have both cylinders the same sign.
6. Proceed to solve the crossed-cylinders.
7. The result is the precise lens power difference of the lenses.
8. Since the point (N.V.P.) is not on the axis 90, compensation for decentration in for the reading distance (8 mm down, 2 mm in) rotates the axis 15°.

This procedure is altogether too time consuming with a customer waiting at the fitting table to justify the small improvement in the accuracy of the calculation. The whole consideration is whether the power difference is 1.00D. or more. For borderline differences it may be wise to ask your customer's permission to have a consultation with another dispenser. In any event a discussion of compensation should be held with the customer with a proviso that if a drawing-board analysis discloses that the difference is less than it seems by an approximation the work will not be done.

Have demonstrator lenses (Univis R and slab-off) handy to show to the customer. Do not set the stage for a misunderstanding at delivery time.

With this whole procedure in effect you have added to the quality of your service as a dispenser. Do not move into this work in silence, talk about it to your doctor friends. Get their enthusiasm, then wait for the complimentary remarks from doctors' patients to their doctors to let the program mature. It is a business builder.

IRRELEVANCE OF SYMMETRIC EXTRA-AXIAL PRISM EFFECTS

Some writers have attempted to show how the characteristic prism displacement of prescription lenses at extra-axial points enters into the changes of the patient's habits. Assuming the patient has worn glasses before his first bifocals, he is already well acquainted with the particular prismatic effect (or image displacement) of his distance or even reading lenses about 6 or 8 mm below the centers of the lenses. It has previously been convenient for him to look through that part of his lenses for a good deal of his reading at all times. The eyes which have worn glasses are already acquainted with and have shown an ability to compensate for symmetric prism displacement.

The wearer of an asymmetric prescription in single vision lenses has always had the option to tip his head forward and return to the axial section of his lenses if an area below center became fatiguing. The introduction of bifocals ends that freedom. Now the eyes must turn down to use an area that begins 3 to 5 mm below center and is not actually usable until the eyes have turned to the area about 8 mm below center.

EXAMPLE

$$R + 0.50 + 1.50 \times 120$$
$$L + 1.75 + 0.75 \times 60$$

Spherical equivalents:

$$R +0.50 + \frac{+1.50}{2} = +1.25$$
$$L +1.75 + \frac{0.75}{2} = +2.12$$

The left lens is the minuend:

$+1.75 + 0.75 \times 60$

$-0.50 - 1.50 \times 120$

$+1.25 \begin{cases} +0.75 \times 60 \\ -1.50 \times 120 \end{cases}$

Transposed:

$+1.25 \begin{cases} +0.75 \times 60 \\ +1.50 \times 30 \end{cases}$

$+2.00 \times 41$

$+0.12$

$+1.37 \quad +2.00 \times 41$

$A + B = +0.75 + 1.50 = +2.25$

$A + B - C = \dfrac{+2.25 - 2.00}{2} = +0.12$

Sph. $+1.37$

Cyl. $+0.83$ 2.00 at Axis 41 = 0.83

$+2.20$

$\times \; .8$

$1.76^{\triangle}$ prism Base Up Left Eye at 8 below.

The exception is an asymmetric prescription in which an unsurmountable prism is induced in that area of the reading segment. In this case the patient has long since learned that, unlike his experience without glasses when objects were equally blurred in all directions, now he must look through his lenses in the limited area close to the centers of the lenses in order to see comfortably. In other words, he may already have learned to *avoid* looking through his lenses as far as 8 mm below center. Unlike the case described above, *two* things must be accomplished for these problem cases. The bifocal lenses must be so designed as to reduce or obliterate the objectionable prism effect and then the eyes must be taught or encouraged to turn to the formerly uncomfortable area in the distance glasses.

An important change in the patient's visual habits is demanded when accommodative effort is supplanted with plus sphere power. The change in the demands upon accommodative-convergence relationship (A.C.A.) puts the new stress on the Positive Fusion

Reserve, as shall be shown. To review the physiology of near-point vision: If the patient reads at 16 inches (40 cm) he is using 2.50D. of accommodation. If his interocular distance (P.D.) is 60 mm for distance, he uses (2.50 × 6) 15△ of convergence to turn his eyes to the reading point. As his amplitude of accommodation decreases with age, his accustomed accommodative effort does not maintain clear vision at the reading distance, but convergence requirements are the same. Finally, he has greater difficulty and has his eyes examined. The doctor finds that by giving the assistance of a +1.00D. sphere the difficulty of blurred vision is removed.

When the prescription is made up as a reading glass, considerable adjustment must take place. Previously the accommodative mechanism was making great effort to supply the +2.50D. for a 40 cm reading distance. Now the same size reading-type will be seen easily with only 1.50D. accommodation because the remainder is supplied by the reading addition. From the side of convergence, there is also a new experience. Previously when 1.50D. accommodation was in use, only 9△ of convergence was associated (1.5 × 6). Now the eyes are not converged to the accommodative distance of 67 cm (26 inches) for 1.50D. They must continue to converge to 40 cm (16 inches). The previous association was 2.50D. accommodation with 15△ convergence, now it is 1.50D. accommodation with 15△ convergence (instead of 9△), to see singly. The ratio has been changed from 1 : 6 to 1 : 10 ,1.50D. : 15△). At first the reading glasses may feel strange. The type is clear but somehow it seems larger and slightly unsteady. Usually the adjustment is quick. The same effect is over the whole lens field and peripheral fusion helps to orient things. Even the slightly blurred objects at distance are projected properly again.

Why should this readaptation not carry over to bifocals just as easily in all cases? The new bifocal wearer is still not expert in locating the particular reading position required by the segments. He still has considerable accommodative amplitude available, and he can continue to look at many things in the intermediate or reading field through the distance portion of his lenses. By the very design of his bifocals he has an immediate choice. For momentary use he can still summon enough accommodation to see well at the reading distance. Thus he makes a maximum accommodative effort without increased convergence. Then when he deliberately tries to use the reading field, the difficulty he might have had is multiplied. Consider this hypothetical case:

   ℞ O.D. Plano Distance
      O.S. Plano
      O.U. +1.00D. spheres added for reading.

This person sits at his/her desk with some business papers on it and holds a letter in his hands. He looks at a paper on the desktop at 67 cm from his eyes using the upper part of his lenses in which there is no power. Therefore, he uses

    1.50D. accommodation with 9$^\triangle$ convergence for clear binocular vision.

When he looks at a paper 50 cm away, he uses

    2.00D. accommodation with 12$^\triangle$ convergence.

He uses the reading segments of his bifocals to read the letter in his hands at 40 cm and uses only 1.50D. accommodation because the reading addition supplements his requirements with +1.00D. He must continue to converge as much as ever, so he now uses

    +1.50D. accommodation with 15$^\triangle$ convergence.

Now while his eyes are using the reading portions he changes his attention to the paper at 50 cm. The +1.00D. sphere in the segment does half the work of accommodation, so he uses

    +1.00D. accommodation with 12$^\triangle$ convergence.

When his attention turns to the paper farther away he uses

    (+1.50 −1.00D.) 0.50D. accommodation and 9$^\triangle$ convergence.

Table XIX reviews his activities with his new lenses and it is at once apparent that a large latitude in the ratio between accommodation and convergence is necessary for the intended use of the bifocal lenses and greater yet is demanded if the reading portion is used for distances beyond 40 cm.

Such tables are factual optically, but it should never be forgotten that the amplitudes, reserves, and adaptability of eyes are the most individual of functions. It is important though that a dispenser have a full understanding of the challenge presented to the fusion reflex by the replacement of a part of the function (accommodation) by lens power.

TABLE XIX

Distance (cm)	Accom. Required	Lens Rx in Use	Accom. in Use	Conv. in Use	Ratio of Accom. to Conv.
100	1.00D.	0.00	1.00D.	6	1 : 6
67	1.50D.	0.00	1.50D.	9△	1 : 6
50	2.00D.	0.00	2.00D.	12△	1 : 6
40	2.50D.	1.00D.	1.50D.	6△	1 : 10
50	2.00D.	1.00D.	1.00D.	15△	1 : 12
67	1.50D.	1.00D.	0.50D.	12△	1 : 18
100	1.00D.	1.00D.	0.00D.	9△	Indeterminate

The physiologic function that accounts for the required versatility was discussed in Chapter 8 with reference to Percival and the "area of comfort." The name for the function is Positive Relative Convergence (Donders, 1864). This is defined as the amount of convergence that can be stimulated while accommodation is not further stimulated. A healthy pair of young eyes usually has about 12△ Pos. Rel. Conv. During the onset of presbyopia, this function usually diminishes and a number of bifocal problem cases are among those whose fusion convergence is inadequate when accommodative efforts are replaced by plus lenses.

By way of experiment a pair of plano lenses were fitted to a fit-over frame. A pair of plano prism segments 2△ Base Out O.U. were cemented on the lenses. The whole combination had no focal power, but if the eyes viewed objects through the prism segments, it was necessary to increase convergence by 4△ without a corresponding increase in accommodation. For a 60 mm interocular distance (I.O.D.), 6 Prism Diopters of convergence are associated with 1.00 diopter of accommodation. Then 0.67D. accommodation and 4△ convergence are the habitual ratio. If the accommodative effort is replaced by a +0.67D. sphere, 4△ convergence is inhibited. In order to maintain the proper amount of convergence, an additional 4△ outside of the habitual ratio must be stimulated. Thus, the prism segments simulated the effect of an addition of 0.67D. sphere to the convergence function. It was interesting to note how quickly and convincingly this small amount of prism in the fit-over produced "bifocal symptoms" for many young spectacle wearers much before the age of presbyopia.

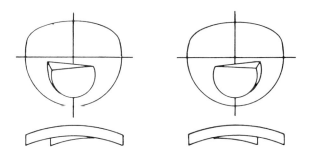

Figure 174. Plano addition prism segments of research bifocals.

A patient with an inadequate fusion reserve may accept a pair of reading glasses with no great difficulty. The demands for change of ratio seem simpler when the whole field of the lens is the same prescription. In much the same way that the special fit-overs can be uncomfortable as the ratio must change with each fixation, so do the first bifocals or a prescription change affect some patients. It is important, however, to appreciate a patient's possible problem and important to know that, although it frequently takes a little longer for some than it does for others, a careful fitting and some patience during the first days usually bring a satisfactory conclusion. A good device to hurry this adjustment is to recommend that the new wearer practice with his lenses while seated at a table or desk. A good exercise is the morning paper at the breakfast table or eating a meal or doing desk work. Avoid using the lenses for work at intermediate distance for a few days. Walking with the lenses will become easier when the near-point problem clears up.

To summarize, the changes of habit that the patient must make in order to use multifocal lenses satisfactorily are (a) learn to move his eyes automatically to a restricted area (porthole) in his visual field when he wishes to see clearly at near-point; (b) become accustomed to a constant angle of depression and a restricted lateral movement for near-point; (c) in some instances, learn to use an area formerly avoided because of induced prism from an asymmetric prescription; and (d) develop new ratio between accommodation and convergence to compensate for accommodation replaced by spherical lens power.

None of these is really too difficult to surmount, even all of them are not a serious hazard. Most problem cases involve optical conditions that we are about to discuss. All too frequently improper lens designs, improperly fitted, are the cause of the patient's discomfort.

In the previous chapter, reference was made to the prodigious amount of research and computation that has been done through the years to open the aperture (useful field) of spectacle lenses. The vast majority of all prescription lenses are almost precisely the same dioptric power over an angle of 60° which practically covers the field of binocular vision. It has been pointed out that a spectacle wearer is able to make sensory revaluation of his spatial perception very shortly after his glasses are fitted. Even the wearers of quite strong prescriptions indiscriminately use the centers or the margins of their lenses and are unaware of any prism displacement so long as the prescriptions for the two eyes are identical or nearly so. In other words, the lens designers have been successful in their part of providing prescription lenses with such curve correction that free ocular movement has become a reality.

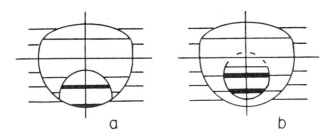

Figure 175. Prism at N.V.P. in round and flat top segments.

In recent years, however, several writers have extolled the advantages and even the necessity of designing and grinding bifocals in such a manner as to produce an optical center at the reading point in the bifocal segment (Fig. 175*a*). The premise in most of these articles is that the displacement induced by the prism effect of the decentered distance portion of the lens at the near vision point (N.V.P.) conflicts with the performance of the reading portion. The fact is that the patient is as well adapted to the use of any portion of the upper part of his lenses as he is to the point about 8 mm below the optical centers. It therefore seems to be open to question whether, because a patient chooses to wear bifocals, he must have bicentric lenses when no thought is given to such a necessity for the same individual's prescriptions for single vision lenses to be used for distance or for reading. It takes little imagination to visualize the confusion that would result if opticians were to attempt through slab-off or by any other means to provide distance and reading centers in all prescriptions whether the lenses were identical or not. There seems to be no particular reason why such an attitude should be adopted for bifocal wearers. Contrariwise, it seems that it would be advantageous to attempt to retain as many of the patient's habits as possible and that the least possible change be made to the displacement or prism effect of the distance prescription at the near-vision point (NVP).

This point of view is satisfied when the optical center of the reading segment is placed at the N.V.P. (Fig. 175b). In this way the prism displacement characteristic of the distance lens at this point is not disturbed. Present-day flat-top bifocal lenses fulfill this requirement admirably. The optical center of the segment is usually 4 to 5 mm below the dividing line and is therefore very near the average reading position. As an added advantage, the proximity of the dividing line to the optical center minimizes "jump." The fact that the eye uses the axial (central) rays of the reading segment causes the least change to the chromatic and other aberrations of the distance lens to which the patient is assumed to be habituated. Only those distance prescriptions that develop prismatic imbalances and interfere with binocular vision in the area from 6 to 10 mm below the geometric centers of the distance lenses require special consideration for optical modification.

In 1937, Lueck clearly presented the prismatic effects of lenses in the Bausch & Lomb Technical Publication No. 18 entitled *Bifocal Analysis in Anisometropia.* His paper covers trigonometric and graphical methods by which the combined prism effects of

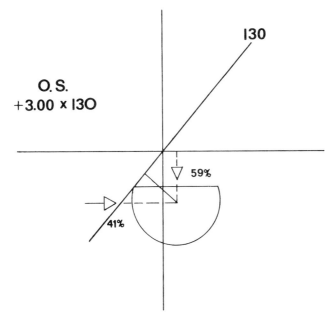

130

**O. S.
+3.00 × 130**

59%

41%

Figure 176.

sphere and cylinder power can be estimated simultaneously. Included at the end of the report is a series of tables to show the precise amounts of vertical prism generated by oblique cylinders with powers up to 6.00D. in which three amounts of depression and an inset of 2 mm for reading are taken into account. The component of horizontal prism is not discussed in this paper.

Two years later, Boeder, the Director of the Bureau of Visual Science at American Optical Company, offered a book entitled *Analysis of Prismatic Effects in Bifocal Lenses.* His illustrations of the zones of prismatic imbalances graphically portray how asymmetric prescriptions limit the areas of usefulness of single vision lenses. As part of the book are four large charts, one of which carefully works out the various factors that affect the optical center of the segment. The table for calculating vertical prismatic effects of cylinders is unique in that it provides a separate consideration of the increment due to segment centers decentration. By increasing or decreasing the amount of this fraction, greater or lesser amounts of inset can be carefully treated.

An approximation of these prism effects in many lenses can be made by arithmetic. An ophthalmic optician should be sufficiently familiar with the methods so that he can make mental calculations for the simpler lens problems. For this reason, a few examples will be discussed. In practice, Boeder's or Lueck's tables should be consulted or the problem plotted or calculated for precise results.

In the investigation of the prism effect at a particular point, removed by some distance from the optical center of the lens, three factors must be taken into consideration: (a) distance of point from lens center, (b) spherical power of lens, and (c) cylindrical power and axis of lens. The prism effect is significant only when the patient has binocular vision. In monocular vision, the prism displacement is not confusing because it is a function of the lens that gradually increases toward the margin of the lens.

In the discussion of Relative Convergence it was noted that the eyes have rather large degrees of tolerance to prisms set either Base In or Base Out. By way of demonstration, one or two diopters of prism either Base Out or Base In can be tolerated by most individuals often imperceptibly. Such latitude does not exist in the vertical field. Compensation for the condition of one image projected above the other is very limited to all persons. A $1^\triangle$ or $2^\triangle$ prism with the Base Up or Down held before the eyes of most persons will produce double images at once, with one image above the other. If the eyes do persist in single vision, there is usually a feeling of intense strain or effort.

When a spherical prescription with differing amounts of power for the two eyes is considered as described Figure 143, the prism effect at any point away from the optical centers is found by the application of Prentice's law of decentration. Restated: Lens power in diopters times decentration in centimeters equals prism diopters. If it is required to find the amount of prism difference in the prescription:

> O.D. +1.25   Optical centers 65/61
> O.S. +0.50   At a point 8 mm below the
>   optical centers.

The difference between the lenses is

$$+1.25 \quad \text{O.D.}$$
$$-(+0.50) \quad \text{O.S.}$$
$$\overline{+0.75} \quad \text{On the right side}$$
$$\times 0.8$$

$$\overline{\qquad}$$

0.6$^\triangle$ Base Up right side.

Whether this small amount of prism Base Up will be tolerated can be predicted only from the doctor's examination record. In a large number of cases it is not significant, but in others it may increase an existing phoria (muscle imbalance) and would be intolerable. The second part of the consideration of the horizontal prism effect is the amount created by the power of the distance prescription when the eyes are converged for reading. In this case, since the centers are to be spaced 65/61, the decentration for each eye is 2 mm. By Prentice's law the total effect is

$$1.25 \times 0.2 = 0.25^\triangle$$
$$0.50 \times 0.2 = 0.10^\triangle$$
$$\overline{\qquad 0.35^\triangle}$$

The optical centers are wider than the projection of the visual axes for near, therefore these plus lenses for distance impose the effect of prism Base Out on the reading segments. A greater convergence effort is required to overcome the effect of Base Out prism and is normally undesirable. The plus lens added to the distance to replace the failing accommodation for the presbyopic patient likewise reduces the habitual effort of associated function of convergence. However, this small prism effect of 0.35$^\triangle$ Base Out is regularly ignored. In the rare instances when it might have significance, it can be neutralized by an additional decentration of the bifocal reading segments. A +1.00D. addition generates 0.35$^\triangle$ by an increased decentration of 3.5 mm. A stronger reading addition would require even a lesser amount of compensation. The subject of prism compensation by increased decentration will be discussed later.

When a cylindrical element is involved in the distance prescription, in many instances the calculation can become more complicated. If the cylinder axis is horizontal (180°), there is no power in that meridian and no lateral prism is generated. The full power of the cylinder through the vertical meridian is added to the spherical power of the lens for computation of vertical prism effect. Cylinder axis 90 conversely has no power vertically but adds to the spherical element of the prescription for lateral prism effect. When the cylinder is oblique, the prism effect is usually resolved into two components in which part of the power is found in both the horizontal and vertical meridians.

The division of power is not a direct arithmetical proportion because it is controlled by the sine of the angle of the cylinder in which the meridian power = cylinder power $\times$ sin² axis. This relationship is reduced to a table (Table IV) which gives the curvature of a 1.00D. cylinder in all meridians. For other cylinder curvatures these factors increase in ratio. One also sees that the curvature of the lens in the meridian at a right angle is the difference between 1.00D. and the power in the required meridian.

For Example

    ℞ O.D. +4.50D. × 35

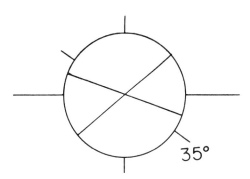

Figure 177. Cylinder effect at oblique axis.

    sin² 35° = .33
    +4.50 × .33 = +1.50D. in the horizontal meridian.
This cylinder axis is at an angle of 55° with the vertical meridian (the complimentary angle to 35°), then
    sin² 55° = .67   +4.50 × .67 = +3.00D.

For example, when using the procedure described on page 130, the power difference in this prescription is:

> ℞ O.D. +4.75 +2.00 × 40
> O.S. +3.75 +1.25 × 80

1. It is unnecessary to reduce these lenses to spherical equivalents because the right lens is plainly the stronger.

2. O.D. +4.75 +2.00 × 40
   O.S. −3.75 −1.25 × 80
   _____
   $+1.00\begin{cases}+2.00 \times 40 \\ -1.25 \times 80\end{cases}$

3.A. Transposing for uniform signs
   −1.25 +1.25 × 170 (a)
   +2.00 × 40   (b)

B. 170° − 40° = 130° × 2 = 260°

C. The diagonal of the parallelogram is approximately +2.25D. long (c)

D. The axis of the diagonal is 56°. But cylinder (A) axis is 170°. Hence the angle between the diagonal and (A) is 66°. Therefore, the midline and combined cylinder axis is 23°.

E. The induced sphere is
   $$\frac{(a+b)-c}{2} = \frac{(+1.25+2.00)-225}{2} = \frac{100}{2} - +0.50D$$

F. Therefore, the total sphere is:
   +1.00 −1.25 +0.50 = +0.25

G. Hence the combination of the oblique cylinders and lens difference is:
   O.D. +0.25 +2.25 × 23 (O.D.)

Figure 178 shows the zones of prism effect for the combined lenses and the optical difference which also shows the "zone of binocular comfort" when the limits previously assumed (0.5$^\triangle$ vertical and 2$^\triangle$ lateral) are applied.

A rapid method to estimate or to check the subtraction of any pair of lenses with a lensometer is described on page 530.

When the eyes converge for reading, the visual axes do not in-

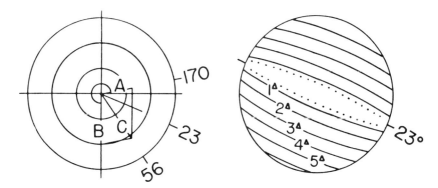

Figure 178. Limited zone of comfort of O.D. +0.25 +2.25 × 23 of lens differences in anisometropia.

tersect identical points in the vertical meridians of the lenses. The combined decentration *down* and *in* for each eye requires different methods than were applied in the cases of single vision lenses or for extra-axial points in the vertical or horizontal meridians. Oblique decentration of a cylindrical or spherocylindrical lens must be resolved into displacements of the two principal meridians of the lens. Precisely, the formula $D_m = D \sin^2 \theta$ should refer to curvature instead of diopters. An oblique meridian of a cylindrical surface is actually a section of an ellipse and does not perform the same as a spherical lens of the same power. The mathematical and graphical methods for the calculation of prism power at the N.V.P. are explained by Bennett, Boeder, and others.* The polar coordinate sheets suggested for crossed-cylinders is useful for the graphical method described by Lueck. For greatest convenience the charts available provide rapid and dependable data for this phase of lens analysis. They present all

*Bennett, A.G.: *Graphical Methods of Solving Optical Problems*. London, Hatton Press, 1948, pp. 20-25.

Boeder, P.: *Analysis of Prismatic Effects in Bifocals*. Southbridge, Mass., American Optical Company, 1939, pp. 22-23.

Emsley, H.H.: *Visual Optics*. London, Hatton Press, 1946, pp. 84-89.

Lueck, I.B.: *Bifocal Analysis in Anisometropia*. Rochester, Bausch & Lomb Optical Company, 1937, pp. 3-15.

Schactschabel, K.: *Dezentration Astigmatischer Brillenglaeser*. Jena, Statlichen Optikerschule, 1927, pp. 43-50.

the information for comparison of the different effects obtainable when both the centers of the distance portions and reading segments are manipulated.

When we return to a consideration of this patient's basic distance prescription, it should be remembered that this individual has worn a pair of lenses approximating this power for a number of years and is therefore acquainted with the zones of prismatic imbalance in the different parts of his lenses. Although this person may have used the marginal parts of his lenses for fleeting glances or for the purpose of orientation, it is altogether unlikely that he has been able to stray very far away from the optical centers for refined vision or any prolonged use of the eyes binocularly. A common practice for wearers of unbalanced prescriptions is to drop the head when reading so that the fixation lines intersect the lenses at points very close to the optical centers. The binocular vision of individuals with anisometropia has been previously discussed. In the case under consideration, this patient can not be expected to use his bifocal segments satisfactorily with a vertical prism of $2^\triangle$. If he has already been wearing ordinary bifocals, he has probably learned to suppress vision in one eye to avoid double vision. Whether it will be advisable to remove the prism effect in the reading segments and risk confusion is a matter that the doctor must decide. The patient's description of the discomfort with his old glasses should be a great help. The prism should be removed from the first pair of bifocals unless the doctor reports that binocular vision is faulty or vision is subnormal in one eye.

The management of centers and prism effects in extra-axial points is called *compensation*. There are several methods available to accomplish this purpose:

1. Compromise of distance lens centers
2. Different segment sizes of same style bifocal
3. Different types or shapes of bifocal segment
4. Slab-off (bicentric surface)
5. Prism in segment only

1. Occasionally the prism effect at the N.V.P. can be brought within the limits of tolerance while a small prism with its base in the opposite direction is induced into the distance lenses.

EXAMPLE

    ℞   O.D. +3.00, O.S. +1.50

         Optical centers 65/61 mm

         N.V.P. 6 mm below the optical centers

         Tolerance $0.5^\triangle$ in the vertical meridian

         Difference = +1.50 (O.D.)

         $1.50 \times .6 = 0.9^\triangle$ Base Up right eye.

Drop the centers of the distance lenses 3 mm O.U. and thereby place N.V.P. only 3 mm below center (Fig. 179). The induced prism is reduced to $0.45^\triangle$ Base Up right eye. The same amount of prism with the Base Down is induced in the distance portion of the lenses because the eyes are above the center of the right lens in primary position. The prism (0.45 Base Down right eye) is barely within the limit.

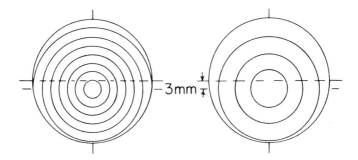

Figure 179. Effect of dropped centers of dissimilar reading lenses.

2. Small amounts of vertical prism are easily corrected by changing the position of the geometric (and optical center) of the segment in the Univis R type of lens. In the pair of lenses under consideration, the +2.00D. addition must be decentered 4.5 mm to produce $0.9^\triangle$, the decentration to be up over the left eye (or down over the right eye) to neutralize the prism Base Up effect before the right eye. If a Univis D is used before the left eye with the center 4 mm below the segment edge and an "R" segment before the right eye ground to place its center 8.5 mm below the top edge of the segment edge, the vertical prism is balanced.

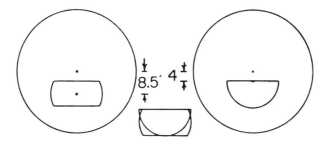

Figure 180. Dissimilar segment centers and shapes to offset vertical prism.

When this patient's eyes converge for near vision, a small amount of prism Base Out is induced (+3.00 × .2 — 0.6ᐃ and +1.50 × 2 = 0.3ᐃ which totals 0.9ᐃ Base Out). The horizontal prism is undesirable but is a factor with which the patient has had to contend all the time he has worn a prescription of this type. Each time he converges his eyes to read at a point on the median line, even without depressing his eyes, he has to overcome a total of 0.9ᐃ due to the fact that his fixation lines are closer than the lens centers of his distance prescription.   If this lateral prism caused undue fatigue in his distance prescription, he could accomplish some compensation by holding his reading matter to the right side or turning his head to the left.

This lateral prism can also be completely overcome if the right eye is turned 4 mm past center to the right thus producing (+3.00D. × 0.4) 1.2ᐃ base to the left while the left eye turns 4 mm of convergence (65/61) plus 4 mm of right vergence (+1.50D. × 0.8) 1.2ᐃ base to the left which neutralizes the right prism.   The position of the bifocal segments often prevents this approach. The patient can hold the vertical prism effect at minimum by tipping his head forward to stay close to the lens centers.   It is impracticable to attempt to overcome the horizontal prism by extra decentration of the segments.   It requires a total of 4.5 mm decentration of the +2.00D. sphere addition to account for 0.9ᐃ. Most of the prism Base Out effect in the reading segments can be obliterated if the optical centers of the distance prescription are set nearer to the near-point measurement. This also tends to pro-

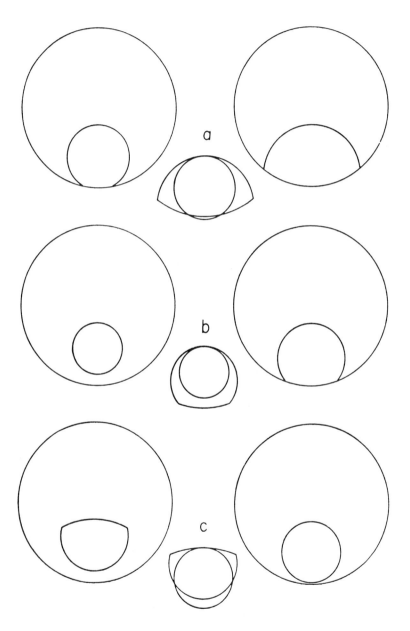

Figure 181. Various dissimilar optical centers and shapes of segments to balance out prism.

mote comfort for the wearer when he converges his eyes for distances less than infinity and uses the upper part of his lenses.

3. The vertical prism in the position of the reading segment also can be corrected by any pair of round segments (fused or one-piece) in which the center of the larger segment is placed 5 mm lower before the left eye and again neutralizes the prism.

These radical treatments of dissimilar segments should be used only as a last resort. They are unsightly and in many cases are not functional because of the small reading area common to the two segments.

a. R. Ultex "B"—22 mm
    L. Ultex "E"—32 mm
    Incidentally, the large segment before the left eye may be decentered to give a total distance between segment centers less than 61 mm and thereby create prism Base In to neutralize some of the prism Base Out induced by the distance prescription.

b. R. Orthogon C—16 mm
    L. Orthogon F—22 mm
    This combination is a slight undercorrection and may not be satisfactory for general use because of the diameter of the right segment.

c. R. Ful-Vue
    L. Tillyer "D"
    This combination is absolutely correct when the left segment is 20 mm in diameter and the center of the segment of the right lens is placed at the dividing line. Again, the only difficulty might be that the segments are smaller than those to which the patient is habituated.

4. A pair of straight-top bifocals in which a slab-off (Fig. 182) prism of 0.9^Δ is ground on the outside curve of the left lens to make the same amount of Base Up prism that is found at the N.V.P. in the right lens balances the vertical error perfectly.

This is the compensation of choice. The only handicap is that it cannot be successfully done for very small amounts of prism because the curves run together and the dividing line becomes badly blurred. If a wide segment like Univis "R" is used, a slight

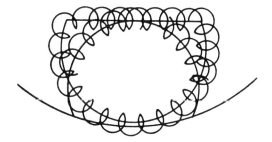

Figure 182. Blur at margins of dissimilar segment shapes.

amount of the prism Base Out can be overcome by extra decentration in.

5. The major manufacturers can grind prism into the one-piece
forms except the flat top Ultex K segment. For the sake of appearance and weight as well as function, it is recommended that
prism segments in one-piece bifocals be confined to the "B" (22
mm) segments. The segment may be ground below or above the
level of the posterior curve according to the prescription for distance and the position of the base of the prism. Prism is available
in Ful-Vue and Univis "R" bifocal segments. It is limited to $3^{\triangle}$
laterally or vertically in each lens.

With any of these compensating (or balancing) methods, the
area at 8 mm below center and 2 mm to the nasal side has been
made optically satisfactory for the patient to use for his bifocal
segments.   In this particular case, in which the addition is
+2.00D. and the distance lenses are rather strong, it is implied
that this person may previously have worn bifocals. In this event,
he already has learned how to find and use the segments of the
lenses even if he did not derive much comfort through the vertical
displacement from the prism effect. If perchance he has had two
pairs of glasses before, and these are his first bifocals, he has an
extra task added to the habit changes necessary for new wearers
of double vision lenses. He not only has to learn how to find the
reading area easily when he wishes to read, he must also *break the
habit* of avoiding this extra-axial field that was formerly an uncomfortable area in both his distance and reading lenses.

Throughout the discussion of compensation for the placement

of optical centers of reading portions of bifocals with dissimilar segments, no reference has been made to the practical effect. It should not be forgotten that the segment of the visual field represented by the reading portion has a fuzzy border. It has been shown that the fields of both the distance and portions of the multifocal segments are invaded by these blurred areas. A large part of the process of becoming acquainted with bifocals is concerned with learning the knack of verging the eyes just the right amount to strike the central area of the fuzzy ring that describes the margin of the reading segment. Some patients are exceedingly reluctant to attempt to change their habits with reference to bifocal segments once they have been learned. A dispenser may unknowingly assume a large risk with these individuals unless their expressed symptoms indicate they are willing to make some effort to rid themselves of discomfort. In binocular vision, the patient has the effect of looking through a porthole that has the composite shape of asymmetric segments. The classical example is a flat-top and round-top combination as shown in Figure 182. The usable field is materially reduced for two reasons. The superimposed shapes leave a small central island for binocular use. The eyes have to be depressed a greater angle for the round-top segment to avoid the blind area caused by the "jump." Altogether the blurred margin is increased to the point, in many cases, in which small segments are used, that the anticipated benefit of the compensation is nullified. The literature is replete with the discussions of this approach to prism correction, but most reports are made from limited numbers of case histories. It is true that individuals with strong binocular function and unbalanced prescriptions have been made so comfortable by the relief from the effects of prism that they have not squabbled with the means, but routine use of asymmetric bifocal segment shapes has usually been curtailed by most advocates after a thorough try.

There are altogether too many factors involved to make broad statements with reference to bicentric (compensated) multifocals in cases of asymmetric distance prescriptions. A first consideration is the *zone of binocular comfort* as determined by the *optical difference* of the lenses and the individual patient's tolerances. The patient's report of his experience with previous multifocals is equally important. When no difficulty is reported, it can be assumed that any or all of several hidden causes may relieve him from the discomfort which the prescription indicates he should experience in this area of his near-vision point. He may have materially reduced vision in one eye of which he may (or even may not) be aware. He may have a poor binocular function—that is, he may unconsciously suppress vision in one eye or the other at the least provocation and thus have no difficulty with diplopia. Many individuals use their eyes monocularly for years before the onset of presbyopia and learn to become easily adapted to the use of one eye while the other retinal image is ignored. Civil engineers, watchmakers and jewelers, microscopists, and many others become habituated to monocular devices. Lastly, visual activities may not involve much near-point seeing and the bifocal segments may be only as a convenience for occasional refined vision. The prospects for success in this type of case like most other things is at its best when an expressed need exists.

Experience shows that one of the first advantages of slab-off is that the compensation can be accomplished in lenses identical with or similar to the lenses worn by other presbyopic patients. Flat top "D" bifocals can be inconspicuously corrected by a slab-off of one lens. Other flat top segments such as "R" can be vertically decentered for small amounts of prism correction. On special factory order, these segments can also be obtained with lateral prism.

The slab-off method is obviously capable of correcting only

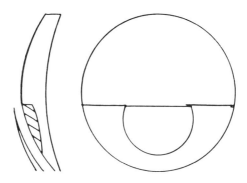

Figure 183. Slab-off at top edge of flat top segment.

vertical prism effects. The bicentric grinding adds prism Base Up effect to the compensated lens. The limit of correction is approximately $3^\triangle$ because of the increase in lens thickness.

A minus prescription in the upper part of bifocal lenses reverses the horizontal prism effect. The decentration from convergence for reading makes prism Base In effect. This prism reduces the stimulation to convergence when the wearer uses the reading portion. Bifocals for myopic eyes ordinarily should have the reading segments set precisely at the measured visual axis separation (O.C.) for reading. The amount added to the near-point optical centers to make the width for distance should be full. The slight amount of prism Base In effect that the lenses produce as the patient uses his eyes for lesser amounts of convergence at distances less than infinity through the upper part of his lenses will ordinarily be advantageous. A record of the exact position of optical centers (O.C.) for near-point should be made on the prescription record and followed by an explanation about any variation to overcome prism effect. A pair of strong plus lens bifocals often produce a better result if the distance optical centers are reduced to the actual near-point measurement without any further decentration in the reading segment. Again, the slight amount of Base In prism in the distance portion of the lenses is tolerated better than an equal amount of Base Out in the reading area.

The position of the top edge of a reading portion or the "height of segment" is the last consideration. An old rule and a good one is to have the top of the segment at the line of the lashes on the lower lid (Fig. 184) when the eyes are looking at the horizon and the head is held in the same posture as used for walking. (This position of the segment is a good point to use for comparison when opticians wish to refer to segments "2 mm higher than average" or "3 mm lower than usual.") When the patient's eyes look straightforward the segment is low enough (with the lenses at an average distance from the eyes) to be almost unnoticed. The blurred streak caused by the upper edge of the reading portion continues around the reading portion. It is the shape of the segment and varies from 2 to 5 inches in width according to the distance it is projected in space. The blur never seems to be as close as the lenses nor as far away as the fixation distance. In the

binocular act of seeing, the fuzzy margins of the two bifocal segments form a composite blur at the margin of the clear reading
area. Any misalignment or maladjustment increases the width of
the blurred area. Reading segments improperly decentered for
the near-point do not accurately superimpose and thereby reduce
the available clear reading field. Dissimilar sized segments as suggested for prism compensation create the same effect.

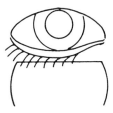

Figure 184. Position of top of flat top segment.

Outside the blur is the distance lens and inside it is the reading
field. This blurred line is connected with much of the confusion
in walking. It must not be forgotten that reading glasses seldom
interfere with surefootedness. It is not always the unfocussed
field that confounds the bifocal wearer. Even prism displacement
must be a large amount in order to be noticeable. When we
realize that the average person's eyes are less than 2 meters from
the ground and that each Prism Diopter means less than 20 mm
(0.8 inch) displacement at his feet, such a small amount of prism
is ordinarily unnoticed. A head movement causes the blurred
line to intercept the line of vision, a small turn to either side
causes a sudden change in the apparent size and position of the
step or curbstone at the wearer's feet. These rapid alterations
create the patient's dilemma. Until the wearer becomes thoroughly familiar with the location of this blurred line, he frequently
may be unsure of his footing. Teach him to avoid the reading
area when he looks at his feet. Have him turn his head to one
side of the segment. Demonstrate how it works by placing a pair
of pliers or a coin on the floor near his feet. Let him move his
head to bring the objects in and out of the reading portion.

The admonition not to change the style of bifocal is associated more with familiarity of the shape and position of the blurred line than with the change in prism effect. When patients are provided more than one bifocal type to accommodate them for vocational vision, as for example, large Ultex for near work and small segment bifocals for outdoor use, one finds that these individuals develop a tolerance or versatility that permits them to change to and fro without confusion. Prolonged use of any particular type of lens often fixes habits that in some instances overshadow improved optical performance.

From the physiological point of view, bifocals should be prescribed as early as possible after the incidence of presbyopia. Each diopter of addition has about 6$^{\triangle}$ of convergence associated with it. Therefore, the shock and the adjustment for it are greater with each advancing year. The longer separate reading glasses are worn, the more difficult it may become to develop a habit to read in a restricted area of the lens field. As accommodative amplitude diminishes, the eyes cannot use the distance portion of the lenses so freely for intermediate distances as is the case in early presbyopia. At the time of +1.00D. addition, the eyes can momentarily read most type for short periods through the distance portion. Conversely, objects can be quite clear for distances up to 1 meter (40 inches), the focal distance of the addition. Even the floor at one's feet is not badly blurred. This overlapping of fields diminishes as the need for increased addition develops. This is a further complication in the adaptation to bifocals later in life. The exception to the rule would be the person who seemed very doubtful that he could adjust himself to bifocals at a low addition. The doctor's professional judgment may be that a greater need would provide the motivation for a greater effort on the part of his patient.

One doctor developed a routine for this type of patient that, with a dispensing optician's cooperation, was "sure fire." The doctor wrote the prescription and plainly ordered two pairs of glasses:

1. Distance, clear.
2. Reading.

He then told his patient he was not prescribing bifocals because he thought the patient would have too much trouble getting used to them. The optician was aware of what was going on and did not talk about bifocals unless the patient raised the subject. He told of their convenience but also made some remarks about people not having the patience to learn to use them. The distance glasses were made up in any type of frame, but the optician made every effort to have the reading glasses fitted to a plastic frame. When the glasses were fitted, the optician was especially solicitous of the patient and demonstrated the use of the two pairs of glasses two or three times by taking off one pair, then the other, to show how nicely they performed for their intended uses. He concluded with a strong invitation to return if any difficulties developed.

If there were no difficulties, the doctor was correct in the assumption that two pairs of glasses would fill the need best. The vast majority of these persons were back in less than two weeks with complaints. Now they had not been told that because of their eyes they could not wear bifocals. They had been told they might have too much trouble with bifocals. After the tale of woe was recounted, the patient (or if necessary the optician) brought up the subject of bifocals as a possible solution. The next step was a conversation with the doctor to get his "permission" to change the prescription and try bifocals. By this time the patient had had enough of the business of carrying two pairs of glasses and forever calling attention to his infirmity as well as having great inconvenience as he changed from one pair to the other. He was now ready to make the effort to learn how to use the bifocal lenses. Thus the patient finished with a pair of bifocals in which the optician did not have to set the reading segments too high, because the wearer had a pair of reading glasses to use when his activity was all in the near-point field.

There is a class of individuals for whom bifocals are usually a failure in the early part of presbyopia. These are patients who have weak prescriptions, either myopic or hyperopic, and who have never worn their glasses consistently. For example: O.U. —0.50D. Add +1.00D. They are used to slightly blurred vision at distance or near or both. They have learned all the tricks of how to do without glasses. Sometimes they have flaunted their independence of spectacles. Those in this group who wear plus lenses are ordinarily most happy with two pairs, and if it must be only one pair, they choose the reading glasses. Conversely, the myopes take the distance glasses and do without the weaker lenses for reading. For a long time they will continue to read without glasses. Only vocational demands for alternating clear vision at distance and near will force bifocals on some of these customers.

If the wearer holds his head still and drops his eyes, he will easily engage the segments for reading and the blurred dividing line will be well above the point of fixation. These remarks apply to the round-top bifocals of all types. Flat-top lenses may be fitted 1 to $1\frac{1}{2}$ mm lower with safety. The reduced "jump" and straight dividing line increase the efficiency of the upper part of the reading portion. There are several other factors to consider. A new wearer of bifocals may be highly perplexed and unhappy if the segments are too noticeable when he is trying to use his eyes for distance. It is therefore wise to use a frame or mounting for "first bifocals" patients that can be adjusted to raise the lenses. They can be adjusted a little (1 to $1\frac{1}{2}$ mm) lower than eventually intended and can then be worn for a few days until acceptance has improved. Another device to assist in accustoming the novice to the new lenses is temporarily to tilt them in at the bottom somewhat more than normal. This tends to foreshorten the blurred area in the distance visual field. The patient should have explained to him what is happening and how these temporary adjustments are being made to assist him in the process of learning how to use his new lenses. After a week or two the lenses can be adjusted to set the segments at the height and angle originally intended.

TRIFOCALS

In 1826 Hawkins* divided three round lenses into horizontal slabs in which were fitted sections of +1.25D., +3.00D., and +5.00D. spheres. In 1916, I made a pair of cemented lenses for a landscape artist with three focal powers. A very large segment was cemented on the distance lens with an addition to bring sharp focus on the canvas at the end of her long-handled brushes (prob-

*Von Rohr, M.: *Die Brille als Optische Instrument.* Berlin, Springer, 1921, pp. 309-310.

ably 25 to 30 inches). On top of that segment a smaller segment was cemented with enough more plus effect to give clear vision at her palette. There is no claim to originality. The glasses were clearly described in advance by the patient. Her doctor had explained how they could be made. Surely it must have been an old idea to Doctor Williamson and something that he had prescribed before.

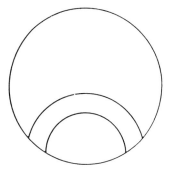

Figure 185. Original Ultex (one-piece) trifocal.

In the years that have elapsed, several manufacturers have experimented with trifocals and repeated articles have been written about them but until about 1940 there was no widespread interest. These lenses are very difficult to manufacture. The investment in research and machinery has been tremendous. The first large-scale production was accomplished in Ultex (one-piece) lenses. The lenses had two curves in the addition, the intermediate portion was about 9 mm wide in an arcuate shape surrounding the reading section (Fig. 185). The power of the intermediate was constant for all reading additions. Those who undertook to wear these lenses fell into either of two widely separated groups—they could not get along without the lenses or they could not wear them at all. Some of the enthusiasts, occasionally a doctor, highly recommended the lenses to large numbers of presbyopes requiring a total reading addition of +2.00D. or more. The percentage of disappointments was very high. Opticians were puzzled at the outcome. Further, they found it necessary to replace a large number of the lenses. In the light of the present development of trifocals it is almost amusing to reread the publicity on the lenses as they were developed. The manufacturer's praise of his product was followed by limited case reports. Optical literature made hasty reference to trifocals usually with broad statements as to their intended uses but no specific recommendations. Frequently the publications reflected a certain amount of fear of the lenses. One writer used as his criteria for screening:

1. Real need (reading addition +2.50D. or more)
2. Special vocational need
3. Sufficient intelligence to follow instructions for the use of the lenses
4. Willingness to assume increased cost of lenses

After anything is reasonably well perfected, it does not take much intelligence to see some of the mistakes made in the development of the idea. From that rather questionable position, a discussion of the trifocal theory will be undertaken. These remarks are intended to give the presbyope's point of view. When the limitations as well as advantages of the lenses are appreciated, better suggestions and advice can be given to the prospective wearer.

A presbyopic patient begins to realize that his vision is not as keen as he would like to have it at a distance of about 25 to 30 inches by the time he is wearing plus 1.50D. add. One of the first instances may be when he is in conversation with a person whose eyes are at or above his own eye level and who is about two feet away from him. His immediate wish is to back farther away from the individual or change his position so that he can approach the person a little closer and get his own eye level high enough to use his bifocal segments comfortably for a good clear image. Similar situations may not present themselves too frequently, but this visual inconvenience at intermediate distance is symptomatic of a new and very real condition that is developing for the presbyopic patient that was not present when his presbyopia was first corrected.

Refraction for middle distance as well as the correcting lens power is a subject separate and distinct from the ordinary reasoning for bifocal and reading lens fitting. The patient who has out-lived the prescription for his last bifocals has arrived at this state. His previous distance prescription is most likely almost correct and in most instances the small accommodative effort required at this point will not be the cause of his principal complaint. His intermediate distance vision will be fair to good depending to what degree his old lenses are outdated. In other words, the more amplitude of accommodation he has lost since his last refraction, the poorer the glasses perform at the reading distance and the better they serve at intermediate points. In his latter days just prior to his eye examination he will have been holding reading matter outside of his normal reading distance much the same as he did just before he was fitted with his first reading correction. His area of sharpest vision extends from 50 to 70 cm (20 to 28 inches). In the patient's opinion, all that is needed is an increased lens power, because that is what solved his problem before.

The new prescription will definitely assist the patient in his reading field, but at the same time, the more his near vision is improved by the addition of plus spheres, the more his vision slightly beyond the focal distance of the addition is blurred. The practice of using the reading segment for reading as well as dis-tances up to an arm's length will be lost and the distance pre-scription will render no assistance. From this reasoning, it is seen that when accommodative amplitude has decreased to the point that as much as $+2.00D.$ is required for reading, the same accom-modative deficiency deprives the patient of the ability to focus his eyes for clear vision at an arm's length of 67 cm. The $+2.00D.$ reading addition blurs his sight just beyond 50 cm and as the patient's age increases, and with it the power of the addition, the gap becomes unavoidably wider. Reference to Table XII and Figure 172 at this time will again impress the incontrovertible fact that unless the presbyope who wears $+2.00D.$ or more addi-tion for reading will be satisfied with clear vision at two and only two distances, he must be assisted by his doctor and optician with lenses for his intermediate distance. Somehow, I feel that it was only the very small lenses in Franklin's glasses that discouraged his usual acuteness and prevented him from also presenting man-kind with trifocals for the prolongation of youth.

Consistent with the characteristics of any optical instrument, the eye has some depth of focus when accommodated for any distance. If blur spots approximating those of 20/40 vision are used as criteria, it is seen in "Focus Depth" in Chapter 17 that when standard photographic lens formulas are applied to the Gullstrand schematic eye accommodated for distances up to 33 cm (3.00D.), some focal depth is found in the near-point field. In the earlier stages of presbyopia, the comparatively larger accommodative amplitude adds to this latitude to give the patient a continuing sharp focus. The shorter object distances tend to diminish the focal depth and more importantly the lack of supporting accommodation reduces the longitude of the reading area.

The probable reasons trifocals were not generally accepted as they were first presented are (a) shape of intermediate field, (b) vertical height of field, (c) "jump" at dividing line, and (d) focal power of intermediate lens. The arcuate shape of the intermediate field of the original one-piece lens is not economic of lens areas. The fact that the optical center of the section is 19 mm from the top edge of the segment causes considerable "jump" at the dividing line. The intermediate fields in the lower corners of the lens are not particularly usable and make it difficult to see the floor near the wearer's feet without tipping the head severely. Since the plane of the lens is about 25 mm from the center of rotation of the eye, 1 mm at the lens equals 27 mm at 67 cm from the lens plane. The width of the intermediate portion was 9 mm. When the pupil is 4 mm in diameter the vertical height of the intermediate field is $(9 - 4 = 5)$ $5 \times 24 = 135$ mm (5.3 inches) when projected to the intermediate distance for which the eye is focussed. At the wearer's feet an average of 150 cm (60 inches) from the eyes, the slightly blurred and somewhat displaced projection of the intermediate segment area is 5×60 equals 30 cm (11.8 inches). The top of the reading segment is necessarily displaced 9 mm lower than the top of the intermediate section.

Objects in the intermediate field are ordinarily at a smaller angle of depression than the reading field—that is, they are usually farther away from the viewer, for example, items some distance away on a desk or table top, instruments in a tray for a surgeon

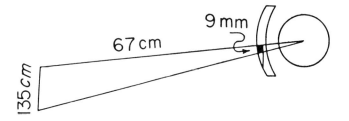

Figure 186. Vertical vista of 9 mm intermediate portion.

or dentist, an automobile instrument board. The top edge (or height) of the trifocal segment can then be set a considerable distance higher than a bifocal reading segment. Obviously it is necessary that this be done or the reading section would be so low that it could be used only with great difficulty.

The width of the intermediate section in the original one-piece trifocal was a great problem in any circumstances. The top edge of the segment was set below the pupillary margin to permit clear distance vision when the eyes were in primary position. The situation was further provoked by the "jump" at the transition from intermediate to near. This "blind area" below the dividing line made it necessary that a rather wide intermediate band be used. The additional displacement of the reading portion often caused the effective near-vision point in the reading segment to be set at an uncomfortable angle of depression.

In the first models of these lenses, the addition in the intermediate field was a fixed amount of +1.37D. Experience shows that this amount proved to be too strong for a large number of patients. The addition substantially replaced all accommodative effort at mid-distance while the total addition required a larger supplement for the near-point. At an intermediate distance of 67 cm, 1.50 diopters of accommodation are required and a +1.37D. addition leaves only 0.12D. in use. A reading distance of 36 cm requires +2.75D. accommodation. When the reading addition is +2.00D., then 0.75D. accommodation is needed.

A view of the task of the accommodative-convergence function in use with this old-style lens shows how great adaptability is required. When a pair of eyes with 60 mm interocular distance fix on an object at 80 cm distance through the distance portion of the lenses, the average ratio between accommodation and convergence, 1 : 6, prevails. Table XX shows how the function must be altered when a trifocal with +1.37D. intermediate and +2.00D. total reading addition is used.

TABLE XX

Fixation Distance (cm)	Accom. Required	Supplied by Lens	Accom. in Use	Converg. in Use	Ratio
		Distance R			
80	1.25D.	0.00	1.25D.	7.5△	1 : 6
		Intermediate Addition			
67	1.50D.	1.37D.	0.12D.	9.0△	1 : 72
		Reading Addition			
36	2.75D.	+2.00D.	0.75D.	16.5△	1 : 22

Practically, there are few persons at the age when +2.00D. addition is required for reading who have such flexibility to the accommodative-convergence function. The trifocal lens should be designed to provide extended clear vision beyond the limit of the depth of focus of the reading addition and inside the depth of focus of distance vision with particular reference to the distance about 67 cm from the eyes. To arbitrarily use such a strong intermediate addition for all cases only sets up the same condition again at a distance of about the far limit of the depth of focus of the +1.37D. addition. Later observations have proved that since the reading addition is a percentage of the dioptric distance to the reading point directly calculated from the loss of accommodative amplitude, it was also proper that the intermediate segment be a percentage of the addition for reading. This lends itself admirably to the fused multifocal lens because the problem of power is simply the choice of proper index of refraction for the two kinds of glass in the segments. Percentages ranging from 37 to 74 of the total reading addition have been used. Experience shows that an amount close to 50 percent is correct for regular uses.

When the intermediate addition is one-half the total reading addition, Table XXI shows the amount of supplementary accommodation that must be supplied at both the intermediate and reading distances outside the focal power provided by the lens. At the extreme right is the total accommodative amplitude of a patient for whom the reading addition provides a reserve of 50 percent.

TABLE XXI

	Intermediate Fixation at 67 cm +1.50D. Accommodation 9△ Convergence			Reading Fixation at 36 cm +2.75D. Accommodation 16.5△ Convergence			Total Accommodative Amplitude
Reading Addition	Lens Supplies	Accom. Supplies	Ratio	Lens Supplies	Accom. Supplies	Ratio	
+1.75	+0.87	+0.62	1 : 14	1.75	1.00	1 : 16	2.00
+2.00	+1.00	+0.50	1 : 18	2.00	0.75	1 : 22	1.50
+2.25	+1.12	+0.37	1 : 24	2.25	0.50	1 : 33	1.00
+2.50	+1.25	+0.25	1 : 36	2.50	0.25	1 : 66	0.50

The gradually diminishing requirements from accommodative amplitude at both distances appear to be consistent with the gradient of the total available amplitude. A comparison of the effect upon the accommodative-convergence effort when this percentage of lens power is supplied to the intermediate correction further clarifies the premise.

Through the distance portion of a pair of trifocals with +2.00D. reading addition fixing at a distance slightly beyond the focus of the calculated intermediate distance, say 80 cm (31 inches), the normal requirements are accommodation 1.25D., convergence 7.5△ with ratio 1 : 6. Table XXII shows the changes in function when the trifocal segments are used.

On the assumption that this beginner with trifocals has previously been wearing +1.50D. added for reading, he is already

TABLE XXII

Fixation Distance (cm)	Accom. Required	Supplied by Lens	Accom. in Use	Converg. in Use	Ratio
67	1.50D.	1.00D.	0.50D.	9.0△	1 : 18
36	2.75D.	2.00D.	0.75D.	16.5△	1 : 25

trained to use $+1.25$D. $(2.75 - 1.50)$ accommodation and 16.5^Δ convergence in the reading portion of the bifocals to his last prescription. To use $+0.50$ accommodation and 9^Δ convergence is almost exactly the same ratio he has been using in reading projected slightly farther from his eyes.

TABLE XXIII

Ful-Vue®	50 and 66% on order
Panoptik®	62%
Univis®	50%
Widesite®	54%
Ultex®	+1.12 up to +2.25 for reading
	+1.37 above +2.25

The percentage of the total reading power to be found in the intermediate addition has varied in the different manufacturers' lens designs. Some of the lensmakers have altered the relationship from time to time as they have sought to meet the requirements of trifocal fitters. Table XXIII, accumulated in 1947, gives the percentages:

Aside from the 50 percent for regular stock blanks, Univis offers to make any of their designs with 37, 67, 75 percent of the reading addition for the intermediate correction. If the prescription had been filled with each of the lens types above, it would have varied as shown in Table XXIV.

TABLE XXIV

	Intermediate Addition	Accommodation Supplied
Full-Vue	+1.00D.	0.50D.
Panoptik	+1.24D.	0.26D.
Univis	+1.00D.	0.50D.
Widesite	+1.08D.	0.42D.
Ultex	+1.12D.	0.37D.

In his new prescription, the major change of the patient's habits will be in the reading section of the lenses at the distance at which his recent difficulties have been the greatest. The problem of becoming acquainted with the intermediate field of trifocals quite obviously will not be physiological, because he has little change of accommodative-convergence pattern at the intermediate distance. When he has become expert (as he one day accomplished with his bifocals) at finding the little window through which he can clearly see at about the distance of his fingertips, he can thank his doctor and/or optician for retention of the ability to see clearly at all distances. It is obvious that bifocals will no longer provide such versatility. The patient's major change of habit is at the reading distance where the recent accommodative effort is being replaced by lenses. Referring again to Table XXIV it is seen that approximately the same amount of accommodation is required at all points.

Experience has proved the desirability of leaving some work for the accommodative mechanism. It has been observed that the very awareness of nearness stimulates some accommodation and convergence. A simple experiment confirms this. Set small type at precisely 25 cm (the focal distance) from a +4.00D. lens. Look at the type through the lens while wearing a full correction for distance. Move the type slightly toward the lens to allow a small portion of accommodation to come into play. The type is usually much clearer and more satisfactorily seen when about 0.50D. accommodation is in use. Stereoscope makers consider the accommodation "at rest" when it has approached 0.50D. while looking at the stereoscopic cards.

A round segment trifocal was among the first developments of the fused type (Fig. 188) Univis. The segment was divided slightly above center with the intermediate section in the upper portion and the reading below. These lenses were more desirable for some wearers because the near-point portion did not consume as great an area as the one-piece model. The optical center of the intermediate portion was still below the intermediate section like the one-piece design, and thus the blind area or "jump" reduced the useful area of the intermediate field. As fusing procedures improved and new glasses became available, the lens makers continued to experiment.

The next step was a flat-top trifocal with the optical centers of the fused portion actually in the intermediate portion. Wearer acceptance improved by leaps and bounds. Further improve-

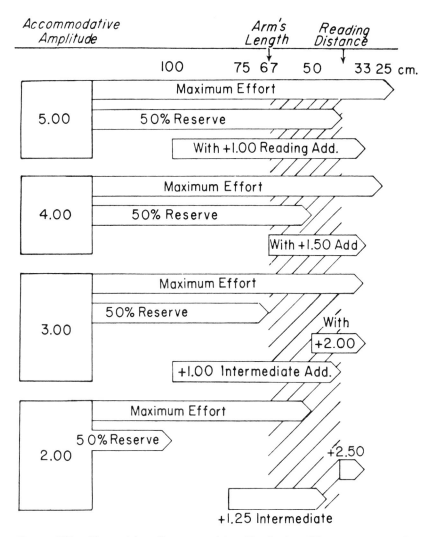

Figure 187. Clear vision distances with trifocals for different accommodative amplitudes.

ments of smaller details, such as width of intermediate section, percentage of power in intermediate addition, etcetera, are bringing these lenses toward perfection. Most of the major fused lens makers have flat-top trifocals and an optician can take ad-

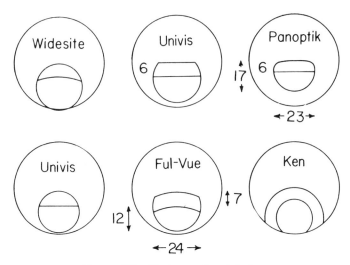

Figure 188. Various trifocal designs.

vantage of the differences in design to interpret each prescription best.

The discussion of depth of focus of presbyopia on page 359 suggests why doctors will infrequently fit any person with a total reading requirement of less than +1.75D. with trifocals. Beyond that point no person who does not have trifocals for regular use is availing himself of all that optical science has to offer—if he wishes to see clearly at all distances. As in all ophthalmic services, the wearer must be in accord with the fact that he has a need for the means by which his eye problem is solved. If he had difficulty with one blurred spot when he adopted himself to bifocals for the convenience gained, he must be ready to again adjust himself, though much easier this time, to another blurred spot. His last pair of bifocals was beginning to fail him for distances just beyond arm's length. He may not know it yet, but his new prescription with +2.00D. addition will cause objects beyond 50 cm (20 inches) to be less distinct. His accommodative amplitude is likely reduced to 1.50D. or less. His new prescription will provide very satisfactory reading vision, but intermediate distances will become rather fuzzy. Therefore, every bifocal wearer whose new prescription is +2.00D or more should have trifocals explained and demonstrated for ordinary use. No one should be beseeched to purchase, but no one should be allowed to regret he did not choose the lenses when his new prescription was filled.

There is a question whether some vocational eyewear should be made as trifocals. Many tinted lenses for outdoor use are really a pair of distance glasses with a reading convenience. Intermediate distance is seldom used. Frequently a pair of bifocal lenses with no more than average size reading area are adequate. However, there will be found outdoorsmen who wish to have keen acuity at all distances and having become accustomed to trifocals will be loathe to discard the convenience at the instrument panels in their automobiles or yachts.

The subject of the placement of the optical distance portion in the vertical meridian with reference to the geometrical center of the lens has previously been discussed. The position of the dividing line of multifocals should be referred to the geometric center of the lens and x-axis to prevent confusion.

This is also a time when progressive addition multifocals perform dramatically. At this point, they are not a cosmetic benefit only. Now is the time when they retrieve the lost accommodative amplitude of youth. No one should be urged to accept a new lens form, but no one should be allowed to regret that he continued with the same bifocals when a change would have made him more comfortable.

The subject of the placement of the optical center of the distance portion in the vertical meridian has been previously discussed in the finding and fixing of the pantoscopic angle. The position of the top edge of all multifocals is specified by its distance above or below the datum line through the geometrical center of the lens.

Because there are some new considerations in the fitting of multifocals, a brief review of pantoscopic angles and the use of Dispensometer will be given:

1. The patient's face is set in primary position, i.e. the chin directly below the brow (see Fig. 189). Ideally the plane of the lenses will now be parallel to the pantoscopic line— upper orbital margin to lower orbital margin. If the eye-

frame does not set the plane of the lenses in this position, effort should be made to alter the temple angles to set the lenses to the proper pantoscopic angle. The angle of the inclinometer is now read on the protractor. This single angle divided by two gives the number of millimeters the optical centers must be set below the centers of the pupils.

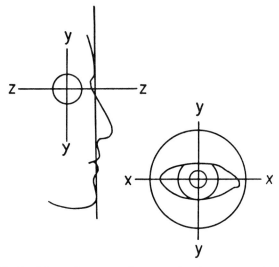

Figure 189. Positions of x-, y-, and z-axes related to center of rotation.

2. Determine the number of millimeters this position of the optical centers is "above" or "below" the x-axis (datum line) of the lenses as the frame holds them before the eyes.
3. Finally, decide the distance the top edges of the segments must be set below the x-axis as the frame is worn.

To summarize:

1. The Dispensometer showed the position of the x-axis (datum line) of the lenses as the eyeframe is worn.

2. The tilt of the lenses was compared with the natural pantoscopic angle of the orbital area.

3. The distance of x-axis set below the pupils was measured on the vertical scale.

4. The inclinometer indicated the tilt of the lenses (pantoscopic angle).

5. The depression of the optical centers below the pupil centers was calculated.

6. The distance of the optical centers above or below the x-axis was found.

7. The position of the top edge of the segment below the x-axis was determined.

By the use of a Dispensometer, all of these measurements are simultaneously and precisely made for the first time. With these easily obtainable data, vertical centers can be manipulated to improve performance of multifocals for lenses with higher powers. The optical centers can be lowered when desirable to place them as close as possible to the N.V.P. and retain the distance and near working areas within the areas of comfortable vision.

When the measurements and observations are completed, the data are used as follows for the laboratory order.

GIVEN: Pupil centers are 3 mm above the datum (180°) line and x-axis.

Angle of inclination, α, of glasses is 8°.

Since the position of the center is dropped 0.5 mm for each degree of tilt (see page 110), the position of the vertical optical centers is

$$+3 - \frac{8}{2} = -1 \text{ mm}$$

In Figure 190 the position of the segment line is —3 mm (the sign is negative because the measurement is below center). Therefore the order would read

O.C. —1

Segment —3 mm

The position of the dividing line of the segment below the geometric center can and must be chosen with considerable care. An ink dot or line in the area of the lower cilia line provides a good point of reference. It may be left on the lens while the patient's reading posture is observed and studied. Routine reference to the position of the segment as a distance above or below the x-axis of a lens is definitive. The position and size of the segment can be measured by several methods that can lead to misinterpretation of orders. The measurement described refers to the original constructions of *eye planes* and *lens planes* and is the tangent of

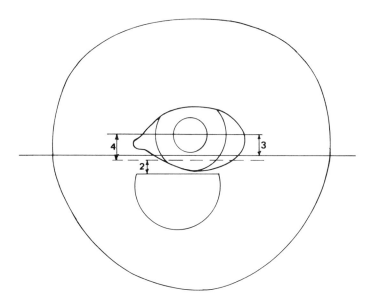

Figure 190. Positions of pupil center, optical center, datum line, and segment top.

the angle of depression or elevation of the eyes. It continues to be easily measured even though the edge of the lens is obscured in the rim of the frame. It is not altered if the shape or size of the lens is changed after the lenses are completed. Endless calculations and measurements in the lens laboratory are avoided when the lens can be "laid out," ground, and finished with only one point of reference—that is, the geometric center or point of origin of the x-axes and y-axes.

In comparison, the placement of the optical center of the distance lens in the vertical meridian varies in importance with the power and type of prescription. The prism displacement and marginal aberrations of weak lenses are so small that symmetric decentrations are insignificant. As power increases, every effort is made to keep the optic axis of the major portion of the lens and the near-vision point as close together as possible. Reference to the center and shape of the *area of binocular comfort* as diagrammed from the optical difference of the lenses of an asymmetric prescription indicates the effect of decentration in the individual case. The benefits of dropping the centers of multifocals judiciously often effect a desirable compromise of vertical prism power as described in the discussion of single vision lens analysis.

REVIEW

1. At what addition is the end of uninterrupted clear intermediate vision?

2. Is the width of the blur around a reading segment one of the causes of a desire for wide reading segments?

3. Find whether prism compensation is required for the following prescriptions. Plot the crossed-cylinders, then check the results with Emsley's table.

    a. —2.00 —2.00 × 55
       —2.50 —1.25 × 120
       Add + 1.75
    b.   —1.00 × 180
    b. —0.50 —1.25 × 35
    c. +0.75 +4.25 × 140
       +1.25 +2.50 × 30
       Add + 1.25

4. Is it essential to obtain optical centers in bifocal segments? Discuss your conclusion.

5. Why are Univis "R" segment bifocals most popular for prism compensation up to $1.00^\triangle$?

6. Do 6 to 7 mm intermediate segments provide adequate vertical width for the intermediate field?

7. Give two reasons why the reading portions of Progressive Addition lenses set higher than ordinary bifocals.

Chapter 12

CATARACT LENS FITTING

✦◆

Cataract surgery, although exceedingly difficult, is one of the most gratifying experiences of an ophthalmic surgeon. By the extraction of the crystalline lens, a patient who has been blinded is able to see again. Since ancient times the subject has had the continued attention of leading scientists. Probably more has been written about cataracts and cataract surgery than any other topic in ophthalmology. In 1899 a book on *The Crystalline Lens System* had a bibliography of over three thousand references! More than seventy years later the production has not decreased while new and improved techniques including cryosurgery, plastic lens implants, and lens emulsification are being used more widely. This surgical act of restoring sight to the blind continues to have the high regard of ophthalmology and the lay public alike.

Spectacle fitting for patients after cataract surgery requires the greatest skill in ophthalmic dispensing. To a much greater extent than in routine work, it is imperative that a high degree of cooperation and a complete understanding exist between doctor and optician. Anything less courts disappointments and disaster for all concerned. Different from an ordinary lens, the lens for an aphakic eye is *actually a final part of the surgery*. Until the best lens has been properly fitted and adjusted, the surgeon's skill is not fully expressed.

In no other experience in spectacle fitting does the patient's prescription change so abruptly. An emmetropic individual may actually become temporarily myopic to the extent of −2.00D. to −4.00D. while the crystalline lens changed shape before surgery. The new prescription is usually more than +10.00D. In other conditions that require strong correcting lenses, the lens power increases by degrees. Hypermetropia above +6.00D. is rarely seen and although myopia may progress to −20.00D., the first correction in childhood was comparatively weak. In all instances the patient gradually adjusts himself to the effects of the lenses. Further, these changes were first experienced during the formative years of childhood and adolescence. The sudden change to cataract glasses for persons past middle age with complications of monocular vision, magnification, curvature of field, chromatic aberration is sometimes almost overwhelming.

A dispensing optician soon learns that many new factors are presented in the fitting and adjusting of cataract lenses that do not enter into the consideration when caring for other eyes. The unusually strong convex lenses involved are problem enough because of weight, but that can become one of the lesser considerations. Misty vision is replaced with glaringly bright objects, all things are magnified and seem startlingly close, colors change from pastels to vivid hues. Frequently the wearer seems to be disappointed with his glasses and makes reference to better vision in the doctor's examination rooms. There is often quite an emotional upheaval at the fitting table. Anticipation of the pleasure with the long-awaited spectacles may have the patient at a high nervous pitch. When the new lenses do not promptly accomplish what has been expected, the disappointment is very keen and requires a great deal of diplomacy on the part of the optician to assure the patient that his glasses will be all right with a little patience on his part. There is what may be called a "settling down" period while the cornea is healing and regaining its previous contour. The lens prescription changes during this process. Ophthalmologists have found that if a prescription is written very soon after surgery that it most likely will have to be changed during the healing of the wound. For this reason some ophthalmologists delay writing a prescription to prevent their patients from having to purchase more than one lens. Despite this caution, however, the lens prescription may still change in small amounts for as long as six months after surgery.

SURGICAL MODIFICATION OF EYE

When the eye is entered and the crystalline lens is removed (Fig. 191), the refracting system of the eye is considerably altered.

In the words of Donders (1864), who originated the use of the word "aphakia": "In the condition of aphakia the eye is, complicated in its normal state, becomes the simplest imaginable dioptric system." As this discussion proceeds, it will be observed, however, that this new simplification rests at the eye. The problem of fitting an appropriate spectacle lens to replace the function of the crystalline lens undoubtedly requires more exacting skill on the part of both the ophthalmologist and the optician than any other type of spectacle lens fitting.

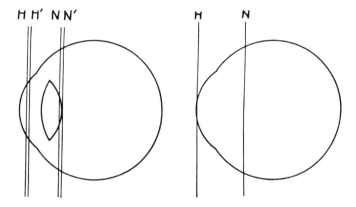

Figure 191. Position of principle and nodal planes.

Ocular imagery is accomplished by the usual laws of physical optics, but if one attempts to investigate all the functions of vision and the eye by the use of physical constants alone, he is certain to be misled. The function of vision is dependent upon psychological and physiological properties which are not explained by physical optics. In this present instance, it is desirable to make a comparison and this can be accomplished only by the use of the accepted data. At the risk of some errors, the data of Gullstrand's schematic eye given in the third edition of Helmholtz's *Handbuch der physiologischen Optik* will be compared as a complete static eye with the same eye from which the crystalline lens has been removed and to which a correcting ophthalmic lens has been added.

Under these conditions the corneal surface is now the only optical surface of the eye. The principal points of the eye that have been within the eye move to the corneal surface. The visual axis approaches the optical axis. This is observed when the corneal reflection is used in the interocular distance measurement. The reflection is no longer on the nasal side of center. It is now exactly in the center of the cornea. The aqueous humor in the anterior part of the eye has the same refractive index $(n = 1.337)$ as the vitreous humor, therefore the curve of the membrane dividing these media (in the absence of the lens) is of no optical importance. If the eye was previously emmetropic, the total refracting power is now $+43.05D$., which is the dioptric power of the cornea alone. A correcting lens with a vertex power of $+10.43D$. placed at 10 mm in front of the cornea corrects the eye for distant vision.

When the correcting lens is optically combined with the aphakic eye and the "eye and lens" combination is considered, one finds that some important changes have taken place. Some writers have made computations with the correcting lens placed at the anterior focal plane of the eye, thus eliminating the magnification of the correcting lens. This distance is considerably greater than spectacles are ordinarily fitted and, in the case of an aphakic eye (23.23 mm), entirely out of practice. It is advantageous to limit the magnification of cataract glasses by placing the lens as close to the eye as possible, therefore a distance of 10 mm is chosen. Possibly this reduction of distance is too conservative. The specifications of the correcting lens are

Total dioptric power	$+10.43D$
Anterior surface	$+12.78D$.
Posterior surface	$-3.00D$.
Center thickness	5.8 mm

It is noted immediately that the focal lengths are considerably increased. If the first focal lengths in Table XXV are compared, 21.4/17.05, it is obvious that the retinal image is increased by 25.47 percent. The principal points of the combination are negative—that is, to the left of the cornea—and the second principal point is now farther from the retina than the first. Although the nodal points are still within the eye, they are much closer to the corneal surface and they too are reversed. The entrance pupil of the uncorrected eye is .55 mm in front of the pupillary plane. The pupillary plane of the combination is more than 2 mm behind the iris of the eye because the additional lens power is now in front of the iris plane.

A pupillary diameter of 3.5 mm is taken. There is no easy way

TABLE XXV

SOME PROPERTIES OF AN APHAKIC EYE WITH CORRECTING LENS COMPARED WITH A NORMAL SCHEMATIC EYE

	Aphakic Eye With Lens	Phakic Eye
Refractive indices:		
Correcting lens	—1.523	
Humors	1.337	Same
Distance from cornea:		
Ant. surface cor. lens	—15.8 mm	
Pos. surface cor. lens	—10.0	
Fovea	24.0	Same
Radii:		
Ant. surface cor. lens	40.95 mm	
Pos. surface cor. lens	174.3	
Cornea	7.8	
Focal lengths:		
First	21.4	17.055
Second	28.6	22.785
Cardinal points from cornea:		
Principal point, first	+3.16	1.75
Principal point, second	—4.16	2.10
Focal point, first	—24.55	—13.74
Focal point, second	24.38	22.82
Nodal point, first	4.03	6.97
Nodal point, second	3.00	7.32
Entrance pupil paraxial	7.01	3.05
Iris (taken)	5.0	3.6
Apertures:		
Iris (taken)	3.5	3.5
Entrance pupil	5.17	3.96
Relative or f: Aper.	5.54	5.24
Definition:		
From infinity to	31.5 feet	20.0 feet
Image size	1.2547	1.0

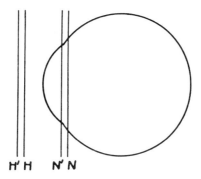

H' H   N' N

Figure 192. Principal planes of correction lens combined with planes of aphakic eye.

in which to assume a normal postsurgical pupil for either shape, size, or plane. It is necessary, if the comparison is to be continued, that a size and position be assumed. Variations caused by iridectomies, adhesions, or other pupillary irregularities can be considered for their optical effects after the simple case has been reviewed. An iris plane of 5 mm is taken as the position of the iris without the support of the crystalline lens or complications at the chamber angle. A comparison of the effects of changes in the iris plane are shown in Table XXVI.

TABLE XXVI
EFFECT OF IRIS PLANE IN "APHAKIC EYE-LENS" COMBINATION

	4.0 mm	5.0 mm	5.7 mm
Distance from cornea:			
Entrance pupil point	5.47	7.01	8.17
Apertures:			
Iris diameter	3.5	3.5	3.5
Entrance pupil	4.91	5.17	5.36
Relative or f'/Aper.	5.82	5.54	5.33

The diameter of the entrance pupil is much wider in the combination, but the increased focal length of the eye still leaves the relative aperture or photographic f: number almost identically the same (f:5.54 compared with f:5.24). These data also show that an enlarged pupil will be compared with the pupil of the other eye in direct ratio of square areas. If one pupil is round and measures 3 mm (Fig. 193), and if the other has an iridectomy the width of the pupil that extends to the limbus and is not covered by the upper lid, then the one eye receives more than twice as much light as the other.

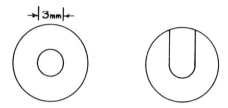

Figure 193. Dissimilar pupils in aphakia.

The cornea may have had a spherical or toroidal surface before surgery, but now an astigmatic effect, due to the incision and the healing process, may be found in the pupillary area that is a referral of the distorted curve at the limbus. Photographic records have been made* that clearly show the early warping at the lip of the wound and the gradual return of the cornea toward a regular curve.

A large number of surgeons do an iridectomy in all cases. Others attempt to leave a round pupil as often as possible. From the aspect of physical optics it would seem that a small centered pupil is more desirable; however, good vision is regularly obtainable after iridectomy. After surgery, the position of rest of the upper lid has considerable bearing upon the refraction and visual acuity. If the lids are spread widely so that the margin of the upper lid rests at or near the upper limbus, the aberrated corneal section is involved. The wider aperture receives a wider bundle of rays from the spectacle lens. Since spherical aberration and coma increase with the square of the aperture, it is obvious that an unusually large pupillary diameter could interfere materially with retinal imagery. In any event, that part of the cornea covered by the upper lid has the most beneficial effect upon the

*Weeks, C.L.: Kerato-photography in keratoconus. *Trans West Ophthmol Soc,* 1940.

optical image because the degeneration of the curve is greatest near the limbus.

With the removal of the crystalline lens the patient has no further accommodation.† This does not mean that the patient can see at only one distance. If the iris has not been involved in the surgery and the pupil is still round and rather small, a surprising depth of field exists (Chap. 17). Some persons who have become proficient at the interpretation of slightly blurred images have demonstrated a faculty that seemed to indicate the existence of a limited accommodation. Donders says, "My investigations have led me to the conviction, that in aphakia not the slightest trace of accommodative power remains." Despite his experimental proof, several hypotheses have been projected (Stricker, 1899; Gibbons, 1904) to account for this phenomenon.

As has been shown, the relative aperture is almost precisely the same under the two conditions with the same size pupil. Further, an increased focal length characteristically should reduce depth of focus and depth of field. At the bottom of Table XXV is shown the calculated disadvantage of the corrected eye. For equal-sized blur-circles, the shorter focussed emmetropic eye corrected for infinity should still see at 20 feet an object that begins to blur at 31 feet for the corrected aphakic eye. This is one of the instances where geometrical optics runs afoul of experience.

If the pupillary diameter is materially reduced after surgery to a centrally located aperture not less than 2 mm (after which diffraction should interfere), then the gain is explained by the pinhole effect of paraxial rays. Some lens forms increase in power toward the periphery. Near-point acuity is sometimes assisted by the marginal astigmatism. Probably one of the best observations is that a person with diminished vision from cataractous eyes learns all the tricks of seeing even beyond what is commonly associated with the measured acuity. When the eye is cleared and a magnifying correcting lens is supplied, he still has the advantages of the devices he has previously learned.

The limits of the normal vision field for a white object found by Roenne are out 93°, in 62°, down 76°, and up 69°. The "lens

†Bettman, J.W.: Apparent accommodation in aphakic eyes. *Am J Ophthmol,* 33:921-928, 1950.

and eye" combination in Table XXV produces a magnification of 25.5 percent. Since the absolute limits of the vision field are substantially the same as the routinely measured relative field,* magnification tends to decrease the angular subtense of the field. This effect is applied to a normal field in Figure 194. Assuming the visual field of the eye reached normal limits before surgery, it is now restricted about 20 percent to out 74°, in 48°, down 61°, and up 55°. Thus an annular scotoma is formed which varies from 14° to 19° in width.

When the eye turns from primary position, visual acuity diminishes as central vision first moves into the spherically aberrated field at the lens margin, then to a band in which objects

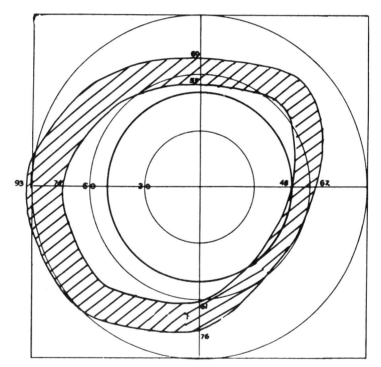

Figure 194. Aphakic lens magnification reduces the visual field by 20%. Reprinted by permission from Duke-Elder, Sir W. S.: Textbook of Ophthalmology, St. Louis, Mosby, 1934. Page 891.

*Duke-Elder, Sir W.S.: *Text-Book of Ophthalmology*, St. Louis, C.V. Mosby Co. p. 891.

disappear. The suddenness with which objects appear at the margin of this new constricted field is sometimes startling to the patient. Dr. A.C. Woods (1952) referred to this occurrence as a "jack-in-the-box effect."

Early small lenses had a vista of less than 37° in the longest dimension. Hence, the entire expanse of the vista through the lens was within the smaller magnified field shown in Figure 194.

The rays in Figure 195 are diagrammatic. They are intended to show the points where object rays reach the retina. Like most illustrations for geometrical optics, they do not trace the actual paths. The ray A shows the limiting ray in the nasal field of vision of an eye before surgery. The ray reaches the visual axis at nodal point N_2 at an angle of 62°. It leaves the second nodal point N' and falls upon the retina at point A'. After the crystalline lens is removed from the eye and a correcting lens added, the nodal points move forward on the visual axis and reverse their order. Now the first nodal point is 4.03 mm from the cornea and the second nodal point only 3.00 mm. This greater separation from the retina reflects the magnifying effect of placing the correcting lens in front of the eye. Because of the magnification, now a ray

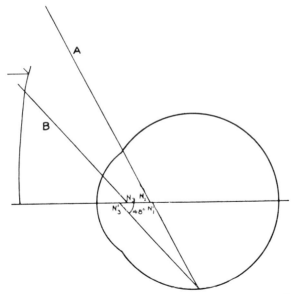

Figure 195. Diagramatic paths of unmagnified and magnified rays.

from 48° in the nasal field falls on the same point as the limiting
ray **A′** fell before surgery.

Let us now inspect the diameter of a correcting lens required
to cover the magnified visual field shown in Figure 195 in which

Upper limit is 53°, lens width 37.16 mm
Lower limit is 61°, lens width 50.52 mm
Nasal limit is 48°, lens width 31.10 mm
Temporal limit is 74°, lens width 97.64 mm

$$a/b = \tan 48°$$
$$a = b \tan 48°$$

$$
\begin{array}{rl}
\log \tan 48° = & .04556 \\
+\log 14 = & 1.14613 \\
\hline
1.19169 = & 15.55 \text{ mm nasal}
\end{array}
$$

$$
\begin{array}{rl}
\log \tan 53° = & 0.12289 \\
+\log 14 = & 0.14613 \\
\hline
0.26902 = & 18.58 \text{ mm upper}
\end{array}
$$

$$
\begin{array}{rl}
\log \tan 61° = & 0.25625 \\
+ \log 14 = & 1.14613 \\
\hline
1.40238 = & 25.26
\end{array}
$$

$$
\begin{array}{rl}
\log \tan 74° = & 0.54250 \\
+ \log 14 = & 1.14613 \\
\hline
1.68863 = & 48.82
\end{array}
$$

Thus it is plain that *no* spectacle lens will cover the entire visual
field on the temporal side since about 49 mm is required on that
radius. This is common knowledge to those who wear glasses.
With eyes in primary position the blurred outer edge and sometimes lower edge of eyewear (even large rimless lenses) are visible.
But because peripheral acuity is so very poor (20/150 or less) and
the continuing uncorrected field beyond is no clearer, the blurred
line (even a heavy plastic rim) is ignored.

It is in these two regions that all lenses for aphakia provide
some temporary torment for the wearer. Although visual acuity
of the aphakic declines toward the lens margin because of normal
decreased retinal sensitivity plus some marginal aberration of

the correcting lens upon the 25 percent magnified image, it is at the lens edge that the unexpected happens. The remaining part of any partly seen object disappears into the annular scotoma previously mentioned. The remaining part of the object is not seen until the head is turned toward it or the object moves across the vacant area toward the center of the visual field.

Latest design lenticular cataract lenses have a prescription area 40 mm round which more than covers most of the visual field, but because the lens has only a 20 mm radius in the temporal field instead of the 22 to 24 mm of a full-field lens, it does present the scotoma about 4° closer on the temporal side. This seems a small price for the great gain in lens weight.

The whole world concerned with cataracts—first aphakic patients, then opticians, lens laboratories, ophthalmic surgeons, lens manufacturers and designers—owes a debt of gratitude to R.C. Welsh, M.D., of Miami, Florida. Before 1961 he found that too many of his patients could not see as well with their prescription lenses as they could with his examining lenses. When he searched for information in the ophthalmic literature there was scarce reward. He started asking questions of lens laboratory men and dispensing opticians, then came upon a copy of the first edition of this book. He used some of the notions presented and continued his research. In 1961 he published a preliminary report. The greatest benefit from it was that because the book was written by a doctor it stirred great numbers of ophthalmologists to think more about the lenses supplied to their patients after cataract surgery. Because Welsh is naturally a crusader type, the whirlwind has not died down. Later he enlisted the help of C.D. Benton, M.D., to turn his report into a book, *Spectacles for Aphakia*, which was published by Charles C Thomas in 1966. As could be expected, since he was a medical doctor and not an optician, he reported elatedly some findings that were new to him and were in the ancient lore of the art to lens makers and dispensers.

Fifty years ago, A. Ray Irvine, M.D., and Archibald Macleish, M.D. (Los Angeles, California) obtained the effect of Welsh's "M.E.D." lenses with four words. They wrote, "Thin lenses, don't decenter." In the days of symmetric lens shapes (before Harlequin) the geometric, mechanical, and optical centers coincided. When these lenses were ground to 1 mm in thickness at the ends, thickness and weight were minimum. The small vertical dimensions of these plus good plier work on saddle bridges assured minimum vertex distance even before the distance was popularly known by that name. A major difficulty in fitting was to obtain adequately substantial temples to sustain x-axis alignment. All bifocals wcrc round top with Kryptoks, the most popular. The ring scotoma problem, never identified by the name, nor frequently referred to, was almost in the paracentral field with 30.5 by 39.5 mm lenses. We should thank Doctor Welsh for leading the return from "cock-eyed" aphakic lens shapes.

Image brightness after cataract surgery is often uncomfortable. Although the f: value of the eye is not materially changed, the iris is frequently inactive. The retina is also conditioned to reduced light after the prolonged dark-adaptation behind the translucent or opaque lens. If iris surgery has been necessary and the square area of the aperture has been increased, the illumination may be two to four times as great.

Coblentz of the Bureau of Standards has made an exhaustive study of the transmission of lenses as shown in his publications since 1918: circular C421, 1938, entitled *Spectral-Transmissive Properties and Use of Colored Eye Protective Glasses.* A paper, *Spectral Absorptive Ophthalmic Lenses and Their Use in Aphakia,* (prepared by Ellerbrock in 1947 and published by Univis Lens Company), also contains authoritative information. Both of these writers emphasize these points: (a) The lower limit of appreciable transmission of ultraviolet light for the normal eye is approximately 380 mμ, while that for an aphakic eye is 295 mμ. (b) Short-wave ultraviolet is irritating and can be injurious to the retina. (c) Ordinary crown glass lenses (as shown in Fig. 190.) transmit all light to about 315 mμ. (d) To remove detrimental short wavelengths, a glass such as Crookes' neutral that absorbs all light below 365 mμ should be used in the presence of ultraviolet light when maximum visible light transmission is desired. (e) A green glass should be worn in sunlight to absorb rays below 400 mμ and reduce the visible spectrum as required.

The feature of even color density is very important in cataract lenses. Glare is largely contributed by excessive stimulation to the *marginal* part of the retina, and when the pupil is eccentric the density of the peripheral portion of the lens is especially significant.

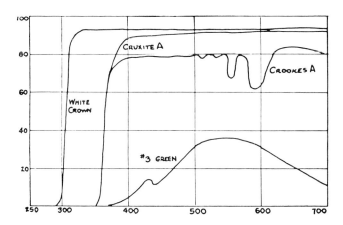

Figure 196. Comparative transmissions of colored protective glasses.

All present models of fused-type lenticular cataract lenses are available in absorption glass to protect in the marginal area where the lens is thin. Outdoor lenses should be fitted as close to the eyes as the lashes and/or brows will permit. The shape of the lens should follow the brow-line to allow minimum light behind the lenses. A plastic or metal frame is very desirable because it creates a shadow across the top and prevents transverse light transmission through the edge of the lens. A longer lens can be fitted to protect the temporal field in the lenticular form without complications of weight and color density. If the posterior edge of the lens or frame can approximate the corneal line, most of the rays will be intercepted. CR39 (hard resin) lenses can be dyed any color or density. A great benefit of this procedure is that the lens becomes even density including the thin marginal portion of lenticular lenses.

PRESCRIPTION TRANSLATION

The translation of the prescription into a lens that gives the *identical* effect of the trial lenses used to arrive at a correction for aphakia has had the attention of many scientists including Gull-strand, von Rohr, Percival, Tillyer, Rayton, Davis, and others. Prescription lenses of +10.00 or more present very difficult problems in geometrical optics. Lens curves, especially the inside curve, thickness, and distance from the center of rotation of the eye, are critical.

The dioptric power of the examining lens is the most important part, but it is not all the significant data the optician must have if he is to undertake to duplicate the effect of the trial lenses used in the refracting room. When he attempts to do the computation, he must also know (a) the distance of the vertex of the posterior surface of the closest trial lens to the corneal apex; (b) if a series of trial lenses is used to make the prescription, what type of lens (profile), the distance between lenses, and their order in the trial frame; (c) the angle of tilt (or inclination) of the lenses in the frame or refracting instrument; (d) the vertical height of the optical centers of the trial lenses; and (e) for the reading prescription, whether the measurement is made with eyes in primary position or depressed toward a normal reading position—that is, whether the test is made through the optical centers of the trial lenses.

1. **Vertex Distance.** A more or less universal understanding is that the posterior surface of the trial lens will be adjusted to the point where it barely misses the lashes. If the back surface of the spectacle lens is placed in the same position, this part of the problem is solved. There are many faces, however, on which the trial frame cannot be adjusted to that position and/or the spectacle cannot or should not be set at that distance. Refracting instruments are designed for a standard vertex distance of 13.75 mm, which is a greater distance from the eye than the length of the lashes. Prescription lenses can be set much closer if the eyes are not too deep-set.

Differences in vertex distance (posterior lens pole to corneal pole) alter the lens effect markedly in cataract prescriptions. When a plus lens is moved from the eye, its effectivity increases, and conversely as the distance between lens and cornea is reduced the effectivity decreases.

If a +15.00D. lens placed at 15 mm from the eye gives best

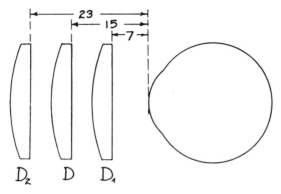

Figure 197. Optical effect of altered vertex distance.

vision, the lens power must be increased to +17.05D. if the lens is placed in the position of D_1, at 7 mm—that is, 8 mm closer to the eye. If the vertex distance is increased to 23 mm with the lens 8 mm farther from the eye as shown by D_2, the power must be reduced to +13.50D. to have the same effect as the original lens. The formulas discussed on page 108 when applied to this problem show:

When D = lens power

  d = displacement in meters

  D_1 = lens moved toward eye

  D_2 = lens moved from eye

$$D_1 = \frac{D}{1 - dD} \qquad D_2 = \frac{D}{1 + dD}$$

$$D_1 = \frac{15}{1 - (.008 \times 15)} = +17.05D.$$

$$D_2 = \frac{15}{1 + (.008 \times 15)} = +13.39D.$$

The power must be reduced to +13.39D. to have the same effect as the original lens. The formulas for these revisions are discussed on page 108.

When the prescription involves a cylindrical element, the dioptric powers of the two principal meridians are considered separately. For example: +10.00D. + 2.00 × 180 is computed first as

+10.00D. and then refigured as + 12.00D. The new amount from the first computation is the compensated sphere. The new sphere is then subtracted from the refigured opposite meridian (+12.00) to find the compensated cylinder. It is obvious that changes in the meridian of the power of the cylinder are increasingly greater than the weaker meridian.

Vertex distances can be satisfactorily measured with the Distometer made by House of Vision (Chicago, Illinois) or the Lens-Corometer made by Austin Belgard (Chicago, Illinois), or the Essel Corneal Reflection Pupillometer. See Figure 105. A convenient scale is included with the apparatus from which the above-mentioned vertex compensation can be read directly.

2. **Trial Lenses Used.** Modern refracting instruments (Green Refractor®, Phoroptor® are equipped with lenses that are additive, and therefore, the power of the lens combination is the same as shown in the indicator. Tillyer, Orthogon, and B & L Precision Trial sets are additive and are correct for one sphere in the rear cell and one cylinder in the cell in front of it, when the lenses are spaced in the trial frame designed for use with them. Any additional lenses interfere with absolute mathematical accuracy, but the small fractional values of the auxiliaries do not ordinarily cause any significant error. Old-style trial sets are accurate as individual lenses but do develop considerable errors when used in combination. An interesting demonstration is to put a +12.00D. sphere, a +1.50D. sphere, and a +3.00D. cylinder of the old style trial set in a trial frame and measure the whole combination in a lensometer. The vertex power of the combination varies noticeably as the order of the lenses in the trial frame cells is changed.

3. **Tilt of Lenses.** Spectacle lenses are ordinarily tilted (see page 328) on the 180 or x-axis in order to be parallel with the line formed by the rims of the orbit. As previously stated, this is the individual pantoscopic angle. The bulkiness of most refracting instruments prevents them from being easily tilted to the position of spectacle lenses. The AO Phoroptor probably makes this adjustment best because the back surface of the instrument is convex. The patient's head must be firmly held by a head-rest if the angle of the instrument is to be maintained through the ex-

amination. Most trial frames can be tilted to the spectacle plane, but again the size of the trial lenses may interfere.

The prescription values of lenses for cataract prescriptions change very rapidly when they are tilted. Table XXVII shows the effects of tilting a +10.00D. sphere when the formula on page 110 is applied.

TABLE XXVII
+10.00D. SPHERE TILTED

$$10° = +10.10 + .21 \times 180$$
$$15° = +10.23 + .31 \times 180$$
$$20° = +10.65 +1.38 \times 180$$
$$25° = +10.65 +2.32 \times 180$$

By way of example, if +10.00D. +2.75 $\times$ 40 is tilted 20°, the obliquity adds +0.41 +1.38 $\times$ 180 to the lens. Since the axes of the prescription cylinder and the induced cylinder may be oblique, one to another, the powers cannot be added directly. By application of the S.P. Thompson formula for the transposition of crossed-cylinders, by the method of plotting on polar coordinate sheets, or Emsley's chart or table previously described, the total effect of the cylinders (+2.75D. $\times$ 40 and +1.38D. $\times$ 180) is +0.43 +3.28 $\times$ 28.

The vertex power of the lens now becomes

$$+10.00$$
$$+ \ 0.41$$
$$+ \quad .43 +3.28 \times 28$$
$$\overline{+10.84 +3.28 \times 28}$$

Thus it is seen that tilting this lens adds more than sphere and cylinder power, it also changes the cylinder axis by 12°.

Repeatedly in the earlier ophthalmic literature when the grinding of cylindrical curves was very difficult, writers explained how astigmatism might be corrected with tilted lenses. Probably nothing emphasizes the effect of tilt any better than the examples given by Percival in his text *Prescribing of Spectacles* (1910). He shows how a strong convex or concave sphere can be made to serve as the prescription lens to correct a sizable amount of astigmatism. The prescription of +11.50 +1.50 axis 180 is obtained from a

+11.00 sphere tilted 20°.

In the days of the popularity of eyeglasses, opticians learned to be cautious about changing the adjustment of a pair of tilted lenses. The glasses may have hung precariously at an angle of 45°. The inclination of the lenses had really become a part of the prescription. If the lenses were set more nearly vertical, they produced a weaker vertex power and were often unsatisfactory.

4. **Compensation.** Compensation for the lens tilt can be made when the angle of the trial lenses with the face plane and the height of optical center with reference to primary position are known. The formula discussed on page 110 in which the lens center is dropped 0.5 mm for each degree of inclination of the pantoscopic angle eliminates the power changes.

5. **Gain and Loss in Vertex Power.** Because of the extreme dioptric power of cataract lenses, there is another effect to be considered which is of no consequence in weak prescription lenses. At the reading distance, the divergent rays from the near-point object cause a reduction in the vertex power. This is an application of the effect of a curved, not parallel, wave front striking a lens as discussed in Chapter 4 on optics. This effect is not significant in minus lenses of equal strength because it is largely a function of lens thickness. If a prescription of +11.00D. sphere is found to be satisfactory for distance vision and a +14.00D. sphere is placed in the frame or refracting instrument (+3.00D. add.) for the reading test, many different effects are obtained if the examining and prescription lenses are not similar in curves (profile).

$$D_v = +14.00$$

$$D_v = D_2 + \cfrac{1}{\cfrac{1}{D_1} - d}$$

$$\frac{1}{D_1} = \frac{1}{D_v - D_2} + d \qquad d = \frac{t}{n} = \frac{.007}{1.523} = .005$$

Lens I is a +14.00D. sphere from a Bausch & Lomb Precision Trial Set. The front surface of the lens is plane. As a distance trial lens, all the refraction takes place at the rear surface. As a reading lens, however, the diverging rays from the near-point

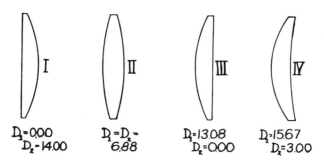

Figure 198. Effect of lens profile on reading lenses.

object cause the lens to perform as if it were a meniscus form with the concave surface away from the eye. The lens is very small and the center thickness is about 2 mm. When the formula for vertex power is applied using an object distance of .333 meter (3.00D.),

$$D_v = D_2 + \cfrac{1}{\cfrac{1}{D_1} - \cfrac{t}{n}} = 14 + \cfrac{1}{\cfrac{1}{-3} - \cfrac{.005}{1.523}} = 11.01D.$$

Thus it is seen that this lens shows an insignificant gain in vertex power over the distance ℞.

Lens II is a symmetric biconvex form of 38 mm diameter and 5 mm center thickness such as may be found in a standard trial lens set. The vertex power is +14.00D., and dioptric power of the surface is +6.88D. When the effect of −3.00D. is applied to this lens for a finite object distance, its vertex power becomes +10.84D., or 0.16D. weaker than intended for use as a distance lens.

$$D_1 = -3.00 + 6.88 = 3.88$$

$$D_v = \cfrac{1}{\cfrac{1}{3.88} - \cfrac{.005}{1.523}} + 6.88 = 10.84$$

Lens III, a planoconvex lens, by the same procedure becomes +10.62D., 0.83D. weaker than the distance ℞.

Lens IV, a meniscus lens with −3.00D. posterior surface, will be +10.53D., 0.47D. weak. This discussion explains some of the differences in the power of reading prescriptions for cataract lenses.

All these lenses measure +14.00D. in a lensometer because the instrument is designed to measure the vertex power of a lens receiving parallel rays. It follows that if the refraction is done with Lens I and the prescription is filled with a lens like Lens IV, although the lenses measure the same, the prescription is almost 0.50D. weak in the paraxial region. It is also evident that this error is only further increased when the prescription lens is thicker and has a deeper base curve. The new precision trial sets (Tillyer and Orthogon) as well as the corrected refracting instruments show much the same effect because the front curves of these lenses are shallow and the lenses are very thin. To conclude that the reading glass lens must be made the same form as the examining lens for the sake of lens power will not prove consistently satisfactory. The formulas for lenses in combination such as trial sets and refracting instruments are best fulfilled when the strong convex lenses are double convex with the greater curve on the rear surface. Because of the small aperture, the restrained field of vision through these biconvex lenses is unnoticed during the eye examination. All lens designers agree that the best type of cataract lens will have a shallow concave back surface. The power discrepancy, like the compensation for vertex distance, must be computed.

The reading card holder on all refracting instruments makes the measurements for the reading addition with the eyes in the primary position. It has been shown that, aside from an undesirable cylinder effect added to cataract lenses when the lenses are tilted or the wearer looks through the lenses obliquely, the spherical power is also altered. Therefore a change in angle from the position of test to the position of use produces a marked difference in the prescribed reading addition.

If a trial frame is used, the same difficulties previously described may make it impossible for the centers of the lenses to be dropped and the lenses to be appropriately tilted for the reading posture. It is likely, however, that the patient will depress his eyes at least a small amount if the trial lenses are of sufficient aperture.

The dilemma of the reading prescription deserves careful consideration. The most significant complications are as follows:

1. The dioptric power of these lenses is beyond the limits of the formula for marginally corrected lenses; therefore no lens can be absolutely identical at the center with some other point such as the reading area of a bifocal segment.

2. The oblique astigmatism can be sufficient to require a different cylinder correction for distance and near unless the angle of depression and the position of the optical center are included as a part of the computation for the prescription.

3. The central vision of the reading prescription can also vary considerably in spherical power if the profile of the spectacle lens is materially different from the trial lens, as is shown above in the comparison of the +14.00D. lens made in several forms.

Hitherto, the optician and patient have had to experiment with the glasses to find the angle at which the lenses would perform the best for reading. When the prescription was written for a single vision lens, there was a certain amount of latitude in the choice of the angle because the patient uses a limited area of the lenses. Bifocals present a more complicated problem.

After the position of the eyes for reading is measured—that is, segment position of bifocal, or habitual depression of eyes for reading in single vision lens—the proper tilting of trial frame, refracting instrument and spectacle lens can be established:

1. If the reading lens is to be a single vision lens, the trial frame and spectacle lens should be tilted to set the lenses normal (at a right angle) to line of sight as discussed in Chapter 10.

2. Bifocal fitting requires equal consideration of three factors, any of which alters the optical effect of the lens.

   Step No. 1. The top edge of the reading segment is usually placed *no lower than the cilia line* of the lower lid. In Figure 199*b*, that would be 6 mm below the center of the pupil with the eye in primary position.

   Step No. 2. Assuming the bridge fit is satisfactory and since the segment of an Aspheric Aolite® Lenticular lens is 2 mm below center, the optical center of the lens must be 4 mm below the pupil center with the eye in primary position.

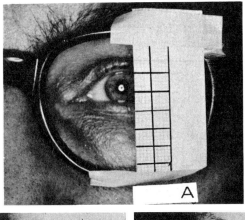

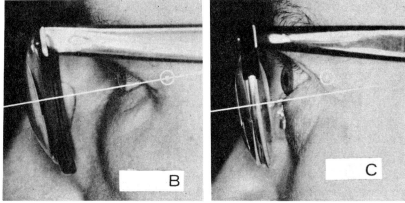

Figure 199. Effect of vertex distance and tilt of aphakia lenses (Davis).

Step No. 3. This position of the axis of the lens requires a pantoscopic angle of $(4 \times 2 =)$ 8° (see page 110).

The lens will be decentered down 0.5 mm for each increase of 1° of angle. There will be a limit to the angle because the segment top will finally be too low for comfortable use.

Let us pause for a moment to consider the ill effect of increasing the pantoscopic angle without modifying the lens center position (Fig. 199*b* shows correct effect while *c* is decentered down).

In the course of designing the Aolite Aspheric Cataract Lens, John K. Davis explored the optical effects of lenses improperly placed before the eyes. He found one of the most common errors in fitting and wearing to be optical centers set too far below the primary position of the eyes. This effect can be created (a) by properly fitted lenses which have slid down the wearer's nose, (b) improper pantoscopic angle, or (c) eyeframes which were originally improperly adjusted. Because the optical effect is the introduction of a spherocylinder axis 180, this fitting defect is frequently much greater than the usual variations caused by alterations of vertex distance. The horizontal cylindrical effect presents the problem of obliquely crossed cylinders. This error is aggravated by the use of full-field lenses. The additional center thickness enlarges the aberration caused by the curvature of the front surfaces of the lenses.

For $+14.00D$. lenses with the z-axes (optical axes) below the center of rotation of the eyes as illustrated in Figure 199c, the induced errors are:

Decentration Down Per mm	Planoconvex		−3.00D. Sph. Base		Aspheric −3.00D. Base	
3	+0.31	−0.26	+0.58	−0.46	+0.31	−0.15
6	+0.99	−0.75	+1.40	−1.03	+0.81	−0.53

Thus an unwanted change to the basic prescription power of the lens is generated by the slippage of a lens of any profile with the aspheric lens showing a slight advantage. The reduced weight of CR39 lenses provides the opportunity for the lenses to be held securely in position without causing discomfort behind the ears. A properly angled and centered lens that slides down the nose 3 mm creates the same error plus a possible vertex distance error by resting farther away from the eye. Thus it is impressed upon us again the *inviolable rule* that the eyeframe must be precisely set at the first delivery and *never* moved from that position.

A part of the necessary fitting table equipment is several men's and women's metal-zyl frames fitted with plastic or glass glazing lenses with the 180 line precisely scratched on the lenses. By this means it is simple to measure the distance of the lens center from the pupil center. From this measurement the whole procedure falls into line. Be certain to record the *temple angle* on the order.

All of this improvising is overcome by the use of a Dispenso-meter. All of the calculations originate from the pupil center in primary position. In view of the many variables in profile of trial lenses, lens spacing, lens order, lens plane (tilt), vertex distance, etc., it is seen than an optician has undertaken a difficult problem even if he has all the data. He approaches an impossibility if his information is incomplete.

In the 1930s, the Green Eye Hospital (San Francisco, California) attempted to overcome these problems by obtaining a large quantity of Carl Zeiss, aspheric Katral lenses as conceived by Gullstrand and designed by von Rohr. When a postcataract refraction was concluded, a large tray of lenses was brought into the refracting room, and the uncut lenses were held before the eye until the proper one was found. The lens was sent to the dispensing optician to fabricate the eyewear. The method was a valiant attempt, but it contained all of the errors described above. There was no means to communicate the position of the lens (vertex distance), center position, or inclination. In a short time, World War II prevented the further importation of the lenses, but by that time, the doctors were discouraged by the inconsistency of their results.

This notion has been perpetuated in Cataract Lens Test Sets. The Tillyer Cataract Trial Set is designed with lens combinations from +8.00D. sphere to +18.00D. sphere and includes all the spherocylindrical combinations to +4.00 Cyl. The lenses are made on −3.00D. base curve, which is the same base curve of the Tillyer cataract spectacle lenses. The thickness of the trial lens is also the standard thickness of the same spectacle lens. When these lenses are used for the examination and the trial frame can be adjusted to the inclination at which the spectacles will be worn, the written prescription can be duplicated accurately in a spectacle lens.

Because of the bulk of the trial frame, the trial lens can seldom be placed in the position in which the prescription lens will be worn. W. A. Boyce, M.D., Los Angeles, California, tried to overcome part of the lens position problem by having the lenses loosened in their trial rings so that he could put them in the back cell of the trial frame and rotate them for axis. But, again, there was no means of communicating the position of the lens (except vertex distance) and this procedure produced inconsistent results.

All of these approaches in which principles of geometrical optics were violated caused doctors to empirically modify their prescriptions and then send their patients to some particular optician with whom they felt their patients seemed most satisfied. This optician had learned the doctor's habits and empirically decreased or increased some of the prescriptions in some cases to provide the best optical effects. This is a sad commentary on the delivery of precise lens effects to patients whose lensless eyes deserve the ultimate in visual care. It was because of all of these uncertainties that I designed the Provisional Lens Plan.

PROVISIONAL LENS PLAN

This procedure simplifies the undertaking for patient, doctor, and optician.

1. No special refraction equipment is required.
2. In essence, it acknowledges that even after arduous mathematical calculation of a perfect lens for the refractive error can be accomplished only by trial and error.
3. It acknowledges that the state of refraction of the eye is unstable during the period early after surgery and the patient's responses are likely to be relatively undependable while reorienting himself to new visual experiences.
4. We do not hopefully approach each new fitting with the expectation that the *first* lens will be totally effective and to be almost regularly disappointed, the case is approached from a tentative attitude.
5. Such a procedure is in no way a doubtful or weak approach.
6. It acknowledges, as has been discussed, that many data relevant to the lens fitting are not, and some cannot be, included in the prescription.
7. It provides a means to keep abreast of prescription lens changes while the ultimate prescription is being worked out.

This is the procedure followed by optical instrument designers. Their original computations are made into lenses. A "mock up" of these lenses is made on an optical bench or other lens holder.

Performance is inspected while the lenses are in a fixed position. Increments of error revealed by the "mock up" inspection are considered in modifying or redesigning the lens system.

This old and proved procedure is the basis for the Provisional Lens Plan.

The cardinal principle of the Provisional Plan is that the selected eyeframe be adjusted to the *ideal* position and serve as the instrument maker's optical bench. Total care must be paid to: pad position, pantoscopic angle, vertical and horizontal optical center position and temple adjustment. No violation of the *ideal* fitting shall be made to improve acuity at the fitting of the first lens. The accuracy of this *ideal* fitting must be verified before the over-refraction for the prescription for the second lens.

Regrettably, this irrefutable lens makers procedure has been basically violated by some who use a temporary frame in an unknown position with temporary lenses not related to the profile of the final lenses. Without one element fixed, it reminds one a simple algebraic statement such as: $x + y = 12$, which has no solution if both elements are simultaneously varying.

Patient Instructions

The patient is told before surgery that he will be provided with temporary glasses soon after surgery. These will serve to help him around. His first refraction after surgery will be done as soon as the doctor feels his eye has "settled down" sufficiently. The patient will be told that it is likely that there may be a change or changes made in the lens prescription to account for the effects of the healing process. New lenses will be supplied as doctor directs.

The Dispenser's Part

Unless the doctor has provided loaners to the patient at the hospital or from his office, the first contact with the patient is supplying temporary lenses. The form of this product may change from time to time but the general form is $+10.00D.$ to $+12.00D.$ for distance and sometimes $+2.50$ add for reading. The lenses are usually plastic.

When the patient brings in his first lens prescription, the selection of the eyeframe is the first consideration. The elements that dictate the choice are (a) whether the frame can be fitted close to the eyes, (b) whether the lens shape places the vertical center satisfactorily, (c) whether it can be angled properly, and (d) whether it is sufficiently substantial to retain its adjustment.

These conditions limit the acceptable frame designs. The frame should have adjustable pads to permit minor adjustments to retain the original position of the frame if or when the tissue on the sides of the nose reshapes under the weight of the eyewear. From the point of weight and adjustability, the Polymil® is supreme. Some patients may not choose it because they feel a rimless style displays the curvature of the lens too freely. Next in line is a metal-zyl frame with a relatively symmetric lens shape often fitted with CC temples for stability.

Interocular Distance

Use the *reading* visual axis separation for the distance for bifocals, thereupon the reading segments will require no further decentration. The usual Base Out effect encountered in convergence is completely overcome by this procedure. The fact that the distance lens centers are deliberately closer than the visual axes produces a small amount of prism Base In which is well received due to the usual convergence problem created by the elimination of angles *alpha* and *kappa* by the removal of crystalline lens.

Lens Selection

After more than thirty years experience in more than twenty-five stores with organized changes in lens styles dispensed in a search for the best lens, CR39 aspheric 40 mm lenticular or full field aspherical lenses have been found to be most completely acceptable.

Since the carrier base of lenticular is nearly afocal, the lens can be decentered, if necessary, without any change in lens weight.

A 40 mm lens spot covers the vertical dimension of the edged lens. The edge of the lenticular section is barely visible in the upper and lower corners of the temporal side of the lens. Because this lens is so very thin, the front surface is close to the eye and produces minimum magnification. The aspheric curvature on the front of this lens reduces marginal aberrations to minimum.

A *large number of base curves* assures accurate application of the lens designer's formula. Several of the largest and best lens manufacturers make these lenses or lens blanks for local processing. Segments are round, oval, or flat-top. The top of the segment is very close to the optical center of the lens.

To the Doctor at the Second Refraction

The reasons why the original prescription must now be modified are (a) the shape of the corneal surface has changed and (b) the position of the spectacle lens is not the same as the examining lens; therefore, undesired spherical and cylindrical optical effects have been induced by the tilt of the lens and the location of the center in the vertical meridian.

Your interest is now to find what sphere and cylinder power added to what your patient is wearing will produce best acuity. Therefore you will do a refraction through the spectacle lens.

Simply place the patient, wearing his glasses, behind your Refractor® and proceed. Be sure to adjust the brow rest so there will be no pressure on the spectacle frame. Do not be dismayed if the increment to be added has a cylinder axis at a wide difference from your first prescription. Tilting the prescription lens and/or reduction of the warped cornea may cause it. Write your new prescription. For example

Add $+0.75 \ -1.25 \ \times \ 65$

In other words, when this lens power is added to the present lens the patient will have his best visual acuity.

By this simple means, all of the variations in the optical effect of the lens supplied to your patient plus any change in the power required by the healing process have been found and measured. Frequently it will be found that no other alterations will be required.

To the Dispenser

When the patient brings in this special "Add to" prescription from the second refraction, take the patient's lenses to the Lensometer and carefully measure them so you can add the new prescription to the present lens as it is (accounting for any small deviations or compensations) from the original lens prescription as written. Return the eyewear to the patient and say that a new lens will be made and that you will telephone when it is ready.

Before writing the new record or laboratory order, observe whether the cylinder axes are the same. If not, combine the crossed-cylinders as described in Chapter 10 by any of the methods given.

Extreme care must be exercised in the removing of the first lens and replacing it with the new one. The frame must not be bent or altered at any point. The fitting of the frame must remain as it was originally set.

Other Methods of Fitting

Experience having demonstrated that the first prescription lens after surgery was very seldom precisely correct, opticians have undertaken to contrive a special reworkable temporary lens for the first prescription.

Austin Belgard prepared a trial set of planoconvex spheres and planoconcave cylinders 40 mm round with the bevel of these lenses like a watch crystal. When the plano sides of the two lenses were faced, a lens with the bevel in the middle was formed. The lenses were fitted into a plain 40 mm round frame.

George McNair had 33×36 lenses made to fit in a specially designed plastic frame. This produced a kind of lenticular effect.

Earl Lewis designed round planoconvex bifocals to be cemented to a planoconcave cylinder and thus construct a custommade, temporary, and also reusable, lens.

Doctor Welsh saved his patients' first pairs of lenses intact to be used as first temporary lenses for others. He reports that he used spherical equivalents for his first prescription to make them more easily reusable. Doctor Joaquin Barraquer (Barcelona, Spain) has a special rack in his refracting rooms for these reusable "Temporaries."

It must not be forgotten that basic to this problem is a linear algebraic equation in which there are two factors; namely, (x) the lens power and (y) lens position. The first lesson in elementary algebra may be $x + y = 8$. The first move toward the solution was to let x or y be some fixed amount. Let $x = 2$, then $y = 6$. But if both x and y were simultaneously changing in value there was no solution.

All of these notions above present the problem in this last form. When the temporary lens is replaced with an intended permanent lens, the frame and usually also the size and shape of the lens was changed so both x and y were simultaneously changed. All that can be said for these procedures is that no lenses were consumed for the first pair, but all the problem of the first lens fitting still faces the fitter.

The instrument makers' approach meets the requirements. Fix x by setting the lens permanently in one position (the proper frame, properly adjusted). Then use that base to find what power needs to be added to a fixed setting to perfect the optical performance of the unit.

Other Lens Forms

In that Doctor Welsh's inquiries began in the 1950s and CR39 had not been developed materially at the time, his whole work was upon the problem of how to make a lightweight *glass* lens. He awakened young lens makers and laboratory operators to how an asymmetrically-shaped lens could be made thinner if the lens were decentered above the lens pattern center. As long as this higher center is compatible with the pantoscopic angle permitting the lens axis to be directed through the center of rotation, the notion is usable, but nowhere in his discussion of Minimum Equivalent Diameter does he correlate these factors. It must not be forgotten that a too high center causes tilted lens effects the same as low lenses. See Figure 165.

It must be remembered that if the lens center is above the pupil center, the lens must be tilted *out* at the bottom to avoid the prescription change incident with a tilted lens.

In Doctor Welsh's observations on the subject of lens thickness, he noted that the knife-edged lens of a spherocylinder lens was the shape of an ellipse with the plus cylinder axis congruent with the major axis of the ellipse. Thus, if the plus axis of the lens were 180° and the lens shape were made oval, the edge of the lens would be uniform thickness at all points. He properly named this "Utopian Center." A limited number of plus cylinder axes are found at 180°, and of these, the amount of cylinder power to make the minor axis of the ellipse compatible with the frame size really approached a "Utopian" incident. The method of visualizing the oval before a laboratory order is written is not difficult:

Take the power in the meridian of the axis and opposite meridian:

+11.00 +5.00 × 160

Use a vertex depth chart to find the shape of the oval:

+11.00 = 5.39 mm center at 42 mm

The same center thickness applied to +16.00 (+11.00 +5.00) is 5.40 mm at 36 mm. Hence the oval would be 36 × 42 axis 160, no thinner than a 42 mm round lens but with less glass across the 70° meridian if 36 mm were not too narrow for the particular pattern. The oval shape of the knife-edge lens could be a handicap if the axis were 90°.

Fused lenticular lenses have virtually passed into oblivion since the development of CR39 lenses. Reduced weight and aspheric surfaces of plastic lenses have been the main reasons.

Doctor Welsh became concerned with the prism Base Out generated in multifocal segments when eyes converged for reading. To offset the prism, he obtained wide segment lenses (even wider than Univis R) so they could be decentered as much as 6 mm each eye. We tried a few of such lenses then changed to centering all cataract lenses at the near interocular distance. This device removed the prism for near-point and caused 2$^\triangle$ to 3$^\triangle$ Base In for distance. This prism is more comfortable than centered lenses because it replaces some of the additional convergence effort now required because of the loss of angle gamma with the removal of the crystalline lens.

Our first attempt to provide an alterable lens for the Provisional Lens Plan was to use very high base semifinished plus cylinders, on which we ground a shallow, concave, inside curve. Cemented segments were used for bifocals. It was our assumption that at the first prescription change, we would regrind the inside surface and make a new cement segment. In practice, each cylinder power change or axis change required a new lens. After the volume of cases of Provisional Plan cases increased, the lens making for prescription changes became a burden.

We were rescued from our plight when A0 introduced the Aspheric Lenticular. In a short time, we originated the grinding and polishing procedure to alter the inside curve of these lenses. We soon ordered semifinished blanks which A0 had not expected to have to make. From our first special order of semifinished blanks has grown the stock item of all CR39 cataract lens makers. The original concept of a factory molded CR39 cataract prescription lens is now a minute portion of the whole market.

It would be remiss to neglect to give the organized fitting table method developed in the dispensing of thousands of lenses for aphakic patients.

Progress of Lens Designs

The design of spectacle lenses to reduce the astigmatic error of oblique rays has attracted the attention of scientists for many years. Tscherning's ellipse, which is seen in most texts on physiological optics, plots those lenses which can be marginally corrected. The convex limit is slightly less than +8.00D. Therefore, the whole cataract lens series is not amenable to the same marginal correction of weaker plus lenses. Some lenses designed by Gullstrand have been made in Europe by Carl Zeiss, Inc., with an aspherical rear surface, known as Katral lenses. The lenses had to be produced to order and, of course, were single vision lenses. The complications and expense prevented a sufficiently large use of the lenses to prove their clinical value.

Percival, von Rohr, Tillyer, Rayton, Davis, and others have studied the best profile. Their independent studies show that the back curve of a lens for aphakia must be concave. Mathematician Percival prefers −5.00D. Without too much compromise, the others agree that a shallower, less bulgy lens with less magnification having a −3.00D. curve is a very satisfactory form. Marginal errors grow at an astounding rate as the curve approaches plano. A convex curve on the posterior surface is unthinkable. In Table XXVIII, the correcting lens (+10.43D.) for the eye under consideration has been computed for an angle of 30°. This is close to the margin of the prescription portion of a lenticular lens.

The axis of the cylinder varies with the direction of gaze down or up the axis is 180°, right or left the axis is 90°.

TABLE XXVIII
LENS FORMS COMPARED

+10.43D. *Sphere at 30°*		
I. Biconvex	+12.01	+16.19 ×
II. Planoconvex	+10.27	+2.09 ×
III. —3.00 Base	+10.00	+1.01 ×
IV. —6.00 Base	+ 9.93	+0.59 ×

1. The gross amount of power increase of a biconvex lens away from the lens axis limits the usefulness of the lens to the paraxial region.

2. The planoconvex lens has a larger field, partly because the secondary focus (+10.27D.) is slightly less than the prescription. The circle of least confusion is closer to the retina than in the case of the first lens where both meridians overcorrect the eye.

3. The —3.00 base lens still has some cylindrical power but the focal lines are almost equidistant from the retina. It is about the effect of a 0.50D. crossed-cylinder added to the prescription.

4. This lens has the least cylindrical error and the sphere is 0.05D. weak. From the viewpoint of geometrical optics, it is the best lens, but it is much more difficult to produce accurately, and cosmetically it is less desirable because of increased bulging and magnification.

First Welch, then Signet, have made extravagant reductions in curvature of the marginal areas of their full field aphakic lenses to reduce the thickness of the lens. In Welch's desire to make an aphakic lens appear as near as possible like an ordinary prescription lens, he has violated the laws of geometrical optics for a good lens of offering only two base curves, namely +12.00D. and +14.00D. This comparative flatness does minimize the magnification of the eye as viewed from the front. These low front curves force any lens above the 14.00D. sphere to have a *convex* inside curve! Some of the extravagantly increased marginal astigmatism becomes absorbed in the weaker marginal power of the lens caused by the flattened curvature.

Disregarding lens optics for the moment, we will evaluate the cosmetic effects of the lenses. Like other full-field lenses, they do not have the juncture and ring at the margin of the prescription area of lenticular lenses. The degeneration of the curvature has produced thin edges and reduced center thickness like lenticulars. Obliteration of the line of demarcation and gradually flattening the marginal curve produces a zone about two-thirds the size of the prescription power of the lenses. From the wearer's side, it widens the vista of the lenses even though the lens correction continues to decline toward the periphery. This gradual diminution of lens correction is accepted by many wearers as an advantage over the abrupt change at the edge of the lenticular center.

The flattening of the lens margin should be a function of the power of the lens base. However, for the advantage of a trade name, Doctor Welsh uses only one curve reduction for all prescriptions. This is admissible since he uses only two front curves for all prescriptions.

Like the amount of "figuring" or parabolizing of the margin of a Newtonian astronomical mirror to obtain a perfect focus, so should the lengthening of the radius of curvature of the aspheric marginal area of a convex surface be a calculated amount. Again, for the sake of a trade name, Signet indicates that an exaggerated flattening of curvature intensifies the optical value of their lens. It should not be forgotten that the original motivation for this lens design was appearance (cosmetic), not improved optics.

This series of lenses is more difficult to produce than a standard lenticular and accordingly must sell at an increased price. It is not our policy to offer it as a first lens when the customer's introduction to the new visual space is very confused. It is presented at the first lens change and can be more easily compared with the lens being worn.

Lenticular type lenses are recommended for all purposes as first choice for single vision and bifocal forms (see Table XXIX).

The first attempts at a convex lenticular lens were cemented form (Fig. 200). The major lens was ordinarily a 6.00D. base toric on which the prescribed cylinder was ground. The cemented section was most frequently a single vision lens; however, a Kryptok bifocal was sometimes prepared for the purpose. The primary aim was accomplished. The lens was very much lighter than a standard lens, but there were two objections: (a) The balsam cement loosened and discolored and finally the edge of the

TABLE XXIX
COMPARISON OF GLASS CATARACT LENSES
All Lenses +12:00D. Sphere, 42 mm Round

| Style | Approximate Curves | | Thickness | | Weight |
	Front	Back	Edge	Center	in Grams
Single Vision					
Planoconvex	+11.50	Plano	1.4	5.9	12.4
Double convex	+6.00	+6.00	1.2	5.9	12.4
Thin-Lite (Flint)	+9.00	Plano	1.1	4.8	16.6
One-piece Lenticular	+14.50	—3.00	1.6	4.4	9.2
Fused Lenticular	+7.75	Plano	1.3	4.1	9.2
Bifocal					
Regular Fused	+11.50	Plano	1.2	5.8	12.6
AO "E" Lenticular					
Cruxite Base	+14.50	—3.00	1.6	4.3	8.9
AO "E" Lenticular					
Calobar Base	+14.50	—3.00	1.6	4.3	8.9
Univis Bilentic	+8.75	+3.00	1.6	4.5	9.1
Univis Bifokat	+9.00	Plano	1.4	4.7	11.0
Old Panoptik Lenticular	+12.00	—2.50	1.9	5.8	15.0
Old Panoptik Lenticular					
Soft-Lite Base	+12.00	—2.50	2.0	5.9	15.8
New Panoptik Lenticular	+10.50	—3.00	1.4	4.3	11.9

central section became irregular and collected dust. (b) The posterior surface of the lens was convex with an average curve of +6.00D. which reduced the field of distinct vision tremendously as is shown in Table XXVIII.

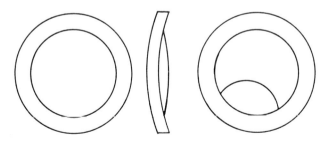

Figure 200. First types of lenticular lenses for aphakia.

The next improvement was accomplished by Continental Optical Company, the one-piece bifocal makers (Fig. 201). The

lenticular was made of a single piece of glass. The first objection
was completely overcome but it could not be made in bifocal
form. The lens was made with a −6.00D. base, so the improvement did not include the optical design. Later the one-piece idea
was made up in better optical forms by American Optical Company and Bausch & Lomb Optical Company. The flat lens has
been made with a center field to give the optical effect of a
planoconvex lens. That part of the prescription above +6.00D. is
ground in the major portion of the lens. This lens is not quite as
light in weight as the others. More recently a one-piece lenticular
lens has been offered with the lenticular portion on the anterior
surface of the lens, and the curves are so chosen that the carrier
lens has an average base curve of −3.00D. This type of single
vision lens is optically and cosmetically very desirable.

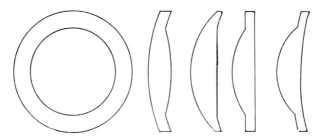

Figure 201.   Progress in lenticular profiles for aphakia lenses.

Monroe* has combined a Tillyer Cataract one-piece bifocal
where the reading portion is on the anterior surface with a
−3.00D. base carrier lens. This lenticular has the advantage that
it can be modified for focal power by changing the base lens only.
A colored base lens usually approximates an even-density lens.
Wooters has projected a means by which an aspheric surface can
be incorporated into aphakic lenses. He reports that the original
Zeiss Katral lens design is improved when the aspheric surface is
on the front surface. He suggests a plastic section onto which the
special surface is molded to be cemented to a regular lens and

---

*Personal Communication, Clark Monroe, Monroe Opticians, Inc., Los Angeles,
Calif.

thus produce a lenticular design similar to the AO "E" or B & L No. 5.

Fused lenticulars followed the one-piece lenses, but they, too, were generally unsuccessful. The principal obstruction aside from manufacturing difficulties was chromatic aberration. If a flint glass segment of n = 1.62 with a v-value near 35 is fused in regular ophthalmic crown n = 1.523, v-value 60, the chromatic aberration of the lens is found as follows:

$$\frac{D_1}{v_1} + \frac{D_2}{v_2} = \text{Diopters of chromatic aberration}$$

If we chose a +10.00D. lens to be made at minimum thickness with a −6.00D. inside curve and the lenticular portion to be made 30 mm diameter, the front surface would be +9.20D. and the fused surface 26.14D. Substituting in the formula

$$\frac{-32.15}{60} + \frac{35.34}{35} = -.536 + 1.010 = +0.474D.$$

Thus, if this lens corrects the refractive error for yellow in the middle of the spectrum, blue is overcorrected by almost 0.25D. and red is undercorrected by a like amount (.475 ÷ 2 = .24). That is, all objects reflecting or transmitting red or blue light are out of focus. Any attempt to favor lighting conditions or surroundings by increasing or decreasing the prescription only hinders the performance of the lens at the other end of the spectrum. Such longitudinal chromatic aberration was intolerable to most people. Color fringes surrounded all objects. One of the most serious effects of these failures was the effect on a large number of doctors. Even to this day there are some who are unduly suspicious of convex lenses in any lenticular form.

About 1925 a new series of high-index glasses were introduced into the ophthalmic field. The first "color-free" or nearly achromatic bifocals were announced. A high-index barium crown glass with almost the same v-value as regular ophthalmic crown was perfected. Many new lens designs were now possible and in the following years a number of important improvements were offered. The cataract lenses now available include several styles described below.

American Optical Company makes the Lenticular "E" Style

Aphakic Lens (Fig. 202). It can be had in a single vision or Ful-
Vue bifocal. The base lens is made of Cruxite® "A" glass to
absorb ultraviolet light. On special order from the factory the
lens is available with darker shades of Cruxite and Calobar.® Only
the base lens is made of absorptive glass, to which is fused a clear
glass lenticular portion; therefore the lens has an *even color
density*. The refractive portion of the lens is 30 mm in diameter.
The top edge of the reading portion is 3 mm below the optical
center of the distance lens. This lens has no chromatic problem
because the power is accomplished as in the one-piece type of
lenticular—that is, by the lens curves. Characteristic of all lenticular lenses, it is much lighter in weight than an ordinary lens.
Cosmetically the lens is also an improvement. The magnification
of the wearer's eye is minimized behind the 30 mm refractive area.

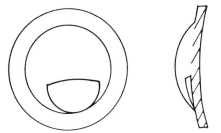

Figure 202. Fused lenticular for aphakia.

Bausch & Lomb make their Panoptik bifocal (Fig. 203) in a
fused lenticular in which barium flint is used for both the lenticular and reading segment portions, thus insuring a "color-free"
lens. The reading segment is 13.5 × 19.5 mm, which sets the top
edge of the segment 1.5 below the geometric center of the distance
portion. The optical center of the reading addition is 3.75 mm
below the segment edge. The lens is available in white glass and
three shades of Soft-Lite® glass. The recently improved model of
this lens in which the lenticular portion is made of a barium
flint glass, n = 1.616, is an especially desirable lens both from the
standpoints of appearance and weight. (See Table XXIX.) It
may be obtained in lens sizes up to 80 mm. The central section
can be had in diameters up to 38 mm but the manufacturers do

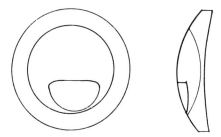

Figure 203. Panoptic lenticular for aphakia.

not recommend them because of added thickness and weight.

Continental Optical Company, the original one-piece bifocal makers, offers two lens forms applicable to cataract cases. The lenticular portion is a +6.00D. curve (Fig. 201) applied to a −6.00D. base with a 28 mm refractive area. This, of course, is a single vision lens. For bifocal wearers, they make the "A" segment 38 mm diameter bifocal on a flat base (Fig. 204) to provide a means for a planoconvex lens. All of the segment sizes 22, 32, 38 mm, and the flat-top "K" can be had with −4.00D. base curves for the conventional type of lenses. Some one-piece cataract bifocals are made with the segment on the front surface (Fig. 204) .

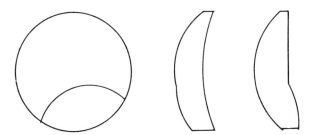

Figure 204. Ultex lenticular for aphakia.

The Univis Lens Company, which specializes in multifocal lenses, offers several lenses especially for cataract cases. The finest lens of the series is their Bilentic Cataract Bifocal (Fig. 205). It is a combination of one-piece and fused construction. The distance portion is a 30 mm field on the posterior side of the lens and has either a −1.00D. or +3.00D. base curve, according to the strength of the distance prescription. The base (or carrier) lens has an inside curve of −6.00D. The reading portion is 17 × 9 mm and set 3 mm below the geometric center of the distance portion. The optical center of the reading portion is at the dividing line, therefore the "jump" is eliminated. This lens is available in white or Crookes glass.

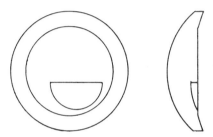

Figure 205.   Bilentic lenticular for aphakia.

The Bifokat® type is an all fused lenticular lens (Fig. 206). This is a planoconvex design with the reading segment and distance portion fused to the posterior surface. The central field is 25 mm diameter and the reading segment 18 mm wide. By its design the top edge of this segment is about 5 mm below the geometric center of the distance circle. The barium glass makes a 6.00D. gain in the reading portion. Therefore the reduction in curvature of the upper portion is 6.00D. minus the addition, e.g. 6.00D. − 2.50D. add = 3.50D. A + 10.00D. Sph. which would be ground with +6.50D., compensated for thickness on the front curve.

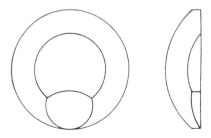

Figure 206. Univis Bifoka for aphakia.

Univis' widely used "D" segment bifocal is available on a flat base. When the segment is turned toward the eye, this blank provides a planoconvex lens of regular design. Their general purpose trifocal (Fig. 207) is also made on a flat base to provide a lens with an intermediate field for those whose activities require sharp vision at an "arm's length." The intermediate field is 6 mm wide and is regularly 50 percent of the power of the reading addition. However, they are able to supply on special order the intermediate portion at 37, 67, or 75 percent of the total reading addition.

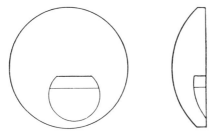

Figure 207. Planoconvex Univis trifocal for aphakia.

A single vision lenticular like the distance portion of the Bifokat is also available (Fig. 208). It finishes as a planoconvex lens. The gain is 6.00D. in the outside curve.

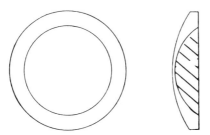

Figure 208. Single vision planoconvenx lenticular for aphakia.

When we refer to the formula on page 113 which shows that magnification is effected by both power and shape, it is apparent that some lenticular lenses may give optical effects slightly different from those of ordinary lenses. The patient's visual acuity is partially dependent upon the magnification induced by the correcting lens before the aphakic eye. Occasionally a patient may observe slightly reduced acuity when the front curve and lens thickness are reduced in the better form lens. The comfort and appearance usually more than offset this small loss from magnification.

FITTING THE MONOCULAR PROVISIONAL LENS

If this is the first eye, the optician must find out whether there are plans to operate on the other eye at some future time. The patient's story about his other eye is very significant in the fitting to follow. For one extreme, the eye may be considered totally blind and no effort is to be made to correct it with surgery and lenses. In such a case, the balancing lens is chosen for cosmetic purposes only and the centers of the correcting lens are set for monocular vision. If the patient seems to be indefinite about the other eye, it is important to explain the reason for the question. It is not difficult to describe to the patient the difference in eye habits of the person who uses only one eye as compared with an individual with binocular vision. It is also necessary to know something about the vision in the unoperated eye. Frequently the prescription reads "Balance" instead of a prescribed lens power. The degree of vision in the eye reveals whether the "fogging effect" of the plus lens is important. If the patient indicates that he has any reasonable amount of perception, it is a good rule to use a sphere in front of the eye that approximates the spherical equivalent of the correcting lens. If the eye has the least indirect vision, the patient usually holds his head and eyes similarly to a person with binocular vision. A person who has only monocular vision often turns his head slightly toward the defective eye to increase his nasal field of vision. For example, if the right eye is used, he turns his head to the left and thus turns his nose out of the way to improve the visual field to the left. There is no definite rule. He may have developed a habit with an opposite compensation for cosmetic reasons. All that one can do is to watch the patient and try to observe his habits. A simple way is to put a vertical mark on the 90 meridian of his (or a fitting) lens up from the bottom to a distance of about 5 mm below the pupil. The position of the line with reference to the patient's pupil as he sits at ease at the fitting table should indicate whether he tends to keep his eye in primary position for distance vision or verges to right or left. When the center is located, the optical center of the distance prescription should be set at that point with the reading segment center set directly below it. In rare instances, the reading center might be decentered slightly nasalward, but the amount will seldom be as much as is found in binocular vision. The same rule obtains in these cases that directs the fitting of all bifocals: *Do not change the wearer's habits any more than absolutely necessary!*

The person who has had one eye operated upon and will now be given binocular vision or the one who will shortly have the other eye operated upon is an altogether different case. In the first instance, the prescription itself may offer quite a dilemma to the optician. The doctor may have written an order to change one lens only. A careful examination of the other lens may disclose that, although it may have served as a correction for one eye, the old lens is centered and fits in such a way that it cannot be properly paired with another lens for binocular vision. It may follow that the visual acuity of the first eye is bad and deteriorating and that the doctor is not expecting the eyes to function together. There is only one thing that an optician can do in such a case. When the old lens has been analyzed and found to be optically deficient, discuss the matter with the doctor. In some cases, the Provisional Lens can be worked out by using the old lens to find the "Add" to produce a better prescription than a conventional *first* lens and, when the final prescription is reached, both lenses can be replaced. In the second instance, the correcting lens will be as carefully placed with reference to pupillary distance and reading position as if both eyes were in use. The patient will then not have to make any further adjustments when the other eye is operated upon.

Interocular distance in corrected aphakia is somewhat different from that in normal eyes. Before surgery, the visual axis of the eye was not the same as the optical axis. The angle between these lines at the center of rotation (angle *gamma*) was about 5 arc degrees or 9 Prism Diopters. When the crystalline lens was removed, the visual axis closely approaches the optical axis and the eye must be turned nasalward. No extra effort is required so long as the patient has only monocular vision. However, when the other eye is operated upon, a new habit of additional convergence must be established at once for all distances. This is not quite the same physiological effort of a person with normal eyes because there can be no associated stimulation to accommodation. If one eye has been in disuse for any considerable length of time, the interruption to the use of fusion many have allowed the eyes to turn out of alignment (usually divergent). The patient's dilemma is caused by the effort to reestablish fusion, that is, to increase his convergence for the visual axis effect, but not to overconverge for the magnified (apparently closer) objects which he sees through his corrected lenses. It will therefore be important that the optical centers of the distance lenses be not too wide and thereby add prism Base Out. Because the vast majority of the activities of those who are operated upon for cataract are at distances well inside infinity, the eyes are converging slightly most of the time. It is therefore recommended that all distance or reading glasses and all bifocals be set at the near-point pupillary distance. The distance portion of the lenses (near $+$ 10.00D.) induces about 1 Prism Diopter for each millimeter of convergence. For an average reading distance this is at least $3^{\triangle}$, an amount too great to offset by decentration of the reading portion. In view of the new demands on convergence to overcome the loss of angle *gamma,* any small amount of prism Base In should be welcome.

The proper position of the reading portion is as high as possible, to avoid marginal aberrations. The use of a flat-top reading segment reduces the "jump" or blind area at the top of the segment so that the eyes do not have to be depressed much below the dividing line to have effective use of the reading field. The distance between the optical center of the distance part of the lens and the top edge of the reading segment as found with the Provisional Lens will indicate the type of lenticular lens to be selected. For those cases requiring the smallest separation, the Panoptik, which is set 1.5 mm below center, is chosen. American Optical "E" and Univis Bilentic are both designed with the segment set 3 mm below the center of the disc. By the construction of the Univis Bifokat, the segment is 5 mm below the geometric center

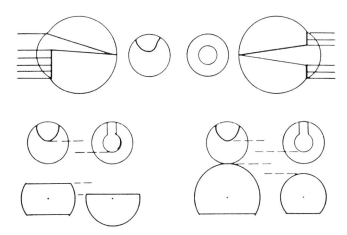

Figure 209. Segment placements for dissimilar pupils in aphakia.

of the distance portion.   The Aolite Aspheric Lenticular segment is set 2 mm below center.

Following cataract surgery, the pupils are occasionally ill-shapen and/or eccentric. The defects have no significance in the fitting of single vision lenses. They must be carefully considered, though, for bifocal fitting, if the bottoms of the pupillary margins are not the same distances from the corneal centers. As has been discussed, the optical and visual axes are nearly coincident in the aphakic eye. Therefore, the interocular distance is the distance between the corneal centers when the eyes are fixed at infinity whether the pupillary apertures are centered or eccentric. If the centers of the distance portions of the lenses are set in front of the corneal centers, it follows that the centers of the reading portions must be symmetric with the distance centers because the depression of the eyes to the reading position is a conjugate movement. It is necessary, however, that one segment top be as much lower than the other as the difference in the lower margins of the pupillary apertures. This can be easily accomplished by either of the methods illustrated. The flat-top procedure is better because the optical centers of the segments are closer to the top and and thus there is less "jump" and the reading area is optically useful almost as soon as the pupillary center has crossed the dividing line.

Single vision lenses do not require quite the same study as multifocals because the wearer will tend to center his vision through a single small area of the lens.

Because of the extreme weight of regular single vision glass lenses, they should not ordinarily be made in lens sizes over 42 mm long. Larger sizes often require decentration and become intolerably heavy. The fragile tissue of the nose is irritated and breaks down because of the weight. Denser glasses such as barium crown or flint glass offer no relief. However, Hilite® glass is advantageous. The increased refractive index does make it possible to grind shallower curves on these lenses, but the increased specific gravity of flint glass much more than offsets the gain. Spectacle crown, n = 1.523, Sp. Gr. 2.52; Flint, n = 1.69, Sp. Gr. 4.23). With the same edge thickness, a flint glass lens is about 20 percent thinner in the center but weighs almost 33 percent more than an ordinary crown glass lens. Regular lenses can be made lightweight if they are fitted to McNair frames which have 33 × 36 mm lens size. This is the type of glass used for some "Loan Glasses."

Plastic lenticular lenses are to be preferred for permanent spectacles because of weight as well as appearance. They should be used in all instances where large lenses are required. Some opththalmologists feel that the slight restriction to eye movements may be beneficial. They think there may be less cause for retinal detachment if the patient turns his head more and reduces the number of wide ocular vergences.

The combined fused and one-piece type is especially desirable for outdoor glasses. The carrier lens (Fig. 202) can be made of green or neutral-colored glass to control both the quantity and quality of the light transmitted. The carrier lens is almost plano and therefore the color is practically even color density. This is particularly desirable because a sufficiently dense glass to give adequate protection to the peripheral field is extremely dark in the central area of ordinary lenses. Since all plastic lenses are tinted by dyeing, they are automatically of even density. Further, by redyeing, the tint can be altered to the wearer's wishes.

An essential publication for a dispenser's library is Albert E. Sloane's *So You Have Cataracts* (Charles C Thomas, Springfield,

1971). The author has had many years experience in the Massachusetts Eye and Ear Infirmary and as an assistant clinical professor of ophthalmology at Harvard University School of Medicine. He has an easy writing style and knows optical and optician's problems in depth.

REVIEW

1. Why is there a blind space at the margin of cataract lenses?

2. Can the size of a cataract lens be chosen to avoid a ring scotoma at the margin? Discuss.

3. Why are ultraviolet absorbing lenses needed after cataract surgery?

4. Which causes the larger difference in lens effectivity, a cataract lens tilted 20° or a vertex distance change of 3 mm?

5. Explain the optical principles of the Provisional Lens Plan.

6. The patient's first prescription is $+11.50$ $+1.25$ $\times$ 25. Doctor has prescribed: Add $+0.75$ -1.00 $\times$ 65. What is the new lens power?

7. A patient's final prescription is

$+12.25$ $+1.75$ $\times$ 155 All $+2.75$
$+13.00$ $+1.00$ $\times$ 30

Is the prism effect in the segment area 7 mm below center tolerable?

Answer: Yes, 0.48D. vertical.

8. If $+12.50$D. is centered before an eye in the primary position and then given 10° pantoscopic angle, what is the resultant tilted lens effect? (Table XXVII).

$+12.50$ = $^5/_4 \times$ ($+0.10$ $+0.31$)

Answer: $+12.62$ $+0.39$ $\times$ 180

9. If the prescription were $+15.00$ $+1.00$ $\times$ 40 in problem 8 what is the resultant lens effect?

$+15.00$ $+1.00$ $\times$ 40
Add 0.15 $+0.47$ $\times$ 180 Tilted lens addition
$+15.15$ ($+1.00$ $\times$ 40   A
          ($+0.47$ $\times$ 180 B

Answer: $+15.25$ $+1.25$ $\times$ 28

10. Distance prescription is $+12.00$D., the addition for reading is $+2.50$ using a refracting instrument with the fronts of all

spherical lenses + 5.25D. Would the same patient accept a stronger or weaker addition by this means than if the refraction were done with biconvex Trial Set lenses? Why?

Answer: Stronger addition.

11. Is the adjustment of vertex distance or pantoscopic angle of a frame ever changed after the first Provisional Lens is fitted? Why?

12. Why is the trifocal cataract lenses controversial? What is your opinion?

13. Why are aphakic patients more sensitive to bright light?

14. Is an aphakic patient's prescription likely to have a significant change after the second year after surgery?

15. Describe the steps for the setting of the bifocal segment, lens center, and pantoscopic angle. How many degrees is the angle increased for each millimeter vertical change of lens center?

Chapter 13

VOCATIONAL LENSES

◆◆

A large share of what is called "vocational glasses" involves multifocal lenses. The specifications for such eyewear usually demand that clear, easy vision is available at two or more points other than the regular distance and near-vision points of ordinary lenses. Enterprising lens makers have been alert to develop means of manufacture for a great number of vocational demands. Therefore, what was one day a new departure shortly becomes routine procedure. There are now more than fifty distinctly different multifocal lenses. Each of them has been conceived to solve a patient's visual problem under certain conditions of lens power and use. Even a cursory inspection of the wide assortment of segment shapes and sizes suggests the variety of applications of the lenses. This diversity in multifocal design has encouraged some dispensers to undertake to crowd all of a patient's needs into one pair of glasses. Experience proves this practice is usually unsatisfactory. As in most things, the more the lenses are specialized for a particular purpose, the less valuable they become for general use. At this point a copy of *Guide to Occupational and Other Visual Needs* (1958), Volume I, by Clarke Holmes, is indispensable. On pages 26 to 50, the various multifocal designs by all manufacturers on the market at the time of publication all illustrated with specifications and ranges of curves and powers. Since then there have been some additions, especially in CR39 hard-resin lenses. The progressive addition increase lenses such as Varilux II, Ultravue, and Younger 10/30 have appeared since 1958.

Most vocational lenses involve the thought of eye safety. For the industrial trades, 3 mm industrial tempered glass or CR39 hard resin are mandatory. FDA regulations require that all prescription lenses (a) be either temperature case-hardened or chemically tempered and (b) be able to withstand a specified drop-ball test. California State laws require prescription lenses for children and people with monocular vision to be CR39 lenses.

One of my first experiences with vocational lenses was a pair of one-piece bifocals with the reading portions set at the top to provide a butcher with clear vision of the dial of an early model of Toledo scales. The distance portion was slightly overcorrected to provide sharp-vision for his chopping block and the meat in the counter case. Present-day double segment bifocals make such an improvisation unnecessary.

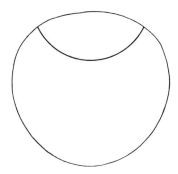

Figure 210. Reversed one-piece vocational lens.

The first part of the investigation must determine these things: (a) the precise distance from eye to each of the points for which vision is to be corrected (tape line measurements are infinitely more satisfactory than estimations) ; (b) the size and location of the object, that is, the area and sector of the visual field involved; and (c) the constancy of the location of the object and the patient's head posture with reference to it.

Frequently, a change in surroundings may cause the patient to be somewhat unsure of distances, location, and so forth. It is recommended that, if there seems to be the least confusion or involvement, the patient be asked to make all measurements carefully with a tapeline. His own survey of the situation, in which he is taking some responsibility, often brings to light factors which might otherwise be overlooked.

For these vocational spectacles, some doctors indicate the distance for which the addition is prescribed as

Add. O.U. +1.00D. for 50 cm

This notation has advantages. If the patient's measured distance varies materially from the prescribed distance, the doctor can be consulted by the dispenser for the possible prescription modifications.

The size and shape of the object and the regularity of the vergence angle determine the dimensions and position of the segment in the lens. With further reference to the case described above, his difficulties caused by early presbyopia when his total reading addition did not exceed +1.25D., could be satisfactorily met by an inverted bifocal. At an arm's length his accommodation would still be adequate. In any event, the doctor would not have to add more than +0.50D. to his distance prescription and with this slight overcorrection his vision would not blur for objects inside a distance somewhat more than 2 meters or almost 7 feet. The area of regard at the reading distance was almost 10 inches long and 4 inches high. This area at 40 cm is covered by a segment only 20 mm wide with an average pupil size. Therefore the reading segment of the one-piece bifocal was unnecessarily large for the purpose. The "jump" at the dividing line should be avoided in this field. A somewhat wider than average flat-top fused bifocal should serve nicely.

In a few years when his accommodative amplitude had reduced to the point where the addition for 40 cm had increased to +1.75D., the lens problem for this person would be quite different. By this time his vision at intermediate distance (67 cm) would not be satisfactory with less than +0.87 to +1.00D. added to his distance prescription (see Fig. 187). If this amount were added to his distance prescription for his working distance, the middle distance would be out of range and his whole distance field would be badly blurred. It is apparent that he now has *three* points at which he must have assistance because of the reduced amount of accommodation available:

1. Distance vision in the central part of his field.
2. Working vision below center (50 to 70 cm).
3. Near-point correction for 33 cm above his horizon.

Double segment bifocal or trifocal lenses can now be individualized to meet these requirements most accurately. The doctor's prescription will show the two additions required and any of several lenses will fill his needs. Figure 211 shows two of the possibilities.

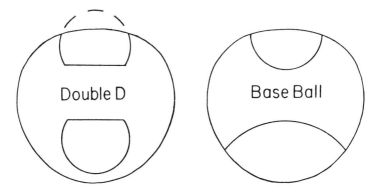

Figure 211.   Double segment bifocals.

A classical case for Double D lenses is a presbyopic dispensing optician. Across the fitting table at intermediate distance at or above the dispenser's eye level sits the customer. It is paramount that he have his best acuity to see details of eyes and lenses at this distance. The lenses provide a perfect demonstration of vocational lenses and are a convincing argument for "lenses to fit eye needs." My firm requires and supplies double segment lenses for all presbyopic dispensers.

An old story is retold of the presbyopic optician who undertook to use regular bifocals and gave his customer an excellent view of the hair in his nose as he tipped his head back to measure interocular centers. When presbyopia arrives do not be ridiculous too!

Research by Ernest Johnson, M.D., and Claire Wolfe, M.D.,* at Ohio State University Medical School has established that the effort to use bifocals for protracted fixation in the area above primary position can result in neck and shoulder pain. Tipping

---

*Johnson, Ernest and Wolfe, Claire: Neck and shoulder pain associated with use of bifocals. *JAMA, 214:*44, 1970.

the head back to read at eye level or above can result in chronic injury to the cervical nerve roots and may cause pain in otherwise asymptomatic spondylopathy. Although heat and traction usually help to relieve the pain, the doctors said that the best therapy is avoidance of hyperextension and extensive rotation of the cervical spine. This indictment of the use of bifocals to read in the upper area of the visual field emphasizes the need for double segment lenses.

Webb Chamberlain, M.D.,* has reported on the restriction of upward gaze with advancing age. By the time that an intermediate addition is needed (ages 55 to 64) the average limitation is 26° upward. The design of double segment lenses (upper segment 12 to 14 mm above the lower) causes the eyes to rotate less than 15° upward even if the optical centers are placed directly in front of the pupils when the eyes are in primary position. Thus the choice of double segment lenses is reinforced by both researches. The power of the additions can vary as required and the separations and positions of the segments can be set in the proper positions. The two-round segment type called "baseball" is obtainable in both one-piece and fused lenses. Ultex E (32 mm) segment lenses with any combination of additions as specified distance between centers are available on special order. An "A" segment one-piece combined with a Tillyer "D" can be obtained from the factory. These larger segments may be important for an individual who has previously worn and become habituated to the larger reading area. Fused lenses—that is, Orthogon "D" and Tillyer "D"—are also obtainable with 20 mm round (or smaller) segments and separated as requested. Ful-Vue and Panoptik bifocals are available with a round segment on the opposite side. The lens can be worn with the flat top segment on either top or bottom. Univis D is made "double D" style. The separation between the segments of this lens is very accurately controlled. It is ordinarily easiest for a patient to learn to wear straight-edged segments because of the reduced "blind areas" and minimum image displacement. Double segment Executive lenses have the advantage of very wide segments. They are available from the

---

*Chamberlain, Webb: Restriction in upward gaze with advancing age. *Am J Ophthalmol,* 71:341, 1971.

manufacturers' stock depots. These lens forms are highly desirable for a great number of patients in *middle presbyopia,* that is, those whose additions range from +1.50D. to +2.25D. On occasion, the additions at top and bottom may be identical. Frequently the working distance is at arm's length at the top and this segment is made with slightly less power; for example, a shoe dealer who must be able to see stock numbers on shelves above eye level, a librarian who must see books on racks above eye level, or a refractionist who looks at his refracting instrument or trial frame above the primary position. In each case the point at which clear vision is required in the upper field is greater distance than an average reading distance. None of these persons can perform his duties satisfactorily with the distance prescription and each has difficulty looking down his nose with his head tipped back while he tries to raise his reading addition (which is focussed too short) into position to see above his horizon.

Occasionally the prescription has complications in power (or otherwise) which preclude the use of lens styles suggested above. Again the shape or location of the vocational field is such that a cemented segment offers the best solution to the problem. There is also the advantage of radical change in shape or position of segment when it is cemented. The major disadvantage of discoloration and loosening can now be overcome. After the exact power, size, and position have been found, the segment can be permanently cemented on with plastic cement. Bausch & Lomb Optical Company Plastic Cement and No. 7026 Cement made by B.B. Chemical Company, Cambridge, Massachusetts, will fix segments securely.

Berens* has had a unique multifocal made for his personal use with three different additions (Fig. 212c). The intermediate and reading portions are obtained from a conventional Panoptik trifocal. Below the reading area, a wafer has been cemented on the front surfaces of his lenses with +4.50D. addition combined with 1.5 Base In O.U. This segment is used for momentary use to view very small objects such as surgical needles at a fixation distance of about 22 cm (8.26 inches). Many professional men can advantageously wear such a segment for those objects that are

---

*Berens, C.: personal communication.

uncomfortably small for a regular reading distance and yet not small enough to justify the use of a loupe or other magnifier.

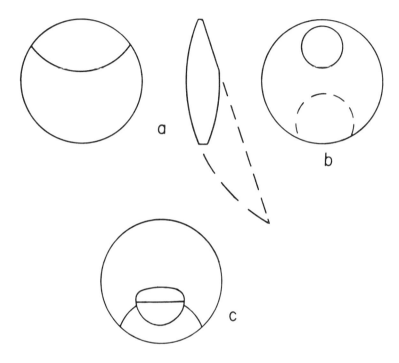

Figure 212. Unusual designs of multifocals for special purposes.

The classical case for a vocational segment in the upper part of a multifocal is the physician who wears a head mirror. A lens is frequently set in the head mirror aperture that gives comfortable vision at the working distance, but this is not always satisfactory because the other eye is not corrected and binocular vision is sacrificed. Cordes* has found that the only dependable means to fit this class of patients satisfactorily is to have them bring in their head mirrors or special equipment and while they are actually performing in the normal working position to mark the area for the segments on the distance lenses. Much like the marksman

---

*Cordes, F.L.: *Instruction Course.* Research Study Club, Los Angeles, January, 1950.

in Figure 226, the head may be turned sharply to one side or the other when it is tipped forward in the operating position.

To return to the case under discussion, when his accommodative amplitude has further diminished to the point that he requires +2.25D. to +2.50D. addition for his reading distance, a single segment in the lower portion of his visual field will be inadequate, as described on page 359. His major vocational activity is still at arm's length, but he must also be able to see critically in the normal reading field and continue to have clear vision at the special point above center. Now a vocational-type trifocal with about 50 percent of the reading addition in a wide intermediate segment and a small segment at the top will provide for his needs. At the intermediate distance, the field of view is about 13 × 44 cm (5 × 17 inches) when a vocational 8 mm Univis trifocal or 4 × 19 inches when Ful-Vue trifocal is used. The extrawide intermediate segment forces a lower reading field, but this patient will likely use the near-point prescription less than his working distance. The special segment at the top will be placed in the habitual position.

The first one-piece bifocal, which was called the Solid Upcurve Bifocal and patented in 1836, is still available as a lens to be used principally for near. It is the opposite effect of a conventional one-piece bifocal (Fig. 81). The segment is depressed and is actually a *subtraction* instead of *addition*. The present-day trade name of the lens is Rede-Rite®. It is limited in use because of the jump and displacement. As a rule it is seldom usable when the difference in powers exceeds 2.00D. It performs best with a weak plus or any minus prescription. If, however, the field of view required is very small and the depression can be centered on the lens as Figure 210, the displacement in the "window" is materially reduced.

The best lens for this type case is a flat-top bifocal style with a *minus* segment. These are available in Ful-Vue, Panoptik, and Univis lenses, and because the optical center of the segment is approximately at the same point through which the patient uses the window, no displacement is noticed. Although the angular subtense of the segment is small, the field of view through it is adequate. At a distance of only 3 meters, the segment of a Panoptik bifocal gives a field approximately 2.22 meters wide by 1.38 high (or 8 feet, 9 inches by 5 feet, 5 inches). Thus, the major portion of the lens for a cosmetician may be fitted for the working distance and the segment above center serve for clear vision when she looks in the wall mirror at the reflection of her client, reaches for her supplies, or greets a person across the room.

Loss of accommodative amplitude finally limits the use of minus segment (or reversed) bifocals for some purposes in much the same way as inverted bifocals. When the total reading addition has increased to $+2.25D.$, intermediate distance is badly blurred through the reading lens and the distance lens is deficient. The size of the field required for the greatest part of the vocational activity determines the power of the three segment areas that now become necessary. The old rule "percentage of area to percentage of use" prevails here. If the greatest need is the intermediate distance, a small concave window can be ground in the segment side of any bifocal to give the effect in Figure 212b. It has been made for a surgeon's use. The former distance portion of the lens becomes the working field with the addition set for his operating distance. The segment at the bottom is used to read charts or inspect small instruments. The small window at the top allows him to see across the operating room. The major part of the lens is the power of the intermediate prescription. The addition in the segment at the bottom is the difference between the intermediate and reading additions. The segment at the top is enough minus sphere to neutralize the intermediate addition.

TABLE XXX
ONE-PIECE BIFOCAL SEGMENT SIZES

		Wide	*High*
A. O. and B & L.	AA	38	30
Shuron Continental	AL	38	24
Robinson Houchin		38	24

The larger segment sizes of one-piece lens segments are really vocational lenses. In all cases, the top edge of the segment is fitted above the patient's horizon and the glasses are not primarily intended for regular use. They are really reading glasses with distance convenience. The one-piece lens does not perform as favorably as the minus segment fused type with some asymmetric prescriptions. A careful prescription analysis is recommended before these lens types are discussed with the patient. Although the fused lenses are slightly more expensive and more difficult to produce, still there are occasions when no other lens will perform as well.

Bifocals have been made for special near-point work as ear, nose, and throat work, with the segment almost squarely in the center of the lens. The segment also fills the aperture of the head mirror when it is in use. At other times the doctor may have distance vision on either side or below to see instruments at arm's length and may see across the room by dropping his head.

A simple modification of the prescription for any pair of bifocals can convert it into vocational glasses. Large numbers of professional persons who work indoors are often at the peak of their careers between the ages of 48 to 55. Through these years, the total reading addition ordinarily ranges from 1.50D. to 2.00D. Accommodative amplitude will not have reduced to the point that an intermediate prescription is imperative; however, a small plus sphere increase to the distance prescription will be readily acceptable. An addition of +0.50D. permits clear vision to a point slightly beyond 2 meters (79 inches) and reduces the accommodative effort at all points by a like amount. By way of example, during his office hours a dentist seldom has occasion to see beyond 2 meters, the focal length of +0.50D. His whole professional activity is within a small room and almost everything is within arm's reach. Therefore, for office use, the doctor may write his prescription:

        Distance: O.U. + 0.75 D.
                Add +1.50 for reading
        For Office Use: O.U. + 1.25 D.
                Add + 1.00 D for reading

Such treatment is really anticipating the benefits of trifocals. The size and position of the segments should be carefully considered. The precise posture and work area should be measured. Do not let the image distance of the dentist's mirror confuse the issue. The object (teeth) is not more than an inch from the reflecting surface. The new series of pages for Volume II of *Occupational and Other Visual Needs* helpfully gives specific suggestions of bifocals for each vocation.

RECUMBENT SPECTACLES

An interesting application of prisms is a device named recumbent spectacles. These are intended for reading or even viewing television while in bed. They have been simply constructed and must be worn over the appropriate prescription lenses (if any) for the distance of the object viewed. Different from the 45° prisms used in binoculars, the prism angles are 30°, 60°, 90°.

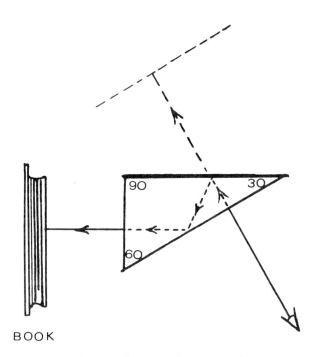

BOOK

Figure 213. Recumbent spectacles.

REVIEW

1. What is the rationale for emphasizing impact resistant lenses for all vocational lenses?

2. Why must a presbyopic dispenser wear double D lenses?

What are the disadvantages if he does not?

3. What are some other vocations that could be advantageously practiced with double D lenses?

4. Give a report on the fixation distances required by a housewife in her daily routine as illustrated by Clarke Holmes.

5. Select another vocation listed in *Occupational and Other Visual Needs* and list the working distances and a satisfactory bifocal.

Chapter 14

PROTECTION LENSES

◆◆◆◆◆◆◆◆◆◆◆◆◆◆◆◆◆◆◆◆◆◆◆◆ ◆◆ ◆◆◆◆◆◆◆◆◆◆◆◆◆◆◆◆◆◆◆◆◆◆◆◆◆

T here are two aspects to this subject. First, there is the matter of an ophthalmic product to protect the eye globe and its adnexa. Second, there is the production of filtering products to prevent the transmission of injurious light into the eye.

SAFETY LENSES

Thin glass in ordinary form is hazardous because if broken by a flying object or other means it may splinter and enter into the eye as well as injure the lids. Through the encouragement of the National Safety Council and the National Society for the Prevention of Blindness, safety glasses have been increasingly used in industry until now they are required by law. Over 50,000 confirmed accidents have occurred in which one or both safety glass lenses have been broken but the wearers' eyes have not been injured.

Development of Safety Glasses

In 1922, when American Optical Company decided to acquire optical wholesale companies and set up their own distributing organization, among firms they purchased was King Optical Company, Cleveland, Ohio. A large portion of Mr. Walter King's business was the sale of case-hardened 3 mm thick clear plano lenses in protective metal frames for the use of employees in hazardous work in the heavy industry plants in his area. To case-harden the lenses, the glass was heated almost to the point of softening, then the lens was placed between two jets of compressed air. The rapid cooling of the lens surfaces caused surface strain by compression. This special product intrigued A.O. Co. management. Mr. King was brought to Southbridge, Massachusetts, to head up a new safety glass department at the factory. This

471

was a new departure in merchandising because the product is not sold to the user. It is sold to the employer.

Legend has it that Mr. King wished to have a dramatic demonstration of the tempered lenses for corporate executives. It was important to develop a test that would regularly break an untreated lens but did not affect the case-hardened lens. A lightweight stand was made which had a ring at the base upon which the lens under test was placed. A small point of impact was desirable and the weight of the object should be consistent. A ball bearing was selected as the object. Successively larger balls were tried until one which fell one meter (40 inches) and broke a regular 3 mm lens but did not break the tempered lens completed the demonstration. This equipment was easily portable and the test could even be made on an executive's desk. The sales artifact was so successful that it was submitted to the Bureau of Standards to analyze and set standards.

Proof that the new safety glass department was not completely informed on the physical principles involved in case-hardened glass was demonstrated in 1927 when the sales department at the factory undertook to supply the new Armorplate® lenses in prescription glass form to the employees of Pullman Co. Thick semifinished cylinders were ground and case-hardened at the factory and distributed to company laboratories across the country to make 3 mm prescription lenses. No thought was apparently given to what would happen when the case-hardened back surface of the semifinished lens was ground away. Actually, such a lens is less impact resistant than an ordinary lens of equal thickness. The virtue of these weakened lenses was that when they broke, they crumbled into a myriad of small particles rather than splinters

In the process of producing these lenses, they spontaneously fractured at every step, including days after the lenses were edged and placed in the frame. No ill-effects or injuries were reported from these unprompted disintegrations. When the factory became aware of the misadventures, the branch office project was discontinued and the lenses were ground and, when completed, airtempered (case-hardened) at the factory.

It is almost amusing that over forty-five years later, the FDA representatives called a meeting of the optical trade and professions in Washington to discuss the spontaneous fracturing of dress prescription lenses. The same physical stresses of almost a half century before were manifesting in lenses made too thin or improperly heated or quenched. Again there was no report of serious eye damage. Practically all of this problem has disappeared with the advent of chemical tempering.

Chemical Tempering

The process of chemical tempering (strengthening) of glass, like many other developments, is a confluence of the work of many, and as usual, widely separated men. Charles Sheard, Ph.D., D.Sc., who was opticianry's greatest leader in education, had many interests. In 1913, he wrote an extensive paper for *The Philosophical Magazine* entitled "The ionization produced by heated salts." Thus he was discussing the principle by which lenses are now being chemically tempered.

Another of the earliest contributors (1920) was A. A. Griffith, a Briton, whose experiments showed that the fracturing of glass was caused by the spreading or opening of almost invisible flaws that opened as cracks under stress. Almost forty years later, Doctors H. P. Hood and D. Stooky of Corning Glass discovered the strength of glass could be increased by inducing an exchange of ions (chemical radicals) of glass which contained sodium or lithium. Some years later (1961), Doctor S. S. Kistler, at the University of Utah, brought the notion closer to fruition by discovering that the surface of alkali-containing glass can be "stuffed" with larger sized alkali ions to create the stress that squeezes the infinitesimal cracks which would, if unrestrained, cause fractures. This is accomplished by immersing lenses in potassium nitrate at 650° for 16 hours. Chemically tempered lenses are acceptable to FDA as impact resistant. Hence, all of the larger lens laboratories have chemical tempering units. The process is more time-consuming than air-tempering but causes much less spoilage in the process. The compression of the surface of the lenses squeezes the cracks or scratches together and inhibits cleavage (breakage). This reasoning is confirmed when a reduced impact is repeatedly applied to a lens (tempered or untempered). This was demonstrated by a motor-driven trip hammer using a small ballpeen hammer. This device was used to attract attention at National Society for the Prevention of Blindness displays. After hundreds of strikes, the glass suddenly crumbled.

Multiple impacts have been investigated on heat-treated and chemically tempered glass lenses and CR39 plastic. Expanding the discussion above, it is reasonable to feel the differences in response could easily have been a comparison of the number and depth of the microscopically small surface scratches on the lenses.

Recently the specifications of case-hardened lenses have been altered for lenses to be worn by the general public. These dress-hardened lenses are 2.2 mm minimum center thickness and are tested by a slightly smaller ball bearing.

Reinforced or laminated glass lenses are made for children or persons in hazardous pursuits. As in automobile glass, there is an insert of cellulose acetate between two thin lenses. These lenses can be obtained in green shade. This glass is somewhat perishable. It must not be heated beyond 140°F. Under any circumstances the cellulose becomes discolored after prolonged exposure to daylight. The torque exerted on the lenses in ordinary handling finally causes the laminations to loosen at the periphery. As is well known, it is a safe lens. Like an automobile windshield, it will not shatter or splinter. The performance of the glass is insured by Lloyds of London. Libby-Owens-Ford have greatly improved the original laminated automobile wind shields. Discoloration and separation have virtually disappeared.

Combined Optical Industries of Slough, England, offer uncut and finished spectacle lenses made of molded methyl-methacrylate called Igard® Safety Lenses. Their stock list includes powers to + 12.00D. and — 13.00D. in regular form lenses. Since these are pressed lenses, they are made of a thermoplastic. The material seems to be somewhat harder than Lucite or Plexiglas® but they can be scratched rather easily. By a later process these lenses have been produced with a harder surface coat which has increased their popularity. Coburn Industries, Inc., Muskogee, Oklahoma, now owns the company. The lenses are less than half the weight of crown glass (specific gravity crown glass 2.52; plastic, 1.18) and when fitted to a rimless mounting make a pair of very light weight spectacles. The lenses are practically unbreakable.

In 1947 a Pittsburg Plate Glass Company subsidiary, the Columbia Chemical Company, developed an allyl diglycol carbonate resin called CR39 which exceeds all other materials in impact resistance. This material was first made into safety lenses by Univis Lens Company but is now made in ophthalmic lenses by several leading lens manufacturers in the United States and Europe. It is available in single vision, bifocal, and trifocal lenses. It is particularly well received for cataract lenses and because of the molding process it can be supplied in aspheric lenses to reduce marginal aberrations. Since the material is only 40 percent the weight of glass, this contributes to its popularity for thick lenses. It is dyed with organic dyes to reduce visible light and contains a material to filter out ultraviolet in all lens forms.

The dramatic results in eye protection by the use of these products has stimulated most of the states to pass laws requiring protective lenses for all schoolchildren in laboratories and machine shops. After two states passed laws that all spectacle lenses must be made in some form of safety lens, on September 30, 1970, Commissioner of Food and Drugs, Charles C. Edwards, M.D., announced that the Food and Drugs Administration was acting to require that only impact-resistant lenses be used in all eyeglasses to protect the public from eye injuries.

From this investigation a regulation was adopted that required all prescription lenses made of glass to be 2.2 mm minimum center thickness and to be tempered and drop-ball tested. A few dispensing opticians led the way by heat-treating all of the glass lenses supplied for almost three years before the FDA regulations. The Guild of Prescription Opticians urged its members to join their Protective Eyewear Plan. The results of all these efforts have been uniformly excellent.

FILTER LENSES

The transmission characteristic of the materials from which prescription lenses are made is a part of the prescription. One absorption lens maker has aptly named the medium the "fourth component" of the prescription. From this point of view, an ophthalmic dispenser is exceeding his authority when he supplies any absorption lens without the doctor's knowledge and endorsement.

Control of the pupillary diameter and the volume of illumination entering the eyes are often important factors in the treatment and care of some eye conditions such as glaucoma and retinitis pigmentosa. In some instances the doctor may not have discussed or at least sufficiently impressed the patient with his desire that only clear lenses should be worn. Some types of lenticular opacities are least objectionable when the pupils are small. Such pathology may cause visual difficulties when the pupils dilate under reduced illumination through colored lenses. A treatment for glaucoma and some other diseases is a miotic—that is, a drug that contracts the pupil. Reduced illumination, and with it dilated pupils, may be injurious or even dangerous in some instances. It is therefore obvious that again we have reached a subject in which an ophthalmic dispenser does not take the initiative. For several reasons, however, it is important that he have some knowledge of the subject. A thorough discussion of it is beyond the limits of this book. Emsley and Swaine, Sheard, Duke-Elder, Verhoeff, Coblenz,* and others have investigated the subject from the physical, physiological, pathological, and even psychological effects of absorption glasses.

It must be remembered that the rate that light is absorbed is not in direct ratio to thickness. Twice as thick is far from twice as dark. In physics the logarithm of the opacity of a medium (the reciprocal of its transmission) is called the *density*. Table XXXI shows how density is related to transmission. Ophthalmic glasses are identified by the transmission at 2 mm thickness. The following formula shows how the transmission of a glass is altered

---

*Emsley, H.H., and Swaine, W.: *Ophthalmic Lenses*. London, Hatton Press, 1946, pp. 123-135.

Sheard, C.: *Ophthalmic Lenses*. Cleveland, Cleveland Pr, 1921.

Duke-Elder, Sir W.S.: *Recent Advances in Ophthalmology*. London, J. & A. Churchill, 1934, pp. 15-63.

Coblenz: *Technical Paper No. C421*. U S Bureau of Standards, Washington, D.C., 1938.

*Bausch & Lomb, Inc.: *Helpful Hints*. Rochester, NY, 1938.

TABLE XXXI

% Transmission*	Density	% Transmission*	Density
100	0.000	9.0	1.045
95	0.022	8.0	1.071
90	0.045	7.0	1.155
85	0.071	6.0	1.222
80	0.097	5.0	1.300
75	0.125	4.0	1.398
70	0.155	3.0	1.523
65	0.187	2.0	1.699
60	0.222	1.0	2.000
55	0.260		
50	0.300	0.9	2.045
45	0.347	0.8	2.071
40	0.398	0.7	2.155
35	0.456	0.6	2.222
30	0.523	0.5	2.300
25	0.602	0.4	2.398
20	0.699	0.3	2.523
15	0.823	0.2	2.699
10	1.000	0.1	3.000

*Precise extrapolation of transmission percentages can be made with a logarithm table.

by a change in thickness.

Density at the altered thickness (D_2) :

$$D_2 = \frac{(D_s - R) t_2}{s} + R$$

Where s = standard 2 mm thickness

t_2 = altered thickness

D_s = density of standard

D_2 = density of altered lens thickness

R = reflection factor for n = 1.523 glass = 0.038

t_2 = altered thickness

EXAMPLE: −6.50D. sph. made 0.6 mm center Ray-Ban® #3, which transmits 31% (density = 0.509). What is the transmission?

$$D_2 = \frac{(0.509 - 0.038) \times 0.6}{2.0} + .038 = 0.1763 = 66.1\%, \text{ about the}$$

transmission of Ray-Ban #1.

Colored Lenses

Color or filter glasses are referred to in the earliest writings on the subject of spectacles. As late as 1914, there were as many as ten shades for each color. Each optical firm attempted to become identified with a special color of glass for its lenses; this promoted a continuing search for a more popular color until most of the shades of the rainbow were represented. During these days, the color of the glass was chosen by the wearer with much the same attitude as the selection of the color of a plastic eyeframe.

The Glass Workers Cataract Committee of the Royal Society of London interested Sir William Crookes in the subject of an investigation of the effect of intense light from pots of molten glass upon the eyes of glass workers who develop glass workers cataract and to design appropriate filter glasses for their eye protection. At the end of four years work, 1909–1913, along with some dense sage-green lenses to be used near the furnaces in glass factories, he described some mildly tinted formulas for ophthalmic purposes. The metals used in this glass filtered out all the short wavelength (ultraviolet) light below 3600 Ångstrom Units, which is barely beyond the limit of visible violet in the spectrum. In its lightest shade the glass was rather violet-colored and transmitted almost as much visible light as clear crown glass in all colors except yellow. At this point in the spectrum it allowed only 70° of the light to pass. Opticians and lens factories were very enthusiastic about this glass because it had a scientific background, was well received by both the professions and the public, and was standardized. After World War I, this unpatented glass was poorly imitated by a large number of European glassmakers and the whole series of lenses went into disrepute.

A few years later, Soft-Lite Lens Co. offered a glass made by the Bausch & Lomb glass factory. Soft-Lite glass contained manganese, which reduces the transmission of visible light to about 88 percent at 2 mm thickness. This glass followed very closely the absorption line of regular crown glass in the short wavelengths. Therefore, the first formula of this glass was not like Sir William Crookes glass and other similar glasses which contain cerium—it did not filter ultraviolet light. American Optical Company developed Cruxite glass,* which absorbs the shorter wave-lengths of visible light and the longer wavelengths of ultraviolet. This glass, like Soft-Lite, has a pinkish color that easily dis-tinguishes it from bluish Crookes A. The new glasses are cos-metically more acceptable and, because they are produced to standard formulas, have regained the advantages originally con-templated with Crookes glass. The formula for Soft-Lite glass has been altered. It now contains cerium and performs like other filter glasses in the short wavelength area of the spectrum.

Several brownish shades of these two glasses were offered for use as sunglass lenses with more or less success. It was not until 1929 when American Optical Company offered a lighter shade of their ferrous iron-containing sage green industrial glass called Calobar that a definite universal acceptance was found. Bausch and Lomb offered a new development named Ray-Ban. These two glasses, which look somewhat like the glass named after Doctor Fieuzel, have been more widely used for prescription purposes than any dense glass ever produced. Characteristic of the filtering properties of a glass containing ferrous iron, infrared is largely absorbed, as well as ultraviolet, and the visible spec-trum has the greatest transmission at the point of greatest visi-bility—that is, yellow-green. Thus the lenses made from these glasses can be made dense enough to absorb a very large per-centage of the total light energy and still permit useful vision. The literature published by the Bureau of Standards as well as the reports of the manufacturers thoroughly discuss the subject and should be carefully read.

Among developments by the American Optical Company and Bausch and Lomb Optical Company is a uniform density blank, on one surface of which is welded a 1 mm layer of Calobar or Ray-Ban glass sufficiently dense in color to give the effect of a standard Calobar D or Ray Ban No. 3 lens 2 mm thick. This lens will be enthusiastically received by patients who wear strong prescriptions. Minus lenses can be made to not have the pale center and dense margin that have hitherto accented the refrac-

---

*The Physical Properties and Physiological Significance of Absorption Lenses. American Optical Company, 1935, pp. 12-17.

tive error. Dark Calobar and Ray Ban high-index glass has been developed for use in fused bifocals. The demarcation of bifocal segments in densely colored lenses has always been unsightly but heretofore there has been no solution to the problem. The segments in the new lenses are practically invisible from the front surface.

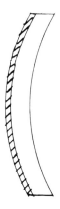

Figure 214.   Fused uniform density lens.

Absorptive glass makers regularly prepare transmission charts of their glasses showing the reduced transmission for denser shades. At the present time, two colors of glass for prescription use have virtually taken the United States market: gray and green. The variations in the transmission characteristics of these lenses from separate makers are trivial. Therefore one chart is adequate for all.

CR39 hard-resin lenses are dyed in organic dyes. Surprisingly, dyed lenses with colors very similar to the glass lenses have transmission curves for visible light that simulate the metal-produced colors in glass. A chart supplied by American Optical Company shows the curves for dyed lenses.

The present trend in young people's glasses is light pastel shades which probably have more aesthetic value than physical effect. Plastic lenses and plastic eyeframes have been dyed after assembled to match the color of clothing.

Thus it is observed that absorption glass is designed to dampen

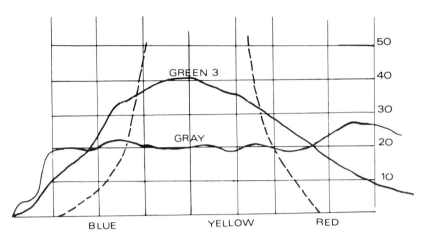

Figure 215. Transmission curves of dyed CR39 lenses.

the whole spectrum as equally as possible (gray glass) to uniformly reduce light intensity. Glass may also be made to selec-

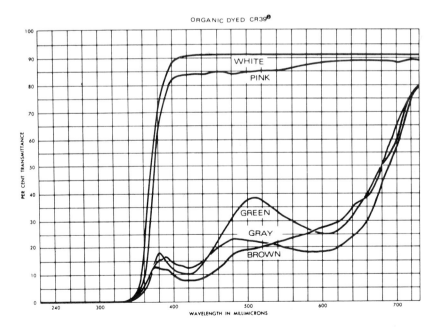

Figure 216. Transmission curves of colored glass lenses.

tively transmit the spectrum (green glass) and follow the relative visibility curve of the eye. Thereby a large percentage of the total spectrum is absorbed, but since the transmission of the glass "peaks" with the sensitivity curve, objects are comfortably visible in very little total transmission. For dazzling light on a snow surface (skiing), a glass that filters out blue and still provides the greatest possible contrast of other colors is required. A glass such as Cosmetan®, a brown glass is the most desirable.*

Glass colors seem to run in cycles. Seventy-five years ago London smoke was very popular. It was followed by blue lenses which were reputed to delay the formation of cataracts. Then Doctor Fieuzel's green glass and its competitors were most used. Crookes glass, a pale amethyst shade, plus two shades of a special gray for outdoor and beach wear caught the profession's and public's fancy for several years. It was followed by ferrous iron green for thirty years.

About 1960 there was a return to gray glass in two densities which has grown very popular. If the cycle continues to turn, pinkish or amethyst glass should return in a few years.

PHOTOCHROMIC GLASS

In the meantime Corning Glass Company has introduced a totally novel glass under the trade name of Photo Gray®. This glass contains silver halides that are affected by ultraviolet light and heat. This causes the glass to turn a mild shade of gray outdoors. Different from the ordinary photographic process involving silver, the process is reversible. When the lenses are brought indoors they begin to fade and shortly have very little color left in them.

The darkening of gelatin or other materials with exposure to light by the use of silver halides has been known and used in photography for more than a century, but to develop a reversal of the action has eluded all men until recent times when it was accomplished for ultraviolet light upon organic products, but this effect was relatively transitory. Doctor Armistead at Corning Glass produced reversible photochromatism in opal glass by the use of silver chloride in the 1940s but could not produce it in a

---

*Tillyer, E.W.: Personal communication, 1971.

clear glass base. In 1960, the project was given to Doctor Stookey who finally developed the right borosilicate glass which accomplished the purpose when some additional elements were added. We know his development is Photo Gray glass which bleaches to about 88° in average temperature and darkens to a little less than 50° transmittance in 77°F temperature after an hour. This reduction in transmission was not found to be adequate for sportsmen and others in very bright sunlight, so a darker shade was produced in the trade name of Photo Sun®, but this glass does not clear up as much indoors as Photo Gray. At first the glass would not tolerate the heat required to produce fused multifocals, but further research produced a new glass formula which was suitable for all of the fused multifocals, hence the service of the glass is complete.

To accommodate spectacle wearers in Europe and other places including (hopefully) the United States, a photochromic glass was developed by Corning named Photo Brown®. It did not become nearly as popular in this country as elsewhere.

Chance-Pilkington, England, has designed a glass from an altogether new formula in which the normal silica (sand) in crown glass is largely replaced by aluminum metaphosphate. This glass is softer than regular crown glass and requires some changes in the grinding and polishing procedures. It is made 2.4 mm thick. The glass is made in two formulas, one for chemical tempering and one for thermal hardening. It passes the FDA test for a $\frac{5}{8}$ inch ball at 50 inches and also of a $\frac{7}{8}$ inch ball at 50 inches. Its trade name is Reactolite® and is made in three density ranges 90° to 20°, 90° to 35°, and 80° to 20°. These glasses have not been introduced in United States as of spring 1978.

January, 1964, can be looked upon as a high point in the history of optical glass technology. It was the date of Corning's announcement of photochromic glass to the world! The transmission chart supplied by Corning Glass Company tells the story.

After a whole night in reduced illumination the glass transmits about 85 percent of visible light. This is slightly less than the transmission of Cruxite A® and slightly more than Cruxite AX®. After one hour in sunlight at 77°F, most of the visible spectrum is transmitted at about 45 percent. Temperature is a considerable factor in the fading or coloring cycles. The activity is more rapid at low temperatures. Because the photo-chromic effect is activated by ultraviolet light, the glass responds surprisingly well on overcast days when the illumination is still rich in ultraviolet.

PHOTOGRAY

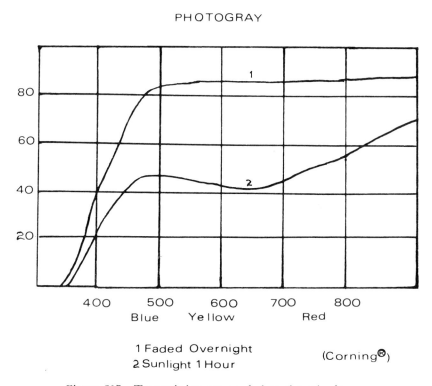

1 Faded Overnight
2 Sunlight 1 Hour

(Corning®)

Figure 217. Transmission curves of photochromic glass.

Photo Gray glass is presented to the purchaser as a "comfort glass." It is not a sunglass. It reduces light to about 45 percent, not 30 or 20 as many outdoor lenses. It cuts noonday sun to less than half its intensity and clears up close to normal for indoor wear. Its popularity is growing. Again too many in the professions and the trade are exceedingly cautious about instigating something new.

The first formula of the glass couldn't be heated to the degree necessary to make fused bifocals. One-piece bifocals are not acceptable by all. The time involved for the glass to make a complete reversal is unpleasant to some. Unlike Minerva, this new product was not born full-blown. When we think about it, the Wright Brothers plane did not have a jet engine. Even the early automobiles did not have air-conditioners, disc brakes, and self-starters.

Subsequently, a new photochromic glass has been developed for the manufacture of fused multifocals. The series now includes Photo Brown and Photo Blue.®

FRESNEL PRISMS AND LENSES

An innovation in lens making has been accomplished by Optical Science Group, Inc. (2201 Webster St., San Francisco, California 94115). They are producing a series of plastic Press-on Fresnel Prisms. These prisms relieve the patient of the unsightliness and weight of strong glass prisms, they have virtually no weight, they can be made adherent to most lens back curves, they can be removed with no injury to the prescription lens when they are no longer needed. They do reduce visual acuity a line or two, but distortion and chromatic aberration are at minimum.

The makers of these prisms propose to expand their product line and add Fresnel lenses in plastic. There seems to be no limit

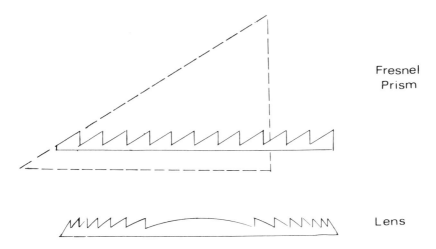

Figure 218. Cross sections of Fresnel prisms and lenses.

to the number of unusual lens systems that can be conjured by the use of these products. They have added a 5 inch +5.50D. reading glass and a series of strong plus lenses to be used as temporary lenses after cataract surgery. These press-on lenses can be applied to the patient's prescription glasses worn before surgery.

It is not trite to say that one who has lost the vision of one eye is more than half-blind. Although the records show that broken spectacles seldom cause the loss of eyes, patients with monocular vision should be routinely fitted with CR39 hard-resin lenses. This is required by law in California. The same law provides that all childrens' lenses must be CR39. These lenses are not only practically unbreakable but, further, are a protection against any flying object. The material is only 40 percent the weight of glass and the lenses can safely be made thinner than glass lenses. A child may scratch the lenses in his daily activities, but there is no fear that he will break his lenses, also the likelihood of any deformity to his nose is obliterated because of the decreased weight. Athletes and patients who require spectacles that are light in weight and free from breakage or fogging are also enthusiastic about these lenses.

REVIEW

1. Differentiate the two separate types of protection that may be implied.

2. "Hard hat area" is "safety glass area." What are the specifications of an industrial safety lens? In how many recorded eye accidents have safety lenses saved eyes?

3. Describe the procedure of case-hardening (heat-treating) a lens. What is the visual test?

4. Give the specifications of the drop ball test for industrial safety and dress safety.

5. Can CR39 be equally safe when compared with case-hardened glass?

6. What was Sir William Crookes' original research that lead to an ophthalmic glass?

7. Give the characteristics of the two most popularly used absorption glasses.

8. Which type of invisible rays receives the most attention in absorption glasses? What are the ill effects of these rays?

9. Although Photo Gray glass is more of a "comfort" glass than a protective, it should be discussed for its benefits. Make the statement you would make to a prospective wearer.

10. Why was Photo Sun glass developed?

Chapter 15

SUBNORMAL VISION LENSES

◆◆

To this point our whole consideration has been with eyes which were assumed to function properly when a satisfactory image fell upon the retina. We shall now inquire into the special case of those eyes which do have less than useful vision with a normal sized retinal image. Aside from an infrequent congenital deformity, these eyes are affected by disease. Logically they are the patients of ophthalmologists who are educated and licensed to do what is to be done to treat the disease. The technical project of selecting a magnifying device to increase image size comes into the sphere of optometrist or optician. But in both instances they are ancillary to the patient's physician who should constantly be informed of what is being done and how the patient is responding to the magnifier. In their enthusiasm over the rehabilitation to acuity some optometrists tend to forget to make sure that the patient is now (or is placed) in the care of an ophthalmologist for medical care concurrent with the fitting of visual aids.

Magnification of image size for distance vision is accomplished with a Gallilean telescope (opera glass or field glass). These devices can seldom be used by an ambulatory person. The magnification and reduction of field of view make motion dangerous. The magnification is usually $2\times$ to $2.5\times$ which means that objects are apparently half as far away. Approaching the object often is a more satisfactory solution. A small opera glass, monocular or binocular, in the pocket or purse which can be used momentarily then returned to the pocket is the safe procedure. The effect of a bifocal has been made by Keeler and Feinbloom with which the wearer has his best distance prescription in the center of a lens with a small telescope in the upper and/or lower margin which can be used by tipping the head. Field glasses on a headband for use at sporting events could also be used and then turned

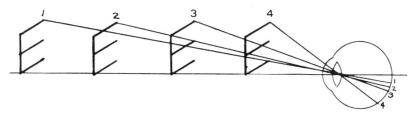

Figure 219. Image size differences caused by object distance.

up out of the visual field. None of these devices is a huge success because of the low magnification. Possibly a 6× would be the exception.

The greatest help for these unfortunate people is improvement of reading. Increased image size provides the help. This often repeated illustration (Fig. 220) in books on refraction is the key to the project.

This example is adapted from K.N. Ogle's book *Optics* (1968), reprinted courtesy of Charles C Thomas, Publisher. A page of

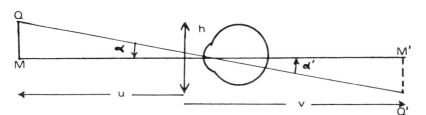

Figure 220. Lens magnification diagram.

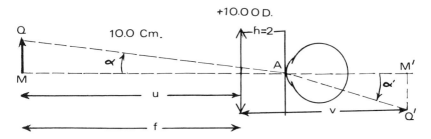

Figure 221. Lens power magnification. Modified from Ogle, K.N.: *Optics,* 1968. Courtesy of Charles C Thomas, Publisher, Springfield, Illinois.

print is held 40 cm (16 inches) from the eye. A +10.00D. lens is placed 2 cm from the eye. The print is moved toward the eye to the focal point of the lens (10 cm). How many times is the size of the print magnified?

1. Angular M (By lens power) $= \dfrac{I}{O} = \dfrac{\tan \alpha'}{\tan \alpha} = \dfrac{\dfrac{I}{v - h}}{\dfrac{O}{u + h}}$

Clearing fractions

$$M = \frac{I\,(u + h)}{O\,(v - h)}$$

Since $I/O = v/u$

$$M = \frac{v}{u} \times \frac{u + h}{v - h} = \frac{vu + vh}{vu - uh}$$

Multiplying by $\dfrac{1/uv}{1/uv}$

$$M = \frac{\dfrac{u}{u} + \dfrac{h}{u}}{\dfrac{v}{v} - \dfrac{h}{v}} = \frac{1 + \dfrac{h}{u}}{1 - \dfrac{h}{v}}$$

If vergences are used

$$\frac{1}{u} = U \text{ and } \frac{1}{v} = V$$

Remember

$$\frac{1}{v} + \frac{1}{u} = \frac{1}{f}$$

Since

$$\frac{1}{f \text{ (in meters)}} = D$$

Then $V + U = D$ and $V = D - U$

Therefore

$$M = \frac{1 + \dfrac{h}{u}}{1 - \dfrac{h}{v}} = \frac{1 + hU}{1 - h\,(D - U)}$$

But when the object is placed at the focal point, $D - U = O$

Then the denominator disappears and

Angular $M = 1 + hD = 1 + (.02 \times 10) = 1.2$

But magnification by a convex lens is a combination of the angular magnification and the increased image size of the object when it is brought from its original position to the focus of the lens.

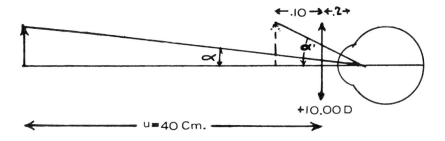

Figure 222. Position magnification.

2. Angular increase (magnification by position)

Original position of card at normal reading distance of 40 cm (16 inches) = .4 meter

f + h = 0.10 + 0.020 = 0.12 meter.

The increase in α' over α is the ratio of the original position to the new position

$$\left[\frac{p}{f + h}\right] = \frac{.40}{.10 + .02} = \frac{.40}{.12} = 3.33$$

But the whole magnification is:

Position Magnification times Lens Magnification.

Therefore

$$A = \left[\frac{p}{f + h}\right] (1 = hF)$$

Multiplying the first factor by F/F to eliminate 1/f

$$A = \left[\frac{pF}{1 + hF}\right] (1 + hF)$$

By cancellation

A = pF = .4 × 10 = 4

Since magnification is a comparison, it is always necessary to retain the reference distance. In this instance, 40 cm (16 inches) is a normal reading distance.

This may seem to have been a long way around to find that the magnification of an object held at the focal length of a lens is the dioptric power of the lens divided by the amount of accommodation in use for a normal reading distance. This could have been stated as a rule, but I feel that to learn, one must know "why." This little exercise may be reviewed if the rule becomes dim from lack of use.

Magnifiers are frequently identified by a reference distance used with microscopes. Since the average old style monocular microscope ocular was about 10 inches (25 cm) from a table and the microscopist copied the image of the slide on a paper on the table top, there followed a false notion that 25 cm was a comfortable reading distance! Hence u became .25 and M became $D \times .25$ or $D/4$.

Most magnifiers are rated by this formula. It actually underrates the dioptric powers or equivalent focal lengths of magnifiers.

OPTICAL AIDS (MAGNIFIERS)

It is preferable to identify all of these devices in terms of diopters, the standard unit in ophthalmic optics. A list in *Optical Aids for Low Acuity** ranges from 3.00D. for a hand-held reading glass to 100.00D. Volk Conoid Ophthalmic lens. These lenses are in three groups according to their support: (a) hand held, (b) stand supported, and (c) head held (in spectacle frame or headband).

1. 4.00D. to 6.00D. For visual acuity near 20/60 to about 20/120.
2. 6.50D. to 8.00D. In the range of 20/120 to 20/160.
3. 8.50D. to 10.00D. About 20/180 to about 20/200.
4. 10.00D. to 13.00D. About 20/200 to near 20/250.
5. 13.00D. to 20.00D. About 20/250 to near 20/400.
6. 25.00D. and stronger. About 20/400 to near 20/800.

These geometric estimations are beset with errors from the beginning, and the range of error expands with the increase in dioptric power.

The reasons for these discrepancies are legion. If the media are irregular, (e.g. keratoconus) or lack transparency (e.g. keratitis, partially developed cataracts), the image is always diffused and

---

*Stimson, R.L.: *Optical Aids for Low Acuity*. Los Angeles, Braille Institute of America, 1957, pp 21-26.

poor quality probably requiring a stronger lens. If, on the other hand, the impairment is at the retina, even a good optical image cannot provide a normal neural stimulation, and the requirement may be almost unpredictable. The most common retinal disease of elderly patients is macular degeneration in which small blind areas (scotomas) are spread irregularly in the area of the fovea centralis and/or whole macular and paramacular area. These patients sometimes may see only part of a word when they look directly at it, but highly motivated individuals learn to look slightly (two or three letters) in front of, behind, above, or below the word to patch together all of the letters. Another disease that produces somewhat similar effect is diabetic retinopathy. Retinal function is hindered by small hemorrhages. Too much magnification can sometimes interfere. Glaucoma reduces the size of the visual field and, in one stage of its development before direct vision has collapsed, the upper part of the visual field close to central vision becomes defective. Too much magnification may extend printed matter into this area of comparative blindness.

Adequate illumination is very important for most everyone with impaired vision. Use an adjustable fixture with a 100-watt lamp. The adjustable arm makes it possible to turn the light on the reading matter without glare.

A reading stand (easel) is a necessity because all magnifiers require the object to be parallel to the lens. The inclined stand allows the patient to assume a rather natural reading position and not have to try to look straight down to a table top. These two accessories are almost equal to the importance of the lens. They are actually analogous to the three legs of a tripod.

In my book I tried to design a specific test for patients with subnormal vision. It is useful in some ways but the best test cards are those designed by Louise Sloan, Ph.D., at Wilmer Institute, John Hopkins University, Baltimore. They are simple to use and consistently lead to the best lens or lenses for the patient.

The cards are sentences, not disconnected letters. The letters have fuzzy margins, similar to enlarged printing. The client's conduct and ability in reading the cards gives a foundation for what improvement can be made.

OUTLINE OF PROCEDURE

The record should of course start with patient's name and address, followed by the referring doctor's name and address. Space should be provided for the distance acuity of both eyes and the cause of impairment if doctor has provided these. This information is valuable in most instances.

Adjust the lamp and reading stand.

Put Doctor Sloan's largest size card: 10M—"It is very hot in the sun today" in top. Some workers start from the smallest. I like to start from success and work toward the threshold, like a Snellen Test Card. The M number of the card multiplied by 2.50, the reading distance being 40 cm, determines the approximate lens power required. Hence if the first card is all that can be read, the magnifier will likely be +25.00D. or somewhat stronger. Try a COIL Plasta Cataract Stand Reader (+20.00D.) for a start. Then go on to a Flash-O-Lens (5×), then a COIL Plasta High Power (+29.00D.) then a Flash-O-Lens (7×). All of these are stand-type readers. If the patient wishes to wear his lens like a spectacle, try a 6× (24.00D.) Ultex in a monocular fit-over over the patient's glasses or 6× Aolite Lenticular in a plastic frame. Draw to his attention that at first the lens was close to the reading matter but now he, like a watchmaker, must get close to his work. Beyond the power of the strongest Aolite Lenticular there are two more stand-type readers called Pre-Coptic, a #10 (approximately 40.00D.) and #20 (approximately 80.00D.). These are doublet lenses and produce a good flat field. They are regularly used by lithographers to inspect plates. They are compact, well built, and not too expensive.

Lower visual acuity than Sloan 10M is not usually going to be easily helped because the very short focal length requires such a short working distance and so few letters can be seen at a time. Keeler Optical Products, Ltd., (39 Wigmore Street, London W.1., England) has two United States offices, one near Philadelphia and another at Palos Verdes, California. They manufacture a number of magnifiers including 10× to 20× illuminated stand magnifiers which are cleverly lighted.

It is of primary importance to become informed about the

Large Type book program in progress. Obtain a sample of *Readers' Digest Large Type*, also a *National Aid to the Visually Handicapped* book (5967 West Third St., Los Angeles, California 90036). Call on your local library and let them tell and show you all that they have to help you. Obtain a free list of forty-eight publishers from Better Vision Institute (230 Park Avenue, New York, N.Y. 10017). Write National Accreditation Council (79 Madison Ave., New York, N.Y. 10016) for the booklet *Standards for Production of Reading Materials for the Blind and Visually Handicapped*. All of these publications are in 18-point type, almost twice the size of most book print (10-point). Therefore with almost twice the size of object it takes about half as much magnification (half as many diopters of lens power). There is a surprising variety of books, magazines, and even *The New York Times* ready and waiting for these unfortunates.

Continuing with the procedure, let the patient continue to read Doctor Sloan's cards until there is some hesitation. Record the M size and distance at which the last card was read. Multiply the M number to have an approximation of the first lens to use. If you have a copy of my "Aids" book, the page of reading types is convenient because the type sizes are identified: 9-point for newspapers, 10-point for books, 12-point for pica typewriter, and so on. The printing job and paper are also better than average. At about 5M the COIL Plasta Stand Readers 8D. and 12D. will be starters. They are very popular. Recently two COIL illuminated stand readers similar to the Flash-O-Lens have been offered. All of these products perform well because they have aspheric surfaces on their plastic lenses. The firm is now owned by Coburn Optical Industries, Inc. Distributing depots are being established.

An inventory to be able to enter into subnormal fitting might start with

3 or 4 B. & L. Hand Readers
    (Different styles and sizes)
COIL Plasta Stand Readers
    8.00, 12.00, 20.00, 29.00 Stand, with two or three hand readers with these lens powers
4 Flash-O-Lens
    2 each 5× and 7×
    Battery and electric

4 to 6 Ultex High Add
4× to top limit
ground with plano uppers mounted in monocular fitovers.
4 Aolite Lenticular microlenses fitted in pairs in plastic frames
3 Fonda half-eye Aolite Prism Base In Readers +6.00D., +8.00D. and +10.00D.
1 Aloe Loupe for Reading
(approximately 10.00D.)
2 Pre-Coptic 1/#10, 1/#20
Sample copies of
   Readers' Digest, Large type
   The New York Times, Large type
   National Aid to the Visually Handicapped book
   Your county library circulars about their catalogue of *Large Type Books*
   Anco #8 Reading Stand from The Lighthouse, New York Association for the Blind, New York, New York.
   Luxo Adjustable Reading Lamp
   Your local electrical fixture dealer.
3 Telesight Clip-on model 4D., 8D., and 12D.
   Telesight Co., 1646 Carroll St., Brooklyn 13, N.Y.
1 Opti Visor with 4, 6, 8 and 10D. Lens cells, Donegan Optical Company, Kansas City, Mo.

Make your records on $8\frac{1}{2}$ by 11 inch paper in duplicate. Send one copy to the referring doctor at once so he may know what has been done.

Thus far no reference has been made to telescopic spectacles. First, they do not provide any more lens power than is available with the simpler lenses described. Second, they are much more expensive than simpler lens systems. Third, the field of vision of all telescopic spectacles is very small. Fourth, they are a monocular device for reading. (Refer to the adjusting of surgical telescopic glasses in Chapter 16 on Miscellaneous Lenses.) Fifth, they have only one advantage, that is a longer working distance.

For example, 10.00D. required working distance, if worn as a spectacle, equals 4 inches; as a stand reader 4 to 12 inches; and as a telescope spectacle $2 \times \bar{c} + 5.00$ add $= 10.D = 8$ inch working distance. The cost is approximately ten times the cost of the magnifiers described. The Aloe Loupe is a production telescopic magnifier that costs the user about $20.00.

Waldemar Friang in Denmark, one of Europe's outstanding

low-vision experts, tries to routinely start with large type and a low-power magnifier, then gradually reduce type size and increase the power of the magnifier with the newspaper as his goal. This procedure may lead to the exchanging and crediting some magnifiers but it does have a good rationale.

Read the following articles:

Sloan and Habel: Reading aids for partially blind. *Am J Ophthalmol 42:863*, 1956.

Sloan and Jablonski: Reading aids for the partially blind. *Arch Ophthalmol (Chicago), 64:465*, 1959.

Sloan and Brown: Reading cards for selection of optical aids for the partially sighted. *Am J Ophthalmol, 55:1187*, 1963.

Fonda, G.: *Management of the Patient with Subnormal Vision*. St. Louis, Mosby, 1965.

Pameijer, J.K.: *An Investigation of Optical Corrections for Enabling Patients with Low Acuity to Read*. Antwerp, N.V. Vitgevers-Maatschappij Ae. E. Kluwer, 1959.

Keeler, C.H.: *Helping the Partially Sighted*. London, Keeler Optical Products, 39 Wigmore Street, 1958. Also contains excellent description of their products.

E. Faye, M.D., has recounted the procedures, aids used, and results at the Lighthouse, New York Association for the Blind, in New York.

It is most profitable to share the experiences of these specialists and glean answers to some of the problems that turn up.

Many firms feel that it is a good policy to permit customers to return a visual aid for full credit within ten days after purchase if it is in good condition. Doctors respond well to this liberal policy when they know that their patients will not be loaded with unusable merchandise. This return privilege does not extend to individually produced eyewear.

Frequently the magnifier does not work as well at home as it did on demonstration. Often the reason is inadequate light. It is well to emphasize the importance of light and be able to supply a Luxo Lamp (or similar) along with the magnifier.

As a parting thought, as long as a dispensing optician is ancillary to an ophthalmologist he should not arbitrarily decide to take care of only part of doctors' patients. Remember that the doctor has spent and continues to spend a large amount of his professional life caring for sick eyes that do not respond to ordinary prescription lenses. Publicize with each doctor that you are trying to assist him and *all* of his patients in any way that lenses in any form can help them.

REVIEW

1. Why is any form of a telescope disadvantageous for distance vision to an ambulatory person?

2. Assume an eye has 20/200 acuity for reading. About how much dioptric power would be needed to see 20/50 size letters? Show the means by which you reached your solution.

3. Name some of the diseases that affect central vision.

4. Name the three increments necessary to provide best visual care for impaired vision.

5. Book type (10-point) can be read with +30.00D. magnifier. About how much lens power would be required for Large Type (18-point) *Readers Digest?*

6. Why do COIL Plasta lenses diopter for diopter perform better than ordinary lenses?

Chapter 16

MISCELLANEOUS LENSES

◆◆

In other chapters, lenses have been considered at all times from the point of view of a therapeutic device to improve vision for some purpose. There are instances when a prescription may be written for a lens or lenses that are intended to reduce or obscure vision or the visual field. Such lenses are used for many pathological conditions including strabismus (crossed-eyes). They are sometimes used in orthoptic and fusion training.

In ophthalmic optics, formulas are derived which accurately analyze the effect of prescription lenses upon retinal image size. For the general case—unless the lenses are placed at an awkward distance (anterior focal plane) in front of the eyes, or are corrected by thickness, profile, and in some cases lenses separated by airspaces—convex lenses magnify the retinal image and concave lenses reduce the image size as described in Chapter 5. Doctors find that in the radically different lenses required for anisometropia or antimetropia, another factor (aside from the induced prism generated at extra-axial points) is the confusion produced by dissimilar retinal images. As we have seen, the function of binocular vision is disturbed by very small differences in image size and quite distressing effects are produced for many persons. Larger differences in the size of the images prevent them from being fused into single images. This leads to double vision (diplopia) and further confusion and discomfort.

A method commonly employed by doctors to avoid these complications is to disregard the wide variation in the two prescriptions and prescribe the correcting lens for one eye only. The acuity of the other eye is then reduced by a lens of such power that the retinal image for this eye is thoroughly blurred.

Stronger plus lenses or weaker concave lenses than the actual requirements are ordinarily used for this purpose to prevent over-stimulation of accommodation in the corrected eye.

On occasion, the patient's refractive error is such that a clear lens deliberately off focus still does not provide sufficient interference with vision. We have also seen that focus depth increases rapidly as retinal function decreases. Chavasse proposed an occluding lens that reduces the acuity of an emmetropic eye to about 20/200. Although the lens is apparently clear when it is in position on the wearer's face, the posterior surface has been made with a pebbled finish that interferes with image formation. This lens blank is made in this country by American Optical Company and Bausch & Lomb Optical Company. As a temporary measure, approximately the same effect can be accomplished by painting the back surface of the regular spectacle lens with clear quick-drying lacquer, such as nail polish. The obvious advantage of this approach is that it can be quickly done at home and when occlusion is no longer necessary, the lacquer can be removed with no ill effects to the lens or glasses.

In Table XXXII are given the light transmissions of various ordinary materials.

TABLE XXXII*

Clear glass	92 down
Ground or frosted glass	43 to 57
Light opal	47
Milk glass	5.5 to 7.4
Smoke glass	20 to 38
Paper, thin	17 to 40
Paper, oiled	10

*Nutting, P.G.: *Outline of Applied Optics.* Philadelphia, Blakiston, 1912, p. 164.

When, in the doctor's judgment, a denser surface is necessary, lenses are "frosted" by grinding the back surface with 180 to 220 grain abrasive. Objects are no longer discernible through such a lens, but there is enough transmission to provide the patient with an appreciation of light and dark or large moving objects. Thus the patient is not limited to the reduced visual field of monocular vision. A frosted plastic or glass lens in a fit-over frame is frequently used when the occluder is to be worn only part time, such as in direct sunlight. The fit-over is often made in a monocular frame.

The diffusion of light in all of these types is often annoying to some patients and finally, total occlusion may be prescribed for one eye. Complete binocular occlusion is ordinarily accomplished with bandages or a postsurgical mask. Black celluloid is most commonly used for monocular occluders. The area of the occluder is determined by the patient's needs. When the doctor wishes to interfere with binocular vision in merely the central part of the visual field, an occluder about the size of the patient's spectacle lens is adequate. Several types are available—an all plastic model that clips over the edge of the spectacle lens, a disc in a metal frame with spring clip to fasten either under or over the spectacle frame, and finally a disc of celluloid can be fitted in place of the spectacle lens in the patient's frame.

When the doctor wishes to prevent most of the light from entering the eye, a wing must extend back on the temporal side. The most successful device manufactured for this purpose, to the present time, is the Bel-occluder made by Watchemocket. It is made in two shapes and several sizes. It is easily attached to and removed from the patient's spectacles and the plastic margin can be reshaped when necessary by heating and bending or by cutting. This occluder can be removed from the metal rim and fitted to a regular plastic or metal spectacle frame.

A rubber model has been made with a suction cup to attach to the under side of the spectacle lens. In many instances the bulkiness of this device is too great for the distance between lens and eye. However, it is safe and because of its size little stray light can get to the eye. Some patients do not like to wear it because perspiration tends to collect under the rubber.

Several means of partial occlusion have been provided to prevent crossed-eyes from receiving images simultaneously. Vertical strips of adhesive tape 5 to 6 mm wide have been attached to the posterior surfaces of the patient's lenses in such a position that when one eye can see between the strips, the other pupil is covered. The strips must be set very accurately to be effective. The glasses must be kept in good adjustment after they are fixed or the angle will be altered. Again, the optical center fixation light and ink stick are helpful to establish the proper placement.

Plastic fit-overs with one-half frosted are sometimes prescribed for cases of squint. The frosted parts are placed on the nasal sides and when the child looks straight ahead with one eye, the turned eye is under the frosted area and therefore receives no clear image in the central field. A variation of this idea is to cut small apertures in the centers of a pair of frosted discs. The fixing eye can use the open space, but the turned eye will be under the frosted area. This type of fit-over is probably not a safe device for outdoor wear because of the serious limitations to the visual field.

On occasion some doctors prescribe a dense-colored lens for treatment of fusion. The dark glass (usually red) is placed before one eye to exaggerate the effect of double vision and, because of the difference in the apparent colors of all objects, to break a habit of suppression of vision in one eye. This procedure apparently has not been highly successful because it is infrequently prescribed.

Occluding devices are also used as means to limit the movement of the eyes. These glasses are called stenopeic glasses because of the narrow apertures. The progress in retinal detachment surgery has increased the use of pinhole glasses. Before surgery and for a considerable period of time after surgery, the patient may be ordered to keep his eyes quiet by the use of spectacles which completely cover the indirect visual field and have a small aperture in the center of the opaque disc.

The aperture is usually placed in the disc before the eye not under treatment. The pinhole should be slightly to the nasal side to let the patient hold his head in a natural position for vision at near-point. For the same reason, the aperture should be 3 or 4 mm below primary position.

Spectacle lenses are not ordinarily worn with these pinhole glasses, but it must be borne in mind that an aperture sufficiently large to allow adequate light to reach the eye is usually larger than the aperture for best results as a pinhole camera. According to the formula given by Abbe* the proper diameter of the aperture of this device is $d = k\sqrt{x}$, where d = the diameter of

---

*Southall, J.P.C.: *Mirrors, Prisms, Lenses.* New York, Macmillan, 1918, p. 5.

the aperture, $k = 0.1275$ (a constant) , and $x =$ the distance from the aperture to sensitive plate (retina) . When this formula is applied to the pinhole disc set at 11 mm in front of the cornea

$x = 25 + 11 = 36$ mm

that is, the length of the eye plus 11 mm

$d = .1275 \sqrt{36} = .7650$ mm

Most prescriptions are written for apertures of 2 to 3 mm and therefore permit the entrance of a larger pencil of light than axial rays. Vision is usually not as good in cases of higher ametropias as would be obtained with a standard trial-case pinhole. For the same reason, the apertures for binocular vision must be very carefully adjusted. The larger pinhole frequently causes the patient to be conscious of two apertures if the visual axes do not intersect the pinholes.

When pinhole goggles are custom made, a Bel-occluder may be fitted to a regular plastic or metal eyeframe. A lens may be set in the frame for the first adjustment and ink lines used to determine the precise position for the aperture. The countersink bit used by a carpenter to countersink a hole for a wood screw makes a fine taper reamer for the pinhole. Ream out the hole by spinning the bit in the fingertips on one side, then the other. The ridge of the aperture will then be midway between the surfaces and will continue to be precisely round. Thereafter the pinhole can be quickly and accurately increased in size as the doctor may prescribe. Pro-Optics, Inc. (Park Ridge, Illinois) makes a whole family of occluders and findings to prepare pinhole glasses. They save much time and produce a good fitting.

An adjustable stenopeic goggle made by Watchemocket for the Air Forces serves handily for some cases for which pinhole lenses are prescribed. The size and position as well as the separation of the apertures are adjustable within limits. This goggle is somewhat heavier than other types but stays in position nicely for bed patients.

ISEIKONIC SPECTACLES

The research at Dartmouth Eye Institute conducted by Ames, Gliddon, and Ogle, and others is probably one of the most extensive studies in physiological optics ever undertaken in this country. The investigation has been centered on the effect of dissimilar ocular images. A very complete literature is available and is worthy of some study.* An ophthalmic dispenser's experience with the lenses for the correction of aniseikonia is limited to the fitting and adjusting of them because they are all produced in the laboratories of the American Optical Company to the special prescriptions of those doctors who have the Ophthalmoeikonometer or other equipment required to make the necessary tests.

The differences in ocular images fall into two classes and their combinations: (a) overall difference in which those things seen by one eye seem to be larger in all directions than the same objects seen by the other eye and (b) meridional difference in which objects seem to be elongated in one meridian—that is, magnification is greater through one meridian than in the opposite. When the variations of a square object are studied in Figure 223 and all the combinations of these variations are contemplated, one realizes that the subject can become quite formidable.

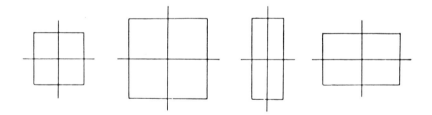

Figure 223. Four aniseikonic projections.

Correction of the condition is generally accomplished by magnification. In other words, the smaller image is increased to the size of the larger in the case of overall magnification. Meridional differences are corrected by using a meridional magnifying lens at

*Ames, A., Glidden, G.H., and Ogle, K.N.: Size and shape of ocular images. *Arch Ophthalmol (Chicago)*, 7:756, 1932; 7:720, 1932; 7:904, 1932.

Ames, A. and Ogle, K.N.: The horopter and corresponding retinal points. *Ann Dist Foundation Opt, 1*:35-45, 1932.

Ames, A., Ogle, K.N., and Glidden, G.H.: Corresponding retinal points, the horopter and size and shape of ocular images. *J Opt Soc Am, 22*:538-574, 575-632, 1932.

the opposite axis. The lens designer has three factors with which he can work to accomplish his purpose. These are lens profile, thickness, and vertex distance from the eye (see Chap. 5). The principal planes of a meniscus lens are in front of the lens; the deeper the curves of the lens, the farther the planes precede the lens. The formulas of ophthalmic optics show that the end result of the combination of one of these lenses with the eye produces magnification. As the lens thickness increases, magnification also increases. The lens position in front of the eye enters importantly into the calculation. Therefore an overall magnifying lens has a rather deep base curve and is much thicker than a standard lens (3 to 5 mm). A meridional lens looks like a bent lens, like a section of a piece of heavy glass tubing, because no magnification is desired through one meridian, Which is flat (or flatter than the opposite), and in the meridian at a right angle there is a strong curve. From the point of view of a lens maker, it is bitoric.

Available to each doctor who has the equipment to test for aneiseikonia there should be an optician available who is familiar with the special requirements of this type of lens fitting. The patients who wear these glasses are instructed to return to the same optician for servicing the glasses from time to time or are referred to other specialists in iseikonic lenses if they leave the community. All ophthalmic dispensers should be ready to assist these patients when it is inconvenient for them to return to their own opticians for servicing. The most common symptom of these patients is headache, usually of the migraine type. When the glasses are put into the proper adjustment, the immediate relief experienced by these patients is often phenomenal.

The same principles that guide an ophthalmic dispenser in the adjusting of all glasses naturally obtain in the case of iseikonic spectacles. The point of reference, however, is the eye-wire and not the posterior vertex of the lenses. The delicacy of fitting these lenses even in instances of little or no refractive power suggests a methodical routine for best results. The patient's prescription (without which little can be accomplished) shows the percent magnification and lens to eye distance. First take a regular lens measure and find the inside curves of the lenses across the horizontal meridian. Refer to a vertex chart such as the one on page 45 of *Ophthalmic Lenses* by Bausch & Lomb to find the depth of the lenses at the centers. By way of example, —7.25D. curve is 3.5 mm deep at 44 mm lens length. If the lenses are set in a plastic frame and the actual edge of the lens is obscured, one must estimate the overhang of the rim. Check the lenses with the prescription copy on a lensometer for cylinder axis. If the lenses are off axis and the tilt of the shape of the lens agrees with the error in axis, the lenses should be carefully corrected for axis without changing the measurements of the bridge or affecting the position of the pads. The lenses should then be dotted for the horizontal, the x-axis, or the Dispensometer used and placed on the patient's face. Let him put the glasses on his nose at the point where he regularly wears them. Correct the tilt of the 180° line to the point where the corneal reflections are aligned with the x-axis, by the necessary minor angling of the endpieces. It is very important to retain the present pantoscopic angle, which is frequently quite vertical. As has been previously shown (Chap. 5), lens power, marginal correction, and spatial projection can be materially affected by the inclination of lenses.

At this point the distance of the lens vertices from the eyes should be measured. If the inside curve of the lenses across the 180° line is found to be —7.25D., the lens length is 44 mm and the posterior edge of the rim of the plastic frame would be about 5 mm closer to the eye than the center of the lens. If the lenses are designed to be set at 12 mm, the edge of the rim should be 7 mm in front of the cornea. To make the measurement, have the patient look straight forward at some chosen point with the face-plane vertical in order to obtain primary fixation. Approach the patient from the side and, with one eye closed to remove parallax, move to the point where only the profile of the lens is seen. From this position find the distance from the back edge of the rim of the frame to the apparent vertex of the cornea. Repeat the measurement on the other side and note whether the average of the two measurements agrees with the prescribed distance. The Essel Corneal Reflection Pupillometer makes this measurement easily and is absolutely precise. If there is considerable difference, such as 2 mm or more, have a discussion about the glasses with the patient. It is significant to know whether the glasses were serviced by an experienced dispenser on the last occasion, whether they felt satisfactory after the last service, whether to the patient's knowledge the glasses have suffered a mishap to get them out of alignment, or whether they had seemed gradually to function less satisfactorily. This interrogation may seem rather lengthy, but it is wise to know everything possible about the case before making *any* changes in the position of the lenses.

Oftentimes, the original fitter may have found empirically that the lenses seemed to perform a little better at a slightly greater or lesser distance from the eyes than originally prescribed by the doctor. He may not have had the temerity to alter the doctor's prescription, as shown on the copy, so the accustomed position may be the position as measured. If a doubt exists, it would be better *not* to change the vertex distance, but to spend the entire effort on the alignment of the glasses. The cylinders (and with them the meridional correction, if any) must be set precisely at the right axis. Considerable care must be exercised to get the planes of the lenses perfectly straight in *all three dimensions* (x-, y- and z-axes) when the eyewear is on the patient's face. Finally check the vertex distances of the two lenses. Despite the fact that the glasses are not precisely in the prescribed plane, still the lenses must be absolutely equidistant from the eyes to the last half millimeter. Let the patient wear the glasses for a period of time, a day if possible, and if the adjustment is subjectively satisfactory, make no further alterations. When the patient is still not quite satisfied, it will then be time to reset the fitting cautiously (at least part if not all of the difference) toward the recorded vertex distance.

There hardly seems to be a limit to the sensitiveness of some of these patients to the proper adjustment of their glasses. A limit of tolerance of as little as a half millimeter is not unusual. Early in the use of iseikonic lenses, I had experience with an unusually critical case. When this patient's glasses were out of adjustment a tremor developed and she could subjectively describe the distortion of her visual field even to a central angle of as little as 20 arc degrees. On this patient's first calls there was considerable doubt as to whether she could sense the infinitesimal discrepancies that were found in the adjustment of the glasses.

For purposes of investigation, any measurable error that existed in the setting of the glasses was increased. If the right lens was 1 mm farther from the eye than the left, the adjustment was changed to set the lens 2 mm away. When the guard-arms had spread apart and the lenses were slightly closer to the eyes than prescribed, the lenses would be adjusted still closer to the eyes. On each occasion the patient emphatically denied any improvement with the "adjustment" although an attitude of great accuracy was assumed. On these occasions, when finally the glasses were set at the prescribed position, the tremor disappeared while the patient was still at the fitting table and an expression of relief came over her face. This was so predictable that it was demonstrated to numerous dispensers and a few doctors over a period of several years. In her early experience with iseikonic lenses, she would allow unknown dispensers to adjust her glasses if she had the misfortune to bend her frames out of line. Early the next day she would regularly return to have the spectacles serviced again. Each time, the new optician who worked on the glasses apparently felt that, because of the patient's great distress, a great amount of bending was necessary. After a few of these experiences in which it took much time to get the lenses back to their accustomed position after the vigorous efforts of others, it became necessary to tell the patient that unless she discontinued the practice of letting inexperienced persons handle her glasses no further work could be done for her.

This story has been told with only one purpose—to give the reason for the following advice. When servicing a pair of iseikonic spectacles, attempt to bring them back to the position from which they apparently have been bent. Do not attempt to improve the fitting by altering the temple angle or to raise or lower the glasses on the patient's face. Calculate the vertex depth from the position of the back edge of the rim and work with the temple spread until the lenses are precisely the *same* distance from the eyes. If the patient is to be seen regularly, make only one of the contemplated "improvements" at each call and keep a record of what has been done, so that the step can be retraced if it does not work.

BALANCING LENSES FOR UNILATERAL APHAKIA

A special case of dissimilar images is the instance of the correcting lens after cataract surgery on one eye and satisfactory vision with little or no refractive error in the unoperated eye. As seen in Table XXV, the correcting lens in combination with an eye from which the crystalline lens has been removed increases the size of the image about 25 percent. This image difference may vary from about 20 to 35 percent according to the patient's ametropia in the eye prior to surgery and the position and form of the correcting lens. In any event, the difference is intolerably great if both eyes are corrected to clear vision. A demonstration of the confusion, although somewhat exaggerated, can be observed if one tube of a low-power opera glass is held before one eye and an attempt is made to walk or see objects at a distance while effort is made to retain vision with both eyes.

Ordinarily a convex sphere approximately the power of the correction lens blurs the vision of the unoperated eye sufficiently to relieve confusion. Under certain circumstances due to the type of lens opacity and/or pupil size, the position of the blurred image takes on some importance. It is therefore not advisable to use a balancing lens in which the vertical center is very much above or below the correcting lens. The enlarged blurred image is somewhat the size of the enlarged clear image, hence vertical diplopia is possible. The classical instance is unilateral traumatic cataract when in the doctor's judgment the lens must be removed. To leave the eye uncorrected may not be satisfactory, but since the other eye is unaffected the unfusable images are intolerable.

Many different methods of balancing the retinal images have been used, several of which are scientifically correct but prove to be clinically impracticable. A contact lens moves the principal planes of the aphakic eye forward a smaller amount than a spectacle lens and the magnification is only 8 to 12 percent in most cases. Most patients obtain useful binocular vision without diplopia with a lenticular corneal contact lens. The normal field of vision is restored. Since the lens moves with the eye, there are none of the difficulties in the peripheral area of aphakic lenses.

The principal contraindication seems to be feebleness.

Experimentally the residual magnification has been neutralized by overcorrecting the lens and using a minus lens to cancel the artificial myopia. Such a course has had very limited success.

A special telescopic trial set has been developed by Austin Belgard in which small amounts of magnification are produced with two lenses after the formula of the Galilean telescope. The changes are at intervals of 5 percent $(0.05\times)$, so it is possible to balance the image sizes rather closely. In the end, the patient has the strong convex lens before the operated eye and a double lens cell before the unoperated eye to magnify all things to the size of the image produced by the cataract lens before the aphakic eye. In actual practice, this is not satisfactory for many patients because of the disturbance to visual projection, the prismatic error induced away from the lens centers, and the considerably reduced visual fields in both eyes. The House of Vision in Chicago has developed a unique solution to this problem. The lens is called Catmin, a contraction of "cataract minifying." The optical design is a Galilean telescope with the objective toward the eye, thus reducing the image size. Sufficient plus power is added to the power of the objective to correct the patient's aphakia. This lens is made of three glass lenses which are cemented together with Canada balsam cement. As shown in Figure 224, the front lens is a large minus lens, the planomeniscus which meets it at the periphery holding the correcting lens before the eye. Despite the small size of the ocular lens, it proves to be quite effective and gives a surprisingly large visual angle because it is set so close to the cornea (usually about 6 mm vertex distance). The only objection to this lens form from the patient is its cosmetic effect. The fact that it is cemented together also makes it rather fragile and it does require

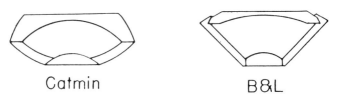

Catmin   B&L

Figure 224. Aphakia minifying lens.

frequent servicing, but it has proved to be the best approach of all. The patient's unoperated eye is not affected, and the vision of the operated eye is corrected and the image size with the prescription lens remains about the same as it had been prior to surgery.

Bausch & Lomb improved upon the idea by designing a combined plastic cell and glass lens that could be finished easily in any well-equipped laboratory. The new lens is lighter and when it is sealed does not collect moisture on its inner surfaces. It has been interesting to watch the growth in the use of this lens. On first sight, many doctors recoil from the glasses because of their appearance and some patients reluctantly accept them. But the performance of the lenses in selected cases has been quite convincing. A patient who has sufficiently reduced vision in the unoperated eye to justify correction of the aphakic eye and who is loath to be deprived of vision in the unoperated eye through the strong balancing lens usually becomes quite enthusiastic about the lens after wearing it for a few days. A few successful cases of this type often alter a doctor's original attitude. The lenses can be fitted with good results to many unilateral cases, but, like the fitting of all cataract lenses as discussed in Chapter 12, there must be a high degree of cooperation between doctor, patient, and dispenser if the best end results are to be obtained.

The problem of image size reduction may have another solution with plastic Fresnel lenses. With them a very thin wide angle

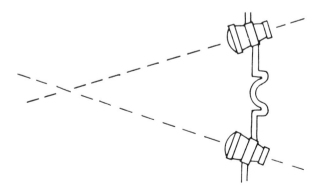

Figure 225. Surgical telescopic spectacles.

reversed Galilean telescope could be produced to balance image size in monocular aphakia.

TELESCOPIC SURGICAL SPECTACLES

First Carl Zeiss and now others have made telescopic magnifiers for surgery (Fig. 225). The lenses in these instruments are necessarily very small for two reasons: they must provide good optical performance without aberration and there must be a large unobstructed field surrounding the magnifiers. The very small field of the instrument, however, demands exceedingly careful adjustment of the spectacle frame.

The first consideration in the servicing of these glasses is whether the lens tubes are rotated on the x-axis, the 180° line, and properly converged on the y-axis as illustrated. In the sunlight or with a distant source of bright light, such as a projecto-chart, let the light enter the telescope through the oculars and form a point image at the working or focal distance in front of the telescopes. Measure the distance from the objective to the focal point. Slide the interocular adjustment in and out to find whether the focal points will superimpose. If one tube is rotated on the x-axis above the other and induces a false hypertropia, one image point will regularly stand above the other. The lens tubes must be aligned either in the framework or in the retaining rings. The spectacles will next be adjusted at the bridge to establish the desired setting for surgery. The oculars should be set far enough away to permit free use of the eyes below the telescopes but still within the exit-pupils of the lens systems.

When the vertex distance is established, the routine procedure for the measurement of optical centers is followed. The regular light-source for interocular distance measurement is held at the focal distance (vertex distance plus distance to focal point previously measured) of the magnifiers. The millimeter rule is held at the vertex distance of the oculars of the spectacle. The telescope is now adjusted to the separation as measured. A crossline drawn on a sheet of paper should now be held by the doctor at the point of clearest focus, while one side of the telescope is occluded. The position of the crossline should be adjusted to the point that places the intersection of the lines precisely in the center of the field of view. While the doctor holds his head and the crossline as steady as possible, move the cover to the other lens. If the separation of the tubes and their angle of convergence is correct, the crossline will be centered as before. If the crossline is not in proper position, either or both of two errors may exist. The ocular lenses may not be properly separated for the visual axes and/or the tubes may not be converged at the proper angle. If there is a question about the optical center separation, the measurement should be repeated. The light test is repeated now to find whether the images are superimposed. If they are crossed at the focal point, the convergence angle must be reduced. When the spots of light are sharply focussed before they come together, the angle should be increased. The adjustment by rotation on the y-axis to correct the convergence angle is necessary for all fittings when the doctor's eyes are separated more or less than average. It takes considerable patience of both doctor and dispenser to get these glasses properly set, but the satisfactory end result is easily worth the effort.

PTOSIS CRUTCHES

A dispensing optician is sometimes involved in the mechanical correction of blepharoptosis,* commonly referred to as ptosis. In this paralysis of the levator of the upper lid, the orbital fold disappears and the lid falls down to cover the eye when the head is in primary position. If the head is tipped back and the lower lid is dropped, the patient can see through the narrow slit between the lid margins. The slit can ordinarily be widened to some degree when the patient exerts the facial muscles to raise his eyebrows. A large number of these cases are corrected surgically. The ones referred to an optician are those that cannot be successfully repaired by surgery or those persons who refuse surgery.

The mechanical correction is obtained by creating a new orbital fold with a piece of wire or other material. The prosthesis for these cases is called ptosis crutch or crutch-glasses. The lid is raised by a semilunar loop of wire attached to the bridge of a

---

*Berens, C.: *The Eye and Its Diseases.* Philadelphia, Saunders, 1936, pp. 1058-1059.

frame or mounting. Many attempts have been made to manufacture an attachment for frames to accomplish this purpose but none has been universally applicable. There are wide variations in the requirements for individual cases that are dependent upon the thickness or bulk of the upper lid, the prominence of the eye globe, and upper margin of the orbit.

The simplest case is the middle-aged person with average prominence of eyes and brows. In these cases the lids are thin to flabby and do not require much support. A piece of solid gold wire (about the gauge and stiffness of a heavy weight wire temple) is bent to the shape of the upper part of the globe at the angle to crease the lid sufficiently to raise the lid margin above the center of the pupil in primary position. The patient's glasses are put in position and the bent wire is put behind the lens and pushed into place. The wire is marked for length, then soldered to the bridge. The outer end of the wire is not attached to the mounting. The resilience of the wire keeps the lid in place and permits the lid to move somewhat when the facial muscles lift the eyebrows.

Most lids require a greater support, which can be affected by a slight modification of the first device in which cases the wire is attached at both ends. It should be made of solid gold to withstand the chemical effect of perspiration. In this design the wire should be soft before fitting. The stiffness will be increased by the necessary plier work in the fitting process. With "S" bends at either end the adjustments are simplified.

Plastic frame makers have made a shelf-like attachment to be cemented to the back surface of the rim of the frame. They have not been widely successful because the pieces have required too much cutting and fitting to be comfortable and effective. It is often advantageous to have the support some distance below the rim of the lens. This adjustment is very difficult with a plastic support.

Occasionally a ptosis may be due to trauma and the area near the lid margin will not tolerate the pressure required for an orbital fold. In such a case the lid may be raised by exerting some pressure directly under the line of the brow. If, after some exploration with the fingertip, a spot is found that will give the desired result, the support can be effected by the pad and arm from a regular pad bridge. The arm is straightened out and soldered to the rim of the frame at the determined point with the length of the pad horizontal. The pad is improved if it is covered with a soft rubber Noscase.® The viscous material holds the lid more securely than plastic. The pressure can be precisely controlled by the size and placement of the pad.

Frames or mountings with lid crutches should be fitted with riding bow temples in all instances. The comfortable support of the lid is dependent upon a critical adjustment of the glasses. If the temples are not well locked into position the slight movement of the bridge destroys the effectiveness of the lid supports.

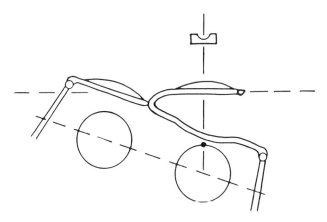

Figure 226. Fry's marksman's spectacles.

SHOOTING GLASSES

A rifleman's shooting posture requires him to drop his head and turn to the side. Expert marksmen who require distance glasses have often had difficulties. There are several contributing factors: (a) The top edge of the spectacle lens must extend above the eyebrow to keep the frame out of the line of sight. The vertex distance is thereby increased 5 to 10 mm. (b) The angle of depression is somewhat beyond the angle for which the spectacle lens is corrected. The pantoscopic angle often causes a tilted lens effect. (c) The supraversion combined with laevo-version (tertiary position) causes a sizable torsion as shown in Table VI. If the lens prescription has a cylindrical component, the axis will not be correct in this direction.

Mr. Max Frey of Lucerne, Switzerland, has devised a workable vocational spectacle (Frey-Schieszbrille) which has been successfully used by a number of international and Olympic champions. The rim of the right lens is attached to the left side of the bridge only to facilitate the necessary decentration of the right lens. As shown in Figure 226, the angle of the lens is adjustable. The temple on the right side is fastened to an endpiece connected to the bridge by the lower half of an eye wire. The marksman assumes his posture with his rifle and the angle of the right lens is adjusted to stand normal (perpendicular) to the fixation axis at the optical center. A knurled endpiece screw makes it easy to turn the lens in the rim or the eyewire can be bent to locate the best cylinder axis subjectively. Mr. Frey, who is an accomplished rifleman himself, finds that a test chart about 100 meters from an open window in his office makes the best test object.

LENSES FOR ARTIFICIAL EYES

Occasionally the appearance of an artificial eye can be improved by the optical effect of the spectacle lens in front of it. The magnifying effect of plus spheres, the minifying effect of minus spheres and the meridional effect of cylinders is useful to change the apparent aperture of the lids. Although the effect is calculable, an easier approach is to hold trial lenses before the eye until the best effect is produced. Oftentimes —3.00 $\times$ 180 reduces the stariness of a new fitting.

FRAME MODIFICATIONS FOR PATIENTS WITH SKIN DISEASED NOSES

Elsewhere a suggestion has been made to substitute a saddle bridge when the area under the pads is affected. In a large number of cases the problem is solved by the transference of the weight of the glasses from the sides to the crest of the nose. A solid gold 5 mm cylinder bridge provides a large contact area and can be shaped to fit the crest angle. Saddle bridge plastic frames are available on factory order in many frame styles.

On occasion the affected area is on one side of the nose and extends up toward the crest of the bridge. In this instance the pad may be retained on the opposite side. A new position of rest for the other pad can often be found in the area of the superciliary ridge at the nasal end of the eyebrow. The guard arm is straightened and reshaped to follow the rim of the lens. A Bausch & Lomb bridge is particularly adaptable because the pad can easily be attached from either side of the arm. One nasal contact point is now below and the other above the lines of the *fitting triangle* but a satisfactory adjustment can be maintained with riding bow temples on a face with average features.

Another approach becomes necessary when no weight can be borne by the nose. A metal frame can be fitted in an ideal case when the frontal bones are advantageously contoured and the tops of the ears are high enough to approximate a horizontal fitting triangle. The simplest case is the one on which a brow-bar from a pair of shooting goggles can be attached to the tops of the rims. A thin strip of "moleskin" padding attached to the acetate center of the arm will increase the adherence of the bar. When the central portion of the forehead will not accept the weight of the spectacles, the support can often be obtained in the areas directly over the eyebrows. A pair of guard arms, with the pads set horizontal, are welded to the back edges of the eyewires at the top. Jumbo pads or the long narrow Shuron pads are required to obtain a large area of contact. The soft rubber pad cover as suggested for the ptosis crutch helps to hold the frame in place. Riding bow temples are necessary to maintain the pressure against the brows.

A plastic frame can be comfortably rebuilt for all of these cases. A piece of clear plastic is shaped to the frontal bone and as far over the temples as may be necessary to hold the spectacles secure. A 150-weight frame should be used for the average case to withhold the weight. Cut a template from manila paper to the shape of the forehead and use this as a pattern for the plastic shield. Complete the fitting and shaping of the clear plastic piece before it is cemented to the spectacles. After the support is attached and the adjusting is perfected, a number of small perforations should be made near the contact edge to promote the circulation of air. A piece of soft rubber tubing like that used for temple covers is split and fitted on the contact edge to add to the comfort and stability of the glasses. Riding bow temples are essential.

REVIEW

1. Why are binocular pinhole lenses worn?

2. What is the best tool to enlarge a pinhole? Why is it more effective than a small rat-tail file?

3. What is the additional dimension that demands greatest precision in the fitting of iseikonic spectacles?

4. What lens applied to the operated eye satisfactorily reduces the aniseikonia induced by cataract surgery? Why is this possible?

5. Discuss the attempts to reduce the magnification of image in the operated eye. Why have these devices had only limited success?

6. How is sunlight used to approximate an adjustment of the telescopic tubes of surgical telescopic magnifying spectacles?

7. Describe the function and fitting of a ptosis crutch.

8. What is the intended accomplishment of Frey-Schieszbrille? Explain fully.

Chapter 17

EVALUATION OF GLASSES

◆◆◆

The analysis and evaluation of a spectacle lens or pair of glasses is no perfunctory task, nor with the assistance of present-day instrumentation is it particularly difficult. It is trite to remark one's judgment does not exceed his knowledge, hence a grasp of some information pertaining to optical lenses and their function with reference to the correction of ametropia is a prime requisite for the appraisal of a pair of spectacles. It is not to be construed that one must be an expert optical technician to be able to determine the quality or value of a pair of ophthalmic lenses. Truly, such ability is not a hindrance, but the inspector's object is to decide the applicability of the product in a particular case, not how to correct a shortcoming nor to know the reason for the dissatisfaction.

AMERICAN NATIONAL STANDARDS INSTITUTE, Z80

In 1963, a committee of all of the professions and functions of the ophthalmic community was formed to set standards for the quality and tolerances of lenses, frames, and sunglasses. The committee is chaired by Arthur Keeney, M.D., Professor of Ophthalmology, University of Louisville, Louisville Kentucky. The first set of standards was dated 1965. These were modified to meet product advances in 1972. The committee is nearing completion of a second revision of standards in 1978. The State of California has written the 1972 standards into a law on lens and frame quality control which went into effect on July 1, 1976.

Paralleling the establishment of tolerances, lensmeters which are a combination of a laser and computer have been produced to measure lenses by electronics and remove possible human error. The Acuity Systems Laboratory Model measures in units of 0.01D. and has an optional print-out of its findings. Thus the quality control of prescription lenses is making another break through.

A pair of spectacles fails in its intended performance unless it successfully passes two examinations. The first consideration is that as a discrete entity: "Are the lenses the power required to fill the prescription?" The second consideration is an evaluation of the *interpretation* of the prescription in which the question is "How do these glasses function—do they accomplish the expectations of the prescription for this patient?" These inspections are as separate and distinct as the methods by which they are made. The analysis of the glasses, as such, is an impersonal examination of the physical and mechanical accuracy of the lenses and frame. An equally important concept is that the prescription lens is about to become one lens in a system of lenses. The question then becomes (a) "How does a measurable deviation from the specifications for this lens affect the whole lens train?" (b) Is it not conceivable that the inspection equipment is able to find and isolate irrelevant imperfections? (c) Has the effort to produce a perfect physical entity obscured the purpose of the lens or the complete eyewear?

EXAMPLE:

 ℞   O.D. + 0.50D. Sph.
      O.S. + 0.50D. Sph.
      Interocular distance 64 mm

Inspection shows centers at 60 mm or centers at 68 mm. In either event, error is 4 mm.

$$0.50D. \times .4 = 0.2^{\Delta} \text{ Prism}$$

But +0.50D. lenses inhibit 0.50D. of accommodation which in the other side of the reflex inhibits 3^{Δ} of accommodative convergence and transfers of stimulation of 3^{Δ} convergence to Positive Fusion Convergence to maintain single binocular vision. The physiological, not physical, question is whether this further or less convergence of 0.2^{Δ} is significant to the function.

These remarks are not an effort to present an apology for inaccurate prescription work. The integrity of each craftsman should impel him to produce workmanship to the limit of the accuracy of his equipment. In the above instance, with meticulous care present-day centering and edge grinding equipment are capable of producing more accurately centered lenses. Surface grinding a pair of flat top lenses using standard 65 mm blanks, caliper grip points will reduce the separation to 62 mm. Half the prism effect on one lens $(0.1^\triangle)$ at 62 mm is a base-apex difference of 0.115 mm. Again, with rigorous attention to calipering, it could have been observed. The problem would have been how to successfully remove such a small error. The case for physical accuracy rests. Are the lenses functionally acceptable? Are some limits of tolerance unreasonably close?

At this point the judgment of an expert optician, not an instrument operator, is required. This is a point in quality control that requires knowledge and experience.

These questions could be accepted as the carping of a cynic or a plea for imperfect workmanship. They are neither. Limits of tolerance should be close enough to assure fine workmanship. The question is that, in the breech, "Should the deviation continue to be viewed only from the view of a physical entity or should it be considered also as a lens added to a system and then evaluated upon its contribution to the whole?" When the performance of the glasses is to be surveyed, they must be placed in position on the patient's face so that the locations of centers, reading portions, and position of the lenses can be considered. After the objective examination, the patient's subjective response and reactions also receive some attention.

Usually the effort required to prepare and fit a perfect pair of glasses is directly proportional to the refractive power of the lenses—that is, the more involved the refractive power, the more difficult the execution and fitting of the glasses. Conversely, a simple prescription, and there are many of them, is easily assayed. Nevertheless, authorities agree that no finished glasses should go unchecked. Thorington* well describes the doctor's risk when he says, "his painstaking efforts and best endeavors may be completely frustrated by poorly fitting glasses." An orderly and thorough seven-point analysis is outlined by him in a following paragraph. An ophthalmic dispenser likes to have his part of the transaction verified; when he has accomplished an unusually good

---

*Thorington, J.: *Methods of Refraction.* Philadelphia, Blakiston, 1947, p. 386.

result, he likes for the doctor to see the beneficial effect on the patient. When the patient seems somewhat unsure of the end results, after the inspection, his questions can often be answered only by the doctor.

The production of precisely made spectacles has been tremendously facilitated. The rapid advances in optical technology and laboratory apparatus are reflected in the uniformly high quality of the prescription work of those laboratories that hold their tolerances to the accuracies possible with present-day materials and equipment. New ophthalmic glasses, abrasives, and polishing materials contribute to better surfaces and lenses. As the professions have accepted and used the improved and "corrected" lenses offered by the several manufacturers, the research departments seem to have been stimulated to develop still finer and better products. Factory finished uncut lenses must pass rigid quality control standards. Semifinished lenses are compensated to provide accurate vertex refraction with standard dioptric curves on the laboratory-ground surfaces. Curve generators (diamond milling machines) and lap-truing machines replace the tedious trial-and-error methods in lens making. The almost universal use of instrument lens measuring devices replaces hand-neutralization and its inherent errors.

The advent of the laser-computer lensmeter which measures lenses to 0.01D. ($^1/_{12}$ the smallest lens unit) closes the gap on lens inaccuracies.

As shall be shown, discrepancies in lenses are measurable that may be imperceptible to a wearer's eyes with keenest vision. These conditions, however, are no argument for laxity. Actually, a laboratory's close attention to small details ordinarily discloses its attitude toward quality of workmanship and materials. However, the criterion of a pair of spectacles is utility. The most precise execution of a prescription written after a most meticulous examination is inconclusive. The desired performance of the glasses is still dependent to a large degree upon the interpretation of the prescription by the ophthalmic dispenser. This latter part of the evaluation of the glasses is made when the finished glasses are inspected on the wearer's face.

Accepted practice in measurements is to include plus or minus one-half of the unit of measurement within the measurement. In other words, if the unit is whole numbers, 3 is considered 3 after the midpoint between 2 and 3 has been passed and continues to be considered as 3 until the midpoint between 3 and 4 is exceeded. Or to say it another way, the measurement is considered 3 or 4, whichever is closer. When this reasoning is applied to ophthalmic products, the first consideration is the unit used in prescription writing and laboratory orders.

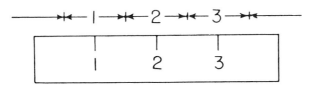

Figure 227. Tolerances in measurements.

The smallest unit of spherical or cylindrical power is 0.12D. Trial lens sets begin at 0.12D. and continue in steps of one-eighth diopter to not more than 2.00D. At that point, the unit becomes 0.25D. to not more than 5.00D. Beginning at 5.50D., a very complete trial set uses 0.50D. as the unit to 10.00D. Single diopters then become the unit to 16.00D., after which 18.00D. and 20.00D. are usually the final lenses. Refracting instruments such as the Greens' Refractor or Phoroptor are designed to increase or decrease 0.25D. to both limits of plus and minus. The changes in units in the trial set and the invariability of the refracting instrument do not hamper the doctor's choice of lenses. He may add fractional amounts of $\pm$0.12D. in the auxiliary disc of the instrument or trial lenses of less than 1.00D. to any lens power and thereby continue to measure as close as 0.12D. through the whole gamut. In practice, the unit tends to increase as the total power increases because the focal lengths of stronger lenses are so close to one another that small differences are not appreciable, as is suggested in Table XXXIII. The distance between the patient's far point and the focal plane of the prescription lens varies about 3 mm (a distance for which spectacle adjustment can compensate) in each instance, although the unit has been doubled in each grouping.

TABLE XXXIII

Diopters	Unit	Focal Length (mm)	Difference (mm)
6.00	0.12D.	166.7	
6.12		163.3	3.4
6.25		160.0	3.3
9.00	0.25D.	111.1	
9.25		108.1	3.0
9.50		105.3	2.8
14.00	0.50D.	71.43	
14.50		68.97	2.46
15.00		66.67	2.30
18.00	1.00D.	55.56	
19.00		52.63	2.93
20.00		50.00	2.63

Tillyer made use of this notion of tolerable error as a function of lens power in his application for the patient* on the series of marginally corrected lenses that bear his name. He said, "I have proceeded on a different principle by setting up a maximum astigmatic variation, less than the difference of proximate lenses of the series and less than will be *noticeable to the eye* (emphasis added) and introducing the variation into the lens to cut down the focal variation. . . ." Then he sets forth a table in which he shows the limits of marginal errors in which the tolerance is a function of the powers in the series. Parts of his chart are included for the sake of comparison with the tolerances of axial errors in Table XXXIV.

The protractors of some trial frames and instruments are divided into intervals of 1° of arc. Most refracting devices, however, are marked for intervals of 5°. Consistent with the comment above, if cylinder prescriptions are found at multiples of 5°, then ±2.5° is included with each measurement.

An outstanding ophthalmologist wrote many prescriptions for the midpoints between the 5° intervals. His explanation was that, on some occasions, at the conclusion of the subjective examination he rotated the cylinder equal distances in opposite directions from the assumed axis. If the blur (from the crossed-cylinder

---

*U.S. Patent No. 1,588,559.

TABLE XXXIV

		B & L	Shuron	A. O	V. A.	Tillyer
Power						
	0.00–2.00	±0.06	±0.06		±0.04	±0.06
	2.25–4.00	±0.06	±0.06		±0.04	±0.12
	4.25–6.00	±0.06	±0.12		±0.04	±0.12
	6.25–9.00	±0.12	±0.12		±0.06	±0.12
	9.25 and above	±0.08	±0.12		±0.12	±0.12
Cylinder axis						
	0.12–0.50	3°	2°		2.5°	
	0.62–0.75	2°	2°		2.5°	
	0.87–1.00	2°	2°		1°	
	1.00–2.00	1°	2°		1°	
	2.00 and above	1°	1°		1°	
Prism power						
	$0.5^\triangle$–$2.00^\triangle$	$0.00^\triangle$	$0.12^\triangle$			
	$2.50^\triangle$ and above	$0.12^\triangle$	$0.12^\triangle$			

effect) was equal, he felt sure that the axis was correct as it stood. However, if the blur was not balanced, the midpoint was not the correct axis. If after repeated tests he found that the patient was finally undecided, that 80° and 85° or that 75° and 90° seem equally blurred, he wrote his prescription for axis $82\frac{1}{2}$°. He anticipated the possibility of some error in the execution and fitting of his prescription and did not wish to prescribe an axis that was somewhat removed from the best position and risk a further difference in the completed spectacles.

Trial case prisms begin at $0.5^\triangle$ and therefore that amount is the smallest unit. On rare occasions a prescription for multiples of $0.25^\triangle$ may be written when a doctor wishes to divide the power of a prism equally between the two eyes (usually a vertical prism). For example, $1.5^\triangle$ may be divided:

O.D. $0.75^\triangle$ Base Down

O.S. $0.75^\triangle$ Base Up

A large number of refractionists would write this same prescription:

O.D. $1.00^\triangle$ Base Down

O.S. $0.50^\triangle$ Base Up

because a lens with the prism base at the top looks much thicker

TABLE XXXV

	Unit	Tolerance
Lens Power		
0.12– 4.00	0.12D.	±0.06
4.25–10.00	0.25D.	±0.12
10.50–20.00	0.50D.	±0.25
Cylinder Axis	5°	2.5°
Prism Power	0.5△	0.25△

than prism Base Down.

When these units are tabulated, the limits become those shown in Table XXXV.

Some of the larger lens manufacturers have prepared tables of tolerances that are about the same as the limits described above. The Veterans Administration has recently included tolerances in a bid for spectacles for the hospitals in which there are instances that the tolerances are closer than either those shown in Table XXXV or the suggested limits of the lens makers.

The most obvious and in many ways the easiest part of the inspection of a pair of glasses is the accuracy of the frame; however, it is usually better to start with the lenses and to use the landmarks established to assist in the observations. As paradoxical as it may seem, large errors are most easily overlooked. Reading lenses may be supplied instead of distance glasses, plus lenses instead of minus, lenses reversed eye for eye, cylinder axis off a right angle—that is, 90° —or prism bases reversed. Such mistakes can go through the hands of several persons when alertness fades. Therefore, the first act upon picking up a pair of glasses is to note whether the glasses are in the general class or category of the doctor's prescription. As described in Chapter 5, look through the lenses held about a foot away from the eyes to observe whether the lenses show "against" motion for plus or "with" motion for minus. If there is a conspicuous difference in the prescriptions of the two lenses, look for the increased sphere or cylinder effect, or the direction of axis. Learn to estimate the axis of a cylinder by looking at a straight line (door or window frame) through the lenses. Practice on rotating the lens slightly on its own center to see "against" or "with" motion that identifies plus or minus cylinder axis. The glasses are now identified to be in the general category of the prescribed lenses.

The next step is to inspect the glass for flaws and the surfaces of the lenses for imperfections, the quality of the bevel and shape of the lens, the size, shape, and dimensions of a multifocal segment. Now the lenses are ready for analysis on the lensometer. At this point, focal powers, axes, prism power, optical centers, and the x-axis of the glasses will be found. Plano lenses, including prisms, have been shown to have no point of reference. Planocylindrical lenses have a *line* of reference—that is, the axis. Only spherical and spherocylindrical lenses have *points* of reference (optical centers) that generate prism by decentration in all directions. For purposes of the location of the x-axis of the pair of glasses, it is necessary to select the proper lens to be measured first when the prescriptions for the two eyes are different. The following are rules (which will be discussed later) by which the first lens is chosen:

1. The stronger of two spheres or spherocylinders
2. The stronger of two planocylinders
3. A sphere or spherocylinder before a cylinder
4. Any lens with power before a plano lens

Place the glasses on the table of the lensometer with the back surfaces of the lenses toward the target. Adjust the table under the glasses until the blurred or focussed image of the target in the chosen lens is centered on the crosslines. This instruction assumes no prism is prescribed in this lens.

The instrument used to determine the focal power of lenses was designed by Abbe. The various applications of his idea have been described by H.F. Kurtz (1923).* In its particular form to measure ophthalmic lenses, it is called Lensometer (American Optical Company) and Vertometer (Bausch & Lomb Optical Company). Before the war (1939), Carl Zeiss distributed an instrument called Refractionometer.® The basic idea of these instruments is rather simple, as is seen in Figure 228. It is convenient to think of the target R as the retina of the eye and the

---

*Kurtz, H.F.: Ophthalmic lens measuring instruments. *J Optic Soc Am*, 7: 123, 1923.

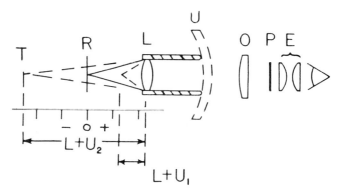

Figure 228. Optical design of Abbe's focimeter.

lens L (Standard Lens) as the optical system of the eye. Parallel
rays through the lens are in focus upon the "retina" R at the focal
length of the lens when the scale on the drum is set at "O."
Through a telescope consisting of objective lens O and eye lens
E focussed at infinity, an observer sees a magnified image of the
target. A protractor is placed at P, the focus of the telescopic
objective, which serves to maintain parallel rays entering the
telescope even if the observer's eye is uncorrected. For convenience, the illumination of the "eye" is reversed. Instead of light
being received on the "retina," a light source behind the target R
causes light to proceed from it and the observer sees an illuminated image.*

The eye lens E of the telescope is adjustable to compensate for
a user's uncorrected refractive error. The instrument must therefore be standardized for the eye of each person using it. When
several individuals use the apparatus, it should be checked by
each user before a measurement is made; or the instrument should
be adjusted to a fixed position and each person learn the necessary plus or minus allowance he must make for his own eye. A
common practice is the use of a colored dot or other mark on the
eyepiece to show the position of the setting.

---

*Waters, E.H.: *Ophthalmic Mechanics*, Vol. I. Ann Arbor, Mich, Edwards
Bros, 1947, pp. 99-101.

Emsley, H.H. and Swaine, W.: *Ophthalmic Lenses*. London, Hatton Press,
1946, pp. 182-185.

To adjust the telescope, set the dioptric drum at zero and un-screw or rack out the eye lens to extend it as far as possible. Look at the blurred image of the target and *slowly* move the eye lens toward the reticle. Stop the adjustment at the *first* point where the image is clear. If the focus is passed, lengthen the telescope again and refocus. To check the accuracy of the adjustment, turn the drum away from zero in either direction. Refocus the lensometer with the drum, and the image should clear up pre-cisely at the point marked zero. If the sharpest focus produces a reading on either side of 'zero, repeat the routine of telescope adjustment.

It was stated in Chapter 5 that when a lens is placed in the anterior focal plane of the eye the lens alters the direction of the rays but does not affect magnification. Hence the target is the same size for any lens power. Therefore, when an unknown oph-thalmic lens is placed against the support in position U (the pri-mary focus of lens L), the instrument is out of focus to the extent of the dioptric power of the lens at the pole (vertex) against the support. If the back focal length of the spectacle lens is behind the target (convex or plus lens), the total optical power $(L + U_1)$ is greater and the target must be moved closer to the lens L. It becomes easy to remember when either of two points of view is taken—(a) a convex lens gives a clear image to a short (hyper-metropic) eye or (b) a short eye has its far-point behind it in the position of the focal point of the convex lens.

Conversely, a concave lens with its primary focal point in front of the "eye"—that is, on the observers' side—reduces the total dioptric power $(L + U_2)$ and the target R must be racked away from lens L to point T. This simulates the elongated eye of myopia. (The effect of a schematic eye and the correction of ametropia as provided by a lensometer can prove to be a very valuable means of demonstrating and studying the effects of lenses. The same formulas used in physiological optics with appropriate changes for the constants can be used throughout.)

An astigmatic lens has two focal lines, and therefore the target R cannot be imaged in both meridians simultaneously. At the focus of each line, the target image is clear in one meridian while the detail of the image at a right angle is badly blurred. When the image is cleared at the axis perpendicular to the first line, the condition is reversed. The algebraic difference of the settings for the opposite axes is the power of the cylinder.

EXAMPLE:

+1.00 and +1.75 indicates 0.75D. cylinder
− 8.75 and − 6.00 indicates 2.75D. cylinder
− 1.25 and +0.75 indicates 2.00D. cylinder

Some differences are found in the designs of the targets R and the protractors and reticles as prepared by the different manufacturers. The instruction manual for each instrument is invaluable if one wishes to avail himself of all the optical and mechanical advantages of the apparatus. However, since their optical designs are essentially the same, some general rules apply to all of them.

When a lens is to be analyzed, either of two conditions exists. Its power is unknown and all particulars must be found, or the lens is expected to have a certain power to fill a known prescription. In the second instance, the undertaking can be quite simple. The easiest measurement is a spherical lens. The drum is set at the prescribed power, the back surface of the lens is placed against the nose in front of the standard, and the table is adjusted to place the image in the center of the reticle. If the target is in sharp focus in all meridians and cannot be improved, the vertex power of the lens is correct. A spherocylindrical lens requires a second setting of the drum and a setting of the protractor. The routine may well be to set the protractor at the prescribed axis, set the drum for either meridian power of the lens, then view the image of the target. To check the accuracy of the axis, the protractor is rotated slightly to note whether the alignment of the target improves with a change of position. No improvement indicates the axis is correct. A cautious movement of the drum to increase and decrease the prescribed power verifies the lens power and, after a similar inspection of the power of the opposite meridian, the power and axis of the lens is known. After a last critical view to set the image of the target in the center ring of the protractor, the lens marking device is used. One dot is on the pole and the others describe the x-axis of the lens. The order in which the meridians of the lens are measured may be affected by the way the prescription is written and/or the habits of use established by the examiner.

A universal procedure that allays confusion will now be described. Many inspectors approach all lenses as if they are completely unknown and thereby hope to avoid errors from presumptions. This routine can be used for all lens prescriptions. It shows all cylinders to have a minus sign:

1. Rotate the drum to a generous overcorrection of plus (or too little minus) and reduce to the point where the image of the target begins to clear up. If the image is not distorted and is equally clear in all meridians, slowly proceed to the sharpest focus of the target. The lens is a sphere and the drum indicates the power and sign. Adjust the lens on the table, if necessary, to center the target in the protractor and apply the ink-marking device.

2. If the blurred image is elongated or distorted, rotate the protractor to align the lines of the target in one meridian.

3. Proceed to reduce the power to obtain a sharply focussed image. Move the lens, if necessary, to center up the target on the protractor.

4. Record the first setting. It is the sphere. The meridian in which the lines are clear is the axis of the minus cylinder.

5. Continue to turn the drum from the original position and stop at the sharpest focus of the image in the opposite meridian. The difference between the settings is the power of the minus cylinder.

6. Readjust the position of the lens on the table, if necessary, to center the image in the protractor and dot the center with the inking device.

EXAMPLE:

First setting: +4.75 165°, second setting +3.00
℞: +4.75 −1.75 axis 165.

First setting: − 0.50 50°, second setting −1.12
℞: − 0.50 −0.62 axis 50.

First setting: +0.75 75°, second setting −1.75
℞: +0.75 −2.50 axis 75.

Sometimes a prescription with a very strong cylinder at an oblique axis or a crossed-cylinder at any axis produces an elongated image difficult to place in the center of the protractor. In such instances, set the instrument at the midpoint between the focal lines and center the blurred circle. This point is quickly found by racking the instrument until the target is clear in one direction and, after noting the reading on the drum, racking it until the target is clearest in the opposite meridian.

EXAMPLE:

(1) +0.50, (2) +3.50, set at +2.00
(1) +4.00, (2) −1.00, set at +1.50
(1) −1.00, (2) −2.00, set at −1.50
(1) +1.25, (2) −1.75, set at −0.25

The point at which the instrument is set in all these cases is the circle of least confusion in the interval of Sturm.* The spherical power at the midpoint is also the *spherical equivalent* of the spherocylinder. This approach is often much more satisfactory than the attempt to estimate the center from the positions of the focal lines alternately seen at right angles to one another.

A precise measurement for cylinder axis is often very difficult for weak cylinders even on the most sensitive lensometers. Choose two or more lines in the target and observe them closely while the protractor is turned 10° or 15°. Visual acuity is very keen in checking alignment of broken lines. When the lines seem to be continuous, read the protractor, then rotate it 10° or 15° in the opposite direction and repeat. With cylinder prescriptions as low as 0.12D. or 0.25D., it may be difficult to find precisely the same measurement repeatedly. When it is difficult to be discriminating under the high magnification of the lensometer, one realizes the difficulty the doctor has had determining his findings and that it was equally difficult for him to get the patient to give him con-

*Southall, J.P.C.: *Mirrors, Prisms, Lenses.* New York, Macmillan, 1918, pp. 310-314.

Laurance, L.: *General and Practical Optics.* London, School of Optics, 1920, pp. 107-109.

Cowan, A.: *Ophthalmic Optics.* Philadelphia, F.A. Davis, 1927, pp. 106-108.

Fincham, W.H.A.: *Optics.* London, Hatton Press, 1942, pp. 138-140.

sistent reports. In other words, tolerances are widest in low lens powers. When the cylinder power is greater, the axis measurement is easier to make and the effect of smaller discrepancies on the patient's acuity is more emphatic. Therefore these lenses must be precisely set in the frame.

When the first lens has been verified and ink-marked, the glasses should be released and the other lens slid into place *without changing the level* of the table. If the lenses are centered correctly, in the vertical meridian, the target should be neither above nor below the center ring when the image is centered laterally. Any vertical prism is visible at once. The sphere, cylinder, and axis of the second lens are measured and compared with the prescription. When the verification is finished, the lens is ink-marked. This completes the use of the lensometer on a pair of single vision lenses without prism.

The reticles of all lensometers are designed to measure small amounts of prism direct. A decentered lens or a lens made with prism prescription displaces the target image toward the base of the prism. For example, if the base-apex line of the prism is lateral (Base In or Base Out) the target is displaced along the 180 line. A compound prism in a lens displaces the target laterally and up or down as the case may be. The prism power may be interpreted as two prisms with their bases in the conventional directions of the x-axes and y-axes or it may be termed a simple prism with the base at a diagonal axis.

Usually the pattern of the reticle is a pair of crossed lines and a series of concentric circles which are spaced to measure prism power in units of $0.5^{\triangle}$ to a maximum of 3 or $4^{\triangle}$. When the prism power of a lens exceeds that amount, an auxiliary trial case prism must be placed in front of the telescope objective to neutralize the deviation a sufficient amount for the light rays from the target to reach the reticle. It will be noted that this trial case prism is set in the direction of *neutralization*—that is, the base is set in the direction opposite to the base of the prism in the lens being analyzed.

A large amount of prism in a lens causes some chromatic aberration which blurs the image of the target in the direction of the base-apex line of the prism. Some instruments have colored targets or fields which tend to filter out the color fringes. A strong prism aso generates some astigmatism in the direction of the base-apex which increases rapidly in meniscus-formed lenses. The cylindrical lens effect from this astigmatism in some instances is sufficient to distort the lens prescription as described next. For the purposes of measurement, these effects can be materially reduced with a neutralizing prism.

It will be remembered that rules were given concerning which lens of a pair must be measured first. If this precaution is not taken, erroneous conclusions are drawn when the lens prescriptions are dissimilar.

EXAMPLE:

$\text{\Bitalic R}$: O.D. + 0.50D.

O.S. + 2.00D.

If the optical center of the right lens is 5 mm below the geometrical center of the lens and the stronger left lens has its optical center at the geometrical center of the lens, two totally different measurements would be made, depending upon which lens is verified first. When the target is centered in the protractor for the right lens, the glasses are analyzed with position "a" as the assumed x-axis, the center of the +2.00D. sphere is 5 mm above that line and the prescription would therefore be measured +2.00D. 1$^\triangle$ Base Up Left Eye. If the left lens is measured first, the true geometric center of the lenses becomes the line of reference, the x-axis. Then the right lens center is 5 mm too low and this decentration produces (.5 $\times$ .5) 0.25$^\triangle$ Base Down Right Eye, which in ordinary circumstances is inconsiderable for a case of this type. Surely this is not a perfect lens, but the error to be considered is 0.25$^\triangle$ and not 1.0$^\triangle$. Further, at a point about 1.25 mm above the geometric centers of the lenses there is approximately 0.25$^\triangle$ Base Down in both lenses. At this particular point, the vertical disparity totally disappears.

In this same vein, it is apparent that a cylindrical lens axis 90 shows no prism effect at any point from top to bottom of lens. If it is paired with a spherical or spherocylindrical lens, a situation is produced similar to the one described.

The protractor on the reticle in the instrument is marked to indicate Prism Diopters in all directions from center. When prism is prescribed in the first lens of a pair to be inspected, the table is adjusted to set the focussed target at the prescribed amount of prism before applying the ink marks; then when the glasses are moved to analyze the second lens, the focussed target should appear at the prescribed point in the field. When the amount of prism exceeds the range of the reticle, supplementary trial case prisms are added.

A pair of unknown lenses may require closer study. The center of the stronger lens is still used as the point of reference. Therefore, it may be necessary to put new ink dots on the lenses if the weaker lens is inadvertently measured first. As was shown in Figure 228, the lens formula can be altered materially when the line of reference is changed. Therefore some judgment is required occasionally to decide whether the position of the lens centers is dictated by the prescription as written or may be the result of haphazard execution. In many cases, however, the findings have notable importance. It must not be forgotten that the patient has worn the lenses and may be habituated to the effect.

When the optical axis of a meniscus lens is not coincident with the optical axis of the lensometer or a patient's fixation axis, some astigmatic and, on occasion, focal error is introduced. As can be seen in Figure 229, a meniscus prism, with or without lens power, is a segment of a larger lens. It demonstrates all the characteristics of the extra-axial point it represents. Aside from the anticipated chromatic aberration, measurable cylinder with the axis perpendicular to the base apex line is found. Like the effect of a tilted lens, the effective prescription is altered materially if the direc-

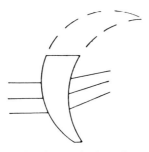

Figure 229. Meniscus prism is marginal section of a large meniscus lens.

tion of the distortion and the prescribed cylinder axis do not correspond. This effect is most conspicuous in prescriptions of this order:

℞: $+0.25 +0.50 \times 135 \bigcirc 5^{\triangle}$ Base Up

Since the prism is Base Up, one meridian of the astigmatism generated by the prism will be 180°. Thus there are crossed-cylinder (135 and 180). This will change the cylinder power and axis of the curves ground on the lens. Many surface-grinders have been severely criticized by an unthinking inspector for this lens effect. To be absolutely precise the astigmatic effect should be combined with the prescription power and compensation made in advance. The only means to estimate the effect of the prism is to neutralize it with a meniscus prism of equal power.

A lensometer is designed to measure the back focal length of a lens, which, by definition, is the distance at which parallel rays come to a focus. In the special case of a lens to be used for near-point, diverging (not parallel) rays strike the prescription lens. It will be shown that in this instance the front focus is the desired measurement. For example, presbyopia makes it necessary that some additional spherical power be added to the distance prescription. Then, as shown in Figure 230, rays of light diverge from the focal point of the reading addition to become parallel before entering the distance lens. Except in the case of a pair of "fit-over" reading lenses, this is not actually seen. In fact, the refraction for the reading prescription probably was done with a single lens representing the total power of distance and reading spheres. In any event the power of the examining lenses was referred to the back surface, therefore the effect of the prescription lens is substantially the same if the profiles of the two lenses are similar. If the front surface of the prescription lens has a greater convexity than the examining lens, the front focus produces somewhat less power than is anticipated.

EXAMPLE:

℞   +2.50D. sphere for distance
      +2.50D. add for reading.

The present-day precision trial lens +5.00D. is approximately a planoconvex and 2 mm in center thickness. A best form pre-

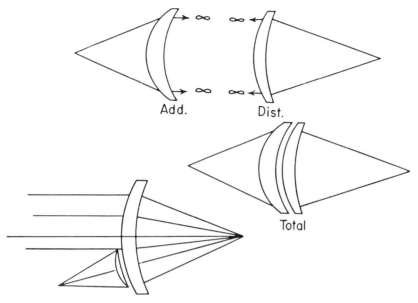

Figure 230. Optical analysis of multifocal lens.

scription lens could have +11.50D. outside curve and be 4 mm thick. The inside curve is then −6.87D. The formula for vertex power is

$$D_v = \frac{1}{\dfrac{1}{D_1} - \dfrac{t}{n}} + D_2$$

When the fixation point is 40 cm the light rays strike the front surface with a −2.50D. wave front, therefore the dioptric value of the refracted rays as they leave the surface is as if the curve were +9.00D.

$$+11.50 - 2.50 = +9.00$$

The value of the lens now becomes

$$D_v = \frac{1}{\dfrac{1}{9.00} - \dfrac{.004}{1.523}} + (-6.87)$$

$$= \frac{1}{.111 - .003} - 6.87 = \frac{1}{.108} - 6.87$$

$$= 9.259 - 6.87 = +2.39D.$$

Therefore, when the lens is used as a reading lens, the power at the back surface is effectively 0.12D. weaker than the distance prescription. In other words, the deeper meniscus lens causes the effective addition to be reduced to +2.37D. instead of +2.50D. Since the difference between the front focus (D_f) and back-focus (D_v) is a function of the convexity of the front surface and thickness of the lens, the comparison is more easily made on the lensometer than by computation. It is apparent at once that the difference is greater with an old style trial set in which all lens curves are flatter.

In the case of reading lenses the front focal power (neutralizing power) often more nearly represents the effects of the lens before the patient's eyes than the back focus (D_v). A close approximation of the difference in lens effectivity can be made by reversing the lens in the lensometer. When the concave surface is turned toward the observer the lens measures +4.88D. instead of +5.00D.

Multifocals represent a special case. In the first place, the powers of the upper and lower portions can be measured separately and thus give an opportunity for comparison which is not possible with a single vision reading lens. This comparison is frequently difficult because of the induced prism and distortion at a distance from the optical axis of the distance portion (Fig. 231). Further, the best forms of fused segments are for front focus measurement and are consistenly off power for those who attempt to measure the back focus of the near-point field.

The proper routine is to:

1. Measure the distance portion of the multifocal with the back

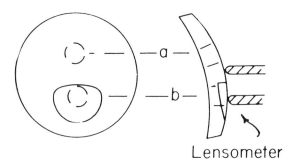

Lensometer

Figure 231. Finding front vertex dioptric power of multifocal lens.

surface of the lens against the nose of the instrument as usual.

2. Reverse the lens and find the distance power in one meridian. Now center the near-vision point of the reading segment in the instrument and measure the same meridian again. The difference in these two readings is the power of the addition.

3. When the power of the distance portion of the lens exceeds 1.00D., measure a corresponding point (Fig. 231*a*) above the optical axis and compare this reading with (Fig. 231*b*) the reading portion. By this method the same amount of prism and aberration is induced in each measurement.

As the power of the distance portion increases, the image in the lensometer becomes so badly displaced and degenerated that the test loses all semblance of a precise measurement. At this point it becomes necessary to use auxiliary neutralizing lenses specially prepared for the purpose. They are planoconvex and concave lenses 42 mm round with 1 mm plastic washers 30 mm in diameter on both sides (Fig. 232). These lenses are plus and minus 4.00D., 6.00D., 8.00D., 10.00D., and 12.00D. They are placed in position in the lensometer with the lens under test in such position as to neutralize the effect of prism and power. Because of the fact that the lenses are separate, the positions of the centers can be adjusted to offset decentration completely. By this means, the same accuracy of measurement is restored to the margins of strong lenses as is possible with weaker prescriptions. The washers are thick enough to allow for 3.00D. difference in curvature between the surfaces in apposition.

These neutralizing lenses serve another important service. The

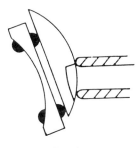

Figure 232. Means to remove prism in segment area of multifocal for aphakia.

marginal aberrations of strong lenses obscure poor optical surfaces and degenerations of curvature from regrinding lenses or excessive polishing. One of the lenses in the set will provide curves that approximate curves of the lens to be inspected and will also reduce the dioptric power of most lenses to such a point that aberration can be easily found by moving the lenses across a straight line, as described in Chapter 5.

At the same time a pair of glasses is looked through for the purpose of classification, an inspector learns to make some other observations. As the lens is moved to and fro to see either a "with" or "against" movement, some notion of the quality of the surfaces of the lenses can be ascertained. The tube of the Lensometer is not more than 6 mm in diameter and therefore it accounts for a very small percentage of the total lens area.

Surface inspection outside an optical laboratory is often quite difficult. It takes considerable time for a person to train his eyes to "see" the quality of the polish of a lens surface, but an observing individual can learn to see an equally important and more frequent defect after a little practice. When a weak spherical lens is held up about a foot in front of the eye in line with a distant straight line such as a door or window frame, and the lens is slowly moved from right to left, the line will move regularly with or against the movement of the lens, as described in Chapter 5. The line may be magnified or reduced somewhat, but it will continue to be straight as the lens is moved. If a cylindrical or spherocylindrical lens is tested, it is necessary to rotate the lens to the position that puts the axis of the lens in the direction of the line.

A lens with a wavy or aberrated surface will cause some distortion to the line. After trial case lenses have been tried and the

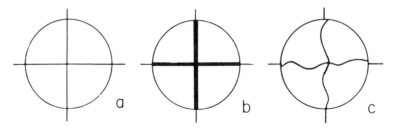

Figure 233. Surface condition inspected by lensometer.

idea of *regularity* of movement is established, a poor quality "novelty store" sunglass should be compared. This defect is usually caused by overpolishing a lens to remove a scratch or surface flaw and is found most frequently on strong convex surfaces —that is, curves of +9.00D. or greater. A cylinder surface is more likely to have an aberration than a sphere. A poorly equipped laboratory where a mechanical lap-cutter is not available may have produced the lens and the surface grinder may have had difficulty cutting the curves on the grinding lap. Aberration of lens curvature that invades the central area of a lens prevents a sharp, crisp focussing of the target of the lensometer. The lens performs like a soiled or badly scratched lens surface. Neutralization of the suspected lens with trial lenses is the critical test for surface irregularities.

LASER LENS METER
Another Breakthrough

The measurement of the dioptric power of lenses is gradually moving into a *new era*. The element of personal opinion in a measurement which has its base in a visual image is ending. A laser-computer measurement obtained by an interrupted laser beam and reported by a minicomputer relieves the former personal element completely. These instruments are available to measure in units of 0.01D., 0.12D., or 0.25D.

The Lens meter is representative of the new instruments. It measures sphere, cylinder, axis, optical axis (center), and prism. It has a dotting device and is available with a print-out.

Surface irregularity (aberration) is automatically printed below the power finding. The absence of "wave" is the assurance that the lens has good surfaces.

Like the expense of an instrument (Vertometer) to replace cost-free hand neutralization, there is also hesitance in some places to invest more than nine-thousand dollars for an instrument of the new era. (1) When laboratories change their production procedure to measure all lenses, that is, uncut lenses and surface ground lenses before they are processed, and (2) when the print-out is placed in the job tray and continues with the order to the one who dispenses the eyewear, there is no reason for further (Lensometer) measure-

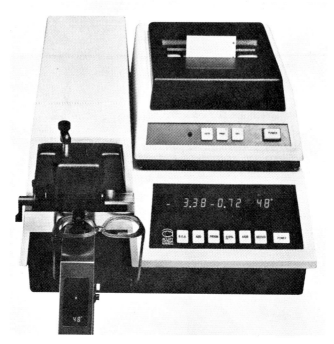

Figure 234. Acuity systems Lensometer with print-out tape.

ments for lens power. The print-out assures each inspector, at any point, the exact power of the lenses. The technicians' time saved, the material cost, and the time spent on incorrect lenses more than pays for the instrument in a reasonably short time. Basic to the whole new step is that it does not require the time of the highest paid technician to precisely operate the instrument. Test lenses are available to provide for a daily calibration. The print-out is evidence in a question on product liability.

At the same time the lenses are cleaned to be measured, it is good practice to check the surfaces of a new pair of lenses for scratches or imperfections. Present-day laboratory and manufacturing control and inspection methods practically preclude the possibility of a defective lens blank or marred surface; however, one more inspection added to the hundreds before is never amiss.

The surfaces of a lens are a conscientious lens grinder's pride.

As an artisan, his accomplishment is the regularity and quality of his lens surfaces. Well-trained, highly skilled technicians, combined with a firm whose business policy is best quality and a willingness to take the material and labor losses of defective and below standard lenses, are a doctor's insurance that his prescriptions will receive the proper care. If an optician undertakes to extract an unfair profit or make enticements with prices, slovenliness in the surface quality of his lenses is one of the greatest "economies" he can effect to support such a practice.

The material loss in the manufacture of ophthalmic lenses is startling. Sterling* made a careful analysis of the loss (or shrinkage) in a pot of glass from the time it left the furnace until it had finally been made into the three most common lens forms. His investigations showed that an almost unbelieveably small percentage (Table XXXVI) of the original batch passed the many inspections and manufacturing processes to finished spectacle lenses. When one realizes the costly materials and equipment and the days of skilled labor, consumed not only on the completed lenses but also those discarded at the many inspections, it is remarkable indeed that lenses of present-day quality can be supplied at a price even near their present cost.

TABLE XXXVI

AMOUNT OF POT OF OPTICAL GLASS IN FINISHED LENSES

(600 pound melt of glass)

	Pounds	%
Regular single vision	52.6	8.8
Fused bifocal	30.0	5:0
Ultex "B" one-piece bifocals	12.0	2.0

REGROUND SURFACES

A common cause of poor lens surfaces is a practice of regrinding lens surfaces to change lens power after the lens has been cut to size. The grinding method for ophthalmic lenses is one that will not produce a good curve to the edge of the lens. The felt or cloth polishing pad is slightly deformed by the pressure of the lens

---

*Sterling, S.: How many lenses in a pot of glass? *Bausch & Lomb Magazine, VIII(3):4-5*, 1931.

against it and thus it rounds off the glass (or as an optician says, "rolls" the edge of the lens). Because of the mechanical support and motion, this action is more severe on convex curves. Regrinding is somewhat less injurious to weak concave curves. In regular procedure, the lens blank is from 4 to 12 mm wider in diameter than the finished lens. The distorted margin is cut away when the lens is reduced to shape. If for any reason the lens is reground after it has been finished, the aberrated curve now extends out toward the optical center and no matter what the quality of the lens at the outset, it is now second quality. A well-trained surface grinder can see the distortion in the curve of a lens by reflected light. It goes without saying that a geometric variation great enough to be seen by such inspection is a much greater amount than can be considered tolerable for ophthalmic purposes.

Regrinding of lenses is a very useful method to make small changes in lens prescriptions for temporary or transitional use. Oftentimes the doctor may wish to make an alteration to a prescription to observe its physiological effect or the functional effect on acuity, then from his findings be ready to write a permanent prescription. Some pathological conditions such as diabetes may show rapid change or vacillation and, again, the doctor may wish to approximate an average correction until the eyes tend to stabilize. Such cases are often cared for as in the Provisional Plan after cataract surgery.

It is seldom advisable to regrind the surfaces of lenses for mars or scratches. Lenses are usually ground as thin as is permitted when they are first produced. Minimum edge thickness of lenses

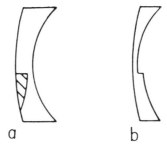

a   b

Figure 235. Cross sections of lenses demonstrating minimum center thickness.

is also controlled by FDA regulations and ANSI-Z80 tolerances.

Some stock must be removed to grind to the bottom of the deepest scratch. Even under magnification it is often difficult to estimate the depth of a fine diamond-like cut. If the thickness of the lens must be reduced too much, the lens is hazardous and violates FDA regulations. The anterior surface most frequently has the abrasions. This surface is more difficult to regrind and accomplish the desired result. Fused bifocal segments are on the front surface and cannot be reworked without changing the size and position of the reading segment. Lenses with weak reading additions may have the segment completely ground away before the scratches are removed. It is the practice of good optical laboratories to make their decisions with reference to reworking the power or surfaces of lenses *before* they are reduced to size and thus avoid compromising the quality of their workmanship. Case-hardened (heat-treated) lenses cannot be reground. When the tempered surface on one side has been reduced in thickness or ground off, the lens is structurally weaker than an untreated lens. It is then hazardous.

The thickness of lenses is controlled as far as possible to provide an edge thickness of 2 mm for all lenses. The edge thickness of all strong concave lenses is controlled by the lens power. The minimum center thickness for eye safety is 2.2 mm. Strong convex lenses to be mounted in plastic rims may be less thick, when weight is a factor. Fused multifocals must be made thick enough to cover the imbedded reading portion. As the power in the addition increases, the lens must be made thicker. A relief to this problem in minus prescriptions is the use of one-piece glass or CR39 (hard resin) lenses.

HILITE GLASS

Schott Optical Glass Company (Duryea, Pennsylvania) has recently made a high index, low density glass to replace the use of flint glass. Lead is replaced by titanium and other chemicals to produce a glass that compares favorably with crown for hardness. Because of the shallower curves, some concave lenses are actually lighter in weight than the same power made of crown glass.

The unsightly concentric rings at the margins of all concave lenses are now effaced in plastic frames by an improved bevel design (hide-a-bevel) and edge coloring (Mayo Rim). These lenses in a plastic frame seem to have edges as thin as ordinary lenses. Sepaniac has proposed to use a rimless-edged lens in a metal frame by grooving or notching the edge of the lens for lenses over —8.00D. He puts an old style zylo rim in the groove to fit the lens to a plastic frame.

Table XXXVII is a condensed manufacturer's thickness chart for standard size spherical lenses. Single vision lenses are held to a tolerance of +0.2 mm from these thicknesses. The table does not refer to bifocal or prism prescriptions.

TABLE XXXVII

Power	Center (mm)	Power	Center (mm)
+1.00D.	2.2	—1.00D.	2.2
+2.00	2.5	—2.00	2.2
+3.00	2.9	—3.00	2.2
+4.00	3.4	—4.00	2.2
+5.00	3.9	—5.00	2.2
+6.00	4.4	—6.00	2.2

To this point in the evaluation of the glasses, the entire consideration has been to inquire into the precision with which the lens prescription has been filled; or, if the glasses are unknown, to learn the characteristics, including the power, of the lenses. Scant mention has been made of the frame. It is assumed that it is properly aligned and holds the lenses true in all three dimensions (x, y, and z). The investigation of how well it performs its other task of supporting the lenses in the proper position is ascertained when the finished eyewear is fitted on the wearer.

For proper placement of the lenses on the z-axis of the eyes, the lenses must be set 1 mm below the line of primary fixation for each 2° of lens tilt. Therefore the average position of the lens centers should be 4 mm below the centers of the pupils when the eyes are in primary position for the average 8° angle.

Oftentimes the patient may be more sensitive to the position of the tops of his multifocal segments than the prism and acuity loss caused by the misalignment of centers and axes. A simple device to check the position of the segments is to have the patient hold his head steady while a card with a single horizontal line on it is slowly lowered to the point where it is seen double with only one eye in use, then shift the occluder to the other side and if the other eye sees the line double without moving the head or the card, the dividing lines are splitting the pupils of both eyes.

The positions of the center dots with reference to the pupils of the eyes provide information whether there is any considerable disparity. A more accurate observation can be easily made with corneal reflections. The special Guibor light for interocular measurement, or an ophthalmoscope held at the reading distance for a fixation point,* provides corneal reflections that should lie equally above or in the x-axis line. If the glasses are designed for reading only, the reflections should be on or near the center dots. This test is very convenient to check the positioning of the reading portions. An ink line through the centers of the segments (Fig. 236) should intersect the corneal reflections if the fixation light is held at the reading distance. Each millimeter of error in the separation of the centers of the segments produces 2 mm of blurred margin to the segments and reduces the average width of the reading field by 1 mm. Irrespective of the position of the optical centers in the reading portions, the frames of the segments must superimpose when the eyes are converged to the reading distance if the full effect of the segment shape is to be enjoyed (Fig. 237).

All of these observations are easily and precisely made with a

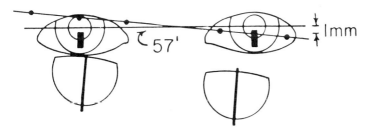

Figure 236. Misalignment of segments when lenses are rotated on the z-axis.

<hr />

*Macleish, Archibald C.: Personal communication, 1936.

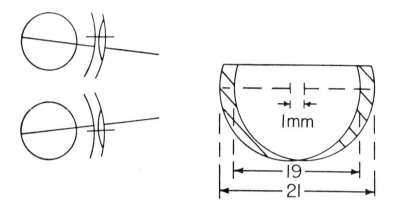

Figure 237. Effect of improperly separated multifocal segments.

Dispensometer. The scales are held in a constant position during the tests.

The importance and tolerance of any disparity that may exist between the optical axes of the lenses and the z-axes of the eyes when the eyes are fixed at infinity, the fixation point for which the lenses were prescribed, can be answered only by the doctor's refraction findings. In any event the erroneous measurement will be converted into horizontal prism and the decision based upon the patient's acceptance of that amount of prism and direction of base as is revealed by the existing fusion or muscle balance.

A special case of the asymmetric prescription is one with a prescription for plano or a planocylinder axis 180 for one eye and a lens of different power for the other. From one point of view, it might be contended that there could be no consideration of optical centers to such a pair of lenses because the one lens has no lateral center. As in the prescription discussed above, this point of view is correct when the center of the lens with power is used for reference. If, however, the eye turns away from the center of that lens or if the spectacles have been made with the optical center of the lens with power away from the position of the intersection of the fixation axis, prism is generated that may seriously interfere with the performance of the prescription. It is apparent that this reasoning is just as applicable to the horizontal meridian as it is to the vertical consideration. It follows, therefore, that a laboratory order for a prescription of this type, whether for single vision lenses or multifocals, should show the same optical center data that it would for lenses of equal power. The lensometer dots for the center of the lens of power should take the same position as they would for an O.U. prescription.

EXAMPLE:

O.D. + 1.50 × 180 for distance
O.S. + 1.25 + 0.05 × 180
I.O.D. 64 mm, DBL 20 mm

The right lens has no focal power through the horizontal meridian and therefore this lens is optically correct when no prism is ground in it across this direction. The left lens has + 1.25D. across the horizontal meridian and if the optical center is properly set it will be 22 mm from the nasal side of the lens. That is, the distance between lenses (DBL) is subtracted from the interocular distance for infinity (I.O.D.): 64 − 20 = 44 mm. Half that amount, or 22 mm, is the distance of the optical center from the nasal side of the bridge. If a pair of large sunglasses were made for this pair of eyes and, through carelessness, the optical center of the left lens were placed at the geometric center of the lens, a large amount of prism Base Out would be possible. Each increase of 8 mm beyond 22 mm generates 1△.

Discrepancies in the position of optical centers of single vision lenses or the distance portions of multifocals should be considered at all times from the viewpoint of the amount of prism created. An error of the location of the optical center of a 0.25D. sphere could be as much as 10 mm and thus produce the effect of 0.25△ without having an undue effect on most eyes. Prism powers are not divided beyond 0.5△ in the trial lens set, therefore half this unit (0.25△) is ordinarily considered within tolerance. Errors in the optical center location of a strong spherocylindrical lens which has an oblique axis will generate prism in both the horizontal and vertical meridians and thus materially interfere with binocular function. The lensometer dots will show the discrepancy when the glasses are in place on the patient's face. The effect of the error can be estimated by calculation or a new pair of center dots can be placed on the lenses and the lenses put back in the lensometer with these dots as points of reference and the prism effect measured on the instrument reticle.

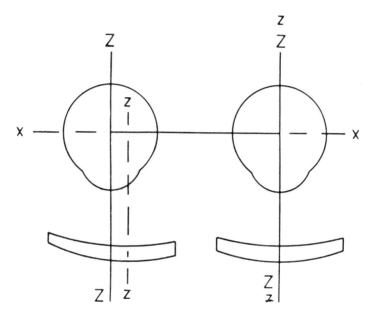

Figure 238. Horizontal prism induced by improper separation of lens centers.

The isobars used by Boeder to show zones of prism power (Chap. 10) are especially helpful in the discussion of discrepancies in the positions of optical centers. In the previous instance when asymmetric prescriptions were analyzed, the optical centers were assumed to be coincident and the resultant optical difference of the two lenses was found by subtracting the power of the weaker lens from the stronger.

The prism effect produced by the decentration of improperly placed optical centers varies widely. Each prescription and the individual wearer's zone of comfortable binocular vision through the lenses must be considered separately. As we shall see, an arbitrary or dogmatic approach to the problem can prove to be disastrous. No single set of specifications can encompass the myriad lens combinations in lens prescriptions. Some representative cases will follow:

1. The simplest instance is identical lens powers—that is, an O.U. prescription. The error is converted into prism power and added to the prescription. If the amount of prism or the direction of the base is significant, the lenses do not pass inspection.

EXAMPLE

O.D. $+2.00 \subset +0.50 \times 90$
O.S. $+2.00 \subset +0.50 \times 90$
I.O.D. $= 60$ mm made with centers at 64 mm

By Prentice's rule, the 250 diopters decentered $0.4 = 1^\triangle$. The lenses are set too wide for the fixation lines, and therefore the prism effect is Base Out. These lenses have the effect of

O.S. $+2.00 \subset +0.50 \times 90 \subset 0.5^\triangle$ Base Out
O.D. $+2.00 \subset +0.50 \times 90 \subset 0.5^\triangle$ Base Out

In this example for the sake of simplicity, the patient's nasal crest is assumed to be at the midpoint between the visual axes, and therefore each eye is measured as symmetrically placed at 30 mm from the nose. In actual practice, many faces do not have such ideally balanced features. Also, only in the rare instance of identical lens prescriptions for the two eyes can individual distances be ignored and the total I.O.D. be used in the analysis of lens centers. The following examples discuss some of the prism effects that are generated when the positions of the lens centers and visual axes differ. It is hoped that these cases emphasize (a) the necessity of careful measurements of the individual positions of patients' eyes and (b) a careful scrutiny of the positions of the optical center marks on the completed spectacles as they are worn by the patient.

2. When the lenses differ in power, an error in the placement of centers produces some new effects. Figure 239 shows a pair of lenses that vary 2.00 diopters in power. When the fixation lines and optical axes are coincident, there is no prism effect. At all extra-axial points, some prism is generated. The prism base is always toward the center of a plus lens. In this instance, $1^\triangle$ is induced for each 5 mm the eyes turn away from the lens centers.

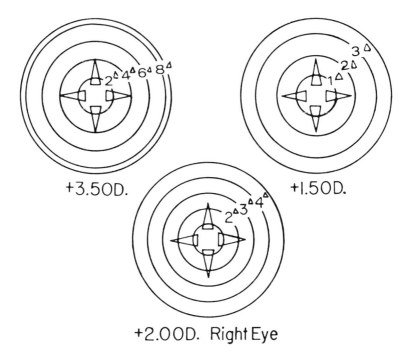

+3.50D. +1.50D.

+2.00D. Right Eye

Figure 239. Optical and prism difference of lenses to correct anisometropia.

The prism effect is before the right eye because the stronger lens is on that side. Therefore, when the eyes are turned into the fields away from primary position, the prism effects are as follows:

$$
\begin{aligned}
\text{To the Right} &= \text{Prism Base In} \\
\text{To the Left} &= \text{Prism Base Out} \\
\text{Up} &= \text{Prism Base Down} \\
\text{Down} &= \text{Prism Base Up}
\end{aligned}
$$

In Figure 240, the position of the centers of the example is shown:

O.D. +3.50D. Sphere
O.S. +1.50D. Sphere

I.O.D. = 65 mm, produced with optical centers at 62 mm and the center of the left lens is also 2 mm below the x-axis.

When the fixation line of the right eye coincides with the optical center of the right lens as illustrated, the center of the left lens

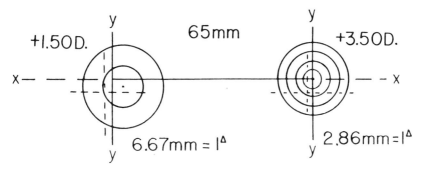

Figure 240.

is 3 mm inside the fixation line of the left eye and also 2 mm below. Two prism effects are generated:

$1.50 \times .3 = 0.45^\triangle$ Base In

$1.50 \times .2 = 0.3^\triangle$ Base Down

If the fixation is shifted 3 mm to the right and 2 mm down to the point that the fixation axis of the left eye and the optical axis of the left lens are coaxial, then the optical center of the right lens is 3 mm inside and 2 mm above the intersection of the x-axes and y-axes. The prism effect is altered, too:

$3.50 \times .3 = 1.05^\triangle$ Base In

$3.50 \times .2 = 0.7^\triangle$ Base Up

On both occasions, the error causes prism Base In. This lateral prism disappears if the eyes converge to the near-point because there is about 3 mm difference between the positions of the optical centers for distance and near vision. We have also noted that when the eyes turn past the center of the left lens into the left side of the visual field, this pair of lenses generates the effect of prism Base Out. Referring to the optical difference of the lenses, we see that $0.2^\triangle$ is generated for each millimeter of decentration. The point of neutralization for the horizontal prism is, therefore, 5.25 mm to the left of the optical center (2.25 mm past the geometrical center) of the left lens. In like manner, the vertical prism is neutralized when the eyes are depressed 1.5 mm below the optical center of the right lens $(2.00 \times .15 = .3)$ to produce

prism Base Up. From these points at the intersection of the dotted
lines in Figure 240 slightly to the left and below the geometric
centers of the lenses, prism effect is the same.

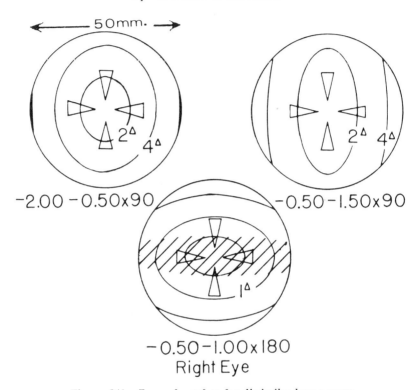

Figure 241. Zone of comfort for dissimilar lens powers.

3. The spherocylindrical lenses in Figure 241 present an altogether different case. Although the prescription is

    O.D. −2.00 −0.50 × 90
    O.S. −0.50 −1.50 × 90

the resultant optical difference is only −0.50 −1.00 × 180, which is
a smaller dioptric value than either of the lenses, and the cylinder
axis is reversed. The zone of comfortable binocular vision is
limited vertically. An error in the locations of the vertical centers
of these lenses produces prism Base Down Right Eye (Base Up
Left Eye) in this pair of lenses, which could be offensive or in-

tolerable in some cases because the disparity is increased when the eyes are depressed for reading or near-point vision. A small amount of prism in the opposite direction would be readily accepted since it would tend to neutralize the prism effect of the optical difference. Optical centers set somewhat below the geometric centers of these lenses, as required for pantoscopic angle, will place the area of comfortable vision more advantageously for multifocal or reading lenses.

4. The following prescription:

O.D. +1.00 +1.00 × 60
O.S. +1.00 +1.00 × 120

is termed "symmetric"* because the cylinder axes are on opposite sides and equidistant from the vertical meridian. The prescription is identical otherwise. Surprisingly, though, the resultant optical difference is a crossed-cylinder axis 45. Characteristic of a crossed-cylinder in this position, there is no focal power in the horizontal or vertical meridians and therefrom prism cannot be neutralized by using the lenses at extra-axial points in these directions. The prism zones (Fig. 242) are hyperbolic functions, not elliptical in this case. It will be noted that the prism bases reverse in each quadrant. The zone of comfortable binocular vision grows very narrow on both sides of the x-axes and y-axes a short distance from center.

5. The prescription in Figure 243 takes an unexpected conformation when the oblique cylinders are subtracted:

O.D. +2.00 +1.00 × 100
O.S. +0.75 +1.50 × 60

The zone of comfortable binocular vision is sizable but restrictive on account of the inclination of the axis. Versions down and to the left or up and to the right produce small prism effect, but movements in all other fields encounter rather strong prisms at rather short distance from center. When additional prism is superimposed from improper placement of lens centers, the zone of comfort is further reduced, a slab-off of 2△ left lens may help.

6. What seems to be a very slight change in powers and axes of

---

*May, C.H.: *Diseases of the Eye*. Baltimore, William Wood, 1900, p. 340.

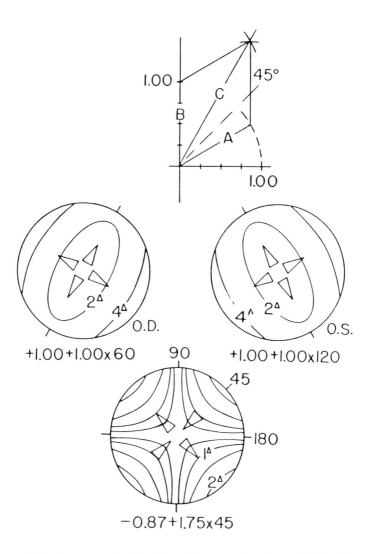

Figure 242. Unexpected prism effect of symmetric spherocylindrical lenses.

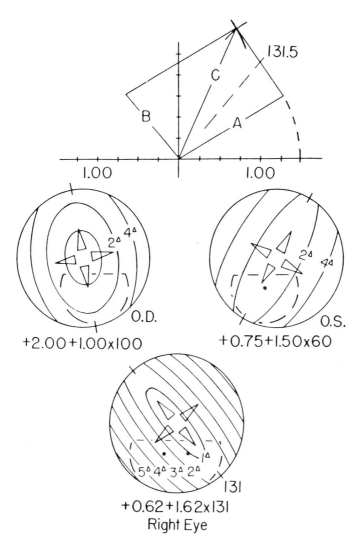

Figure 243. Similar lens powers which individually seem tolerable but as a pair of lenses provide a small and narrow zone of comfort.

the above prescription again provides a striking resultant optical difference. Typically, the axis of the "difference" is not between the meridians of the prescription lenses. The prescription pro-

O.D. −2.00 −1.50 × 65
O.S. −0.50. −1.50 × 20

duces an optical difference of 0.44 −2.12 × 87½ when the powers of the lenses are subtracted. In the vertical meridian, prism from decentration will remain almost constant at almost all points because of the limited focal power (−0.44D.). Across the horizontal meridian the optical difference is about −2.50D. with a correspondingly narrow zone of comfortable binocular vision. Any small error in the placement of the optical centers in this meridian can be quickly neutralized by vergence because each 4 mm of movement generates 1△. Since the lateral vergence to read a typewritten page, approximately 16 cm wide at the normal reading distance, requires an excursion of about 10 mm in the spectacle plane, this patient needs only 2.5△ of Fusion Convergence available to read comfortably with binocular vision.

When the eyes sweep to the left to start a line the effect is prism Base In, as the eyes approach the center of the page the prism effect is neutralized. In the right half of the page, prescription difference induces the effect of prism Base Out that gradually increases. The direction of the base reverses as the eyes sweep back for the next line. It is apparent that if the convergence were deficient in one direction and in good supply in the other, he could induce either prism Base In or Base Out, as the case may require, by turning his head slightly either right or left to use extra-axial points.

After the glasses are finished it is not necessary to diagram a pair of lenses in order to study the prism effects caused by the prescription power or improperly placed optical centers. A very practical investigation can be made with a lensometer. Usually it is too late to help. The lenses can be individually moved into the position where the target is centered on the protractor (no prism) and then ink marked. With this information, one may then set the lenses in the instrument in such position that equal amounts of prism with bases in the same direction are seen in

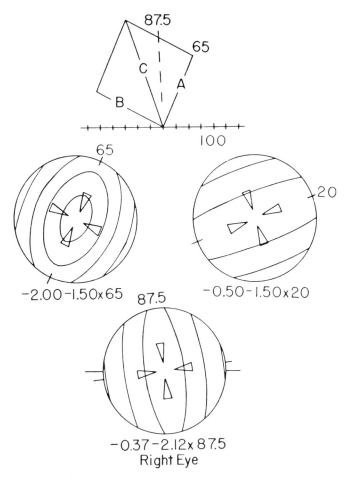

Figure 244. Dissimilar lens powers which combine to provide wide vertical zone in which bifocals should be comfortable.

each lens. The center dots from these points can be compared with the positions of the corneal reflections. If the corneal reflections are markedly above or below the position described in "Prism by Decentration" in Chapter 5), the marginal correction of the lenses is affected and spatial projection may be distorted if the lenses have moderate dioptric power.

Thus we see that when the lenses are identical or nearly so, decentration converted into prism power becomes a fixed error in all fields. The amount of the discrepancy is unaltered at any distance away from center. All variations in the lens prescriptions for the two eyes, whether power and/or cylinder axis, produce changing prism effects at all extra-axial points. Prism effects from improper placement of optical centers superimposed upon this inherent optical difference require individual study, because they may range from an intolerable encumbrance to an effect that is easily neutralized by posture.

The brief reference to refraction in Chapter 8 showed the relationship between accommodation and convergence. If the eyes accommodate for one meter (1.00D.), the eyes converge $6^\triangle$ to be directed to the point at which they are accommodated. It follows that if the accommodative effort is replaced with +1.00D. sphere, there must be a new association, or ratio, established, because the same amount of convergence must be maintained without the accustomed accommodative effort at that distance. In like manner, all prescription changes reflect a modification of the habitual pattern of association between accommodation and convergence. The ratio of 1.00D. of accommodation to $6^\triangle$ convergence represents an average interocular separation of 60 mm.

The Positive and Negative Convergences, that is, the acceptance of prism Base Out or Base In to the first signs of blurred vision at the reading distance is in the order of $10^\triangle$ to $12^\triangle$ for normal eyes. It was seen that, when Percival stimulated or inhibited his patient's convergence by the use of prisms, at some point in the test accommodation was affected.

Spectacle lenses which are indifferently designed or made can likewise add to the burden of physiological adjustment that must be made by the patient at the time a new prescription is fitted. For example, the new prescription is an increase in the amount of plus sphere. When accommodative effort is replaced by lens power, convergence must receive additional stimulation. Any decentration that produces prism Base Out in the spectacle lenses in this case only further complicates the acceptance of the prescription. Conversely, a small error in the opposite direction that adds prism Base In might be highly acceptable. Thus it is seen that the inspection of the position of the optical centers of lenses is an evaluation of the prism effect rather than an investigation of the technical accuracy of the lenses. The locations of the centers are interrelated and, even in the case of no power in one lens, the location of the center of the lens with focal power has significance.

It is the practice of some refractionists to provide slightly better visual acuity for the *dominant** eye for certain patients. This is accomplished by an under- or overcorrection of 0.12D. to 0.25D. sphere to the nondominant eye. It is obvious that a discrepancy in the spherical powers of the prescription lenses that destroys this delicate balance is more significant than the dioptric power involved. A deviation in which both lenses are slightly stronger or weaker than the prescribed amount does not materially affect the intended relationship of visual acuity between the two eyes. A generalization can be made that a symmetrical increase or decrease in lens power is usually more tolerable than an equal discrepancy in one lens only.

Variance between the spherical power of the finished lens and the prescription can be functionally viewed in another way. Inside of or beyond the focal plane of any lens or lens system, the image is blurred. Just how much blur can be tolerated before it affects visual acuity is the limit of tolerance for each individual.† In the discussion to follow, the eye will be considered as an optical instrument in which parallel rays focus at a point and the resolving power of the eye is an angle of 1' (see p. 214). It is well known that because of aberrations and diffraction, rays do not make point images in the eye. However, a large number of eyes see letters that subtend angles much smaller than 5'. All in all, one treads on treacherous footing if he becomes too positive in his statements pertaining to eye function when geometrical optics alone is considered. Nevertheless, eye function is affected in some ways by

---

*Davson, H.: *The Physiology of the Eye.* Philadelphia, Blakiston, 1949, pp. 310-312.

Sheard, C.: *The Sheard Volume.* Philadelphia, Chilton, pp. 31-37.

Duke-Elder, Sir W.S.: *Text-Book of Ophthalmology.* St. Louis, Mosby, 1934, pp. 1044-1046.

†Emsley, H.H.: *Visual Optics.* London, Hatton Press, 1948, pp. 46-55, pp. 538-540.

Hardy, A.C. and Perrin, F.H.: *The Principles of Optics.* New York, McGraw, 1932, pp. 121-134.

optical principles and at least the logic of the calculations is useful if one continues to appreciate that all conclusions are relative.

FOCUS DEPTH

A discussion of *focus depth* and accommodation[†] increases the appreciation of the possible disparities that may exist and how they affect prescription lens tolerances. *Focus depth* (usually associated with photographic lenses) intimately accompanies accommodation. On opposite sides of the focal plane are two planes that represent the limiting distances that rays can focus and still produce blur-circles of object-points so small that they are still recognized as separate image-points. These two planes and their effects upon the optical system of the eye are shown in Figure 245. If we assume that the eye accommodates for object-point **M,** the focus depth is shown in the distance on the z-axis in the first case between **M** and **M₁** and in the second between **M₂ and M₂′.**

$$EG = \text{pupillary diameter} = 2p$$

$$VA = \frac{k}{\gamma}$$

$$\gamma = \text{resolving power}$$

By means of similar triangles, Southall derives a formula in which

$$D = \text{the focus depth} = \frac{k}{2p \times V}$$

when $2p = $ pupillary diameter

$V = $ visual acuity expressed in decimal rating

$k = 0.000291$ radians $= 1'$ angle.

It is apparent that the focus depth is inversely proportionate to both the pupillary diameter and visual acuity. The value of D increases with a decrease in visual acuity and/or decrease in diameter of the entrance pupil.

For ordinary illumination let the diameter of the pupil be taken at 3 mm. (If this measurement is reduced to 2.91 mm, the calculation is simplified since $k = 0.000291$. With these data and normal visual acuity $V = 1$.

$$D = \frac{0.000291}{.00291} = 0.1 \text{ diopter}$$

[†]Southall, J.P.C.: *Am J Phys Optics, 1*:277-316, 1920.

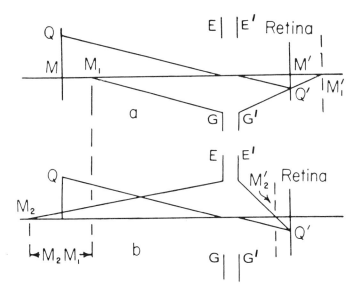

Figure 245. Focus depth as affected by visual acuity.

From these data, it can also be shown that the linear measure of the focus depth is

$$\mathbf{M_2M_1} = \frac{2D}{Z^2 - D^2}$$

where $Z =$ the dioptric distance from object to eye

If a fixation distance of 40 cm $= 2.50$D. is taken in the case above

$$\mathbf{M_2M_1} = \frac{2 \times 0.1}{(2.5 \times 2.5) - (.1 \times .1)} = \frac{.2}{6.25 - .01}$$

$$= \frac{.2}{6.24} = 32.1 \text{ mm}$$

which when converted into diopters of accommodation or addition, becomes

(400 — 16) 382 mm $= 2.62$D.

(400 + 16) 416 mm $= 2.40$D.

Had this patient been able to summon only 20/40 (0.5) visual acuity, or for that matter been satisfied with that reduction in visual acuity, then by the application of the same formula in which

D. now equals 0.2, the linear measurement increases to

$$\mathbf{M_2M_1} = \frac{2D}{Z^2 - D^2} = \frac{.4}{6.21} = 64.4 \text{ mm}$$

This further increase in the focus depth then lengthens the linear distance through which the clarity of the image does not appreciably change:

(400 − 32) 368 mm = 2.72D.
(400 + 32) 432 mm = 2.32D.

A further loss of vision with no changes in other measurements, when visual acuity is 20/60 (V = 0.33), $\mathbf{M_2M_1}$ increases to 97.4 mm. In this instance, with only 2.50D. accommodative amplitude available or +2.50D. added to the distance prescription with no amplitude, the patient would theoretically be able to see almost equally well, as far as blur-circles are concerned, at any point between 31.5 and 44.9 cm. Thus the point of clearest focus becomes increasingly undefined and the patient will search to and fro through some distance in an effort to find his best acuity. He will usually come to rest at the closest point (largest retinal image) at which he can comfortably converge his eyes and hold the object or reading matter.

Another application of these formulas was found by Gleichen (1917) * in the measurements of accommodative amplitude. Since the near-point measurement from which the amplitude is estimated is based upon the first appreciable blur, the point at which the measurement taken is not $\mathbf{M}$ in Figure 245a, it is actually more nearly $\mathbf{M_1}$. Now the distance $\mathbf{MM_1}$ is not dependent upon the accommodative mechanism. It is a fixed distance for all eyes with the same pupillary aperture and visual acuity. As we have seen, this is a small fractional amount for normal eyes. In old age, however, when the pupillary diameter may have reduced materially and the visual acuity decreased, the value of $\mathbf{MM'}$ may become large enough to represent the greater portion of the measurement.

Thus it is seen that under conditions focus depth may have been consumed by the doctor when the prescription was written for the strongest (or weakest) acceptable spherical power. In such an in-

---

*Gleichen, A.: *Theory of Modern Optical Instrument.* Stuttgart, Ferdinand Enke, 1923, sec. 2, pp. 111-112.

stance the tolerance may all be one side of the prescribed sphere—that is, if plus has been fully prescribed, a variance that increases the vertex effect may be intolerable, while a small amount less than the prescription may be quite acceptable to both the doctor and his patient.

From time to time ophthalmic dispensers, laboratory technicians, and some doctors have discussed the advisability of recommending that further information be included with the power of the lenses on the prescription: for instance, in the case of anisometropia, whether the binocular function is of such quality as to justify compensation for prism, or whether subnormal vision in one eye or suppression makes the effort valueless. The same thought has been projected for the problem of lateral imbalances. One suggestion has been made to ask all doctors to indicate the patient's acceptance of small prism effect in one direction and intolerance of it in the other. In the larger present-day lens blanks, it is easy to decenter some lenses to the patient's advantage. This suggested convention to inform the dispenser could be a request for optical centers wider or narrower than actually measured. In other words, if the doctor measures the patient's interocular distance and finds it to be 62 mm and he wishes to have the effect of a small amount of prism Base In and be assured that no prism Base Out effect is found in the glasses, he could arbitrarily prescribe O.C. 58 mm for plus lenses. When the dispenser measures the patient and finds a measurement much wider than the doctor's prescribed optical centers, he would know that decentration for Base In effect is permissible and desirable, but that lenses with any Base Out effect are not acceptable. The use of O.C., (optical centers) was suggested to avoid disagreements when concepts of P.D. are at variance.

These remarks are not to be construed as a vindication of carelessness in the placement of optical centers of lenses. No conscientious optician fits any large number of glasses before he has an experience in which resetting the optical centers of a pair of lenses is the difference between an uncomfortable and comfortable patient. On occasion, the change can be made by a change in the adjustment or exchange of frames with the same lenses. I am convinced that all such small alterations are not psychological, since for experimental purposes I have revived the complaints by resetting the lenses to the improper position.

The relative vertical position of the x-axis (including the optical centers) has little effect upon the muscle balance in weak prescriptions if they are reasonably symmetric. As power increases or lens differences become greater, the setting of the line assumes greater importance. The exact position of the centers in an old pair of glasses in which the lenses are dissimilar can have a great bearing upon a new prescription and new glasses. For example

    ℞: O.D. +1.00 Distance
       O.S. +2.50

If the centers in the old glasses are set very low, the decentration causes varying amounts of prism Base Down Left Eye when the eyes are near the primary position. The optical centers are reached and the prism vanishes only when the eyes are depressed at a large angle. If a new pair of lenses is prepared in which the centers are slightly above the fixation line in primary position, this setting reverses the vertical prism and produces prism Base Up Left Eye, which continues to increase as the eyes are depressed toward a reading position. Another pair of lenses to the new prescription in which the centers are lowered to the habitual position may be the only means by which an uncomfortable patient can be satisfied. Hence it is plainly a matter of wisdom for the positions of the centers of the old lenses are to be located before lenses are made on a new prescription for an anisometropic patient.

The prescription of a pair of lenses to be used for distance vision is altered by the vertex distance formula given in Chapter 5. The vast majority of lenses fitted with a total power of less than 2.00D. are not affected in any way by changes in z-axis (vertex) distance.

Measurable disparities in spherical power for the distance prescription that approach or exceed accepted tolerances are a matter for the doctor's final judgment. He may have prescribed all the plus power that he felt the patient could accept. In such a case, an overcorrection could not be considered, while a pair of lenses slightly under the prescribed amounts may be satisfactory.

The limits of tolerance for the power of the reading portion of a multifocal require separate consideration. The unit of measurement established by the lens manufacturers is 0.25D. It follows that plus or minus slightly less than one-half that amount (0.12D.) is considered an acceptable deviation. However, accommodation is normally an equal effect in both eyes. Assuming the distance prescription has balanced the function of the two eyes, a pair of segments that approach opposite limits, that is, strong in one lens and weak in the other, would approach a difference of 0.25D., which is not acceptable.

Ordinarily a lens prescription for distance vision suspends accommodation and produces clearest vision for infinity. If a small amount of plus is added, vision is blurred; and if minus power is added, accommodation must make up the deficit. For most patients, the amount of near-point addition is determined by a combination of measurement and judgment. Even in the refracting procedure, it is not unexpected that the new experience for the patient's accommodative-convergence relationship (in which accommodation is relaxed by plus lens power) will cause the patient uneasiness. In *Guide to Occupational and Other Visual Needs* by Clark Holmes, there is an excellent discussion of this subject on pages 4 to 6. It is an excellent review of those elements contributing to what experience has developed, what is called good judgment.

When the front focal power of the lens varies from the prescribed amount, the effect on the patient can be viewed from either or a combination of two points: (a) the eyes will perform at the measured near-point distance and accommodative amplitude will make the compensation of overactivity or underactivity or (b) the amount of accommodation will not be varied and the near-point distance will be altered directly according to the variation in lens power. The reading addition is only a supplement to accommodation for the purpose of providing comfortable vision ordinarily at 40 cm. It follows that, no matter what addition is prescribed, the difference is compared with the dioptric effect at the intended fixation distance. In other words, an early presbyope may supply +1.50D. accommodation and the lens adds +1.00D. for use at 40 cm. Later, when the amplitude is diminished, accommodation may supply only +0.25D. and the spectacle lenses supply +2.25D. When the added power in the multifocal varies from the prescription, the working distance of the lenses varies as shown in Table XXXVIII. Thus it is seen that an extreme error of +0.25D. moves the fixation point only 25 to 36 mm toward the patient's eyes. An undercorrection of −0.25D. causes the plane of best focus to move 31 to 44 mm from his eyes if accommodation makes no effort to adjust for the discrepancy.

TABLE XXXVIII

| Accom. | Working | Actual distance when addition for reading is | | | |
		Overcorrected		Undercorrected	
Distance	Distance	0.12D.	0.25D.	0.12D.	0.25D.
3.00D.	33.3 cm	32.0 cm	30.8 cm	34.8 cm	36.4 cm
2.75D.	36.4 cm	34.8 cm	33.3 cm	38.2 cm	40.0 cm
2.50D.	40.0 cm	38.2 cm	36.4 cm	42.2 cm	44.4 cm

The means by which the reading test is made also enters into the optical effectivity of the testing lenses. When the examination is made with a refracting instrument and the suspended reading card holds the eyes in primary position with the fixation axes close to the optical axes of the lenses, the effect of the reading addition in the prescription lenses supplied to the patient may tend to be slightly weaker rather than stronger, if the lenses are fitted in the same plane in front of the eyes. In no way is this error to be compared with the large change in lens power induced when the eyes are depressed to the normal reading position and thereby use the margins of the flat trial lens for a reading test. The tilted lens formula or any of the graphs related to marginally corrected lenses emphasize the terrific disparity between axial and edge power. Prescription lenses which analyze identically with the trial lenses for vertex power in the central area will be effectively weaker. The effect of correction lenses compares more favorably with the prescription when the test has been made with the head tilted forward, so that the plane of the trial frame and lenses is parallel to the test card and the eyes are therefore *normal* to the lenses.

The limits of tolerance for cylinder power are ordinarily unbalanced. That is to say, most refractionists tend to prescribe all the cylinder power that is acceptable to the patient. For this reason, lenses slightly under power are usually passable when cylinder over power are refused. If the lens is to be used for near-point fixation, the cylinder power in it is somewhat reduced in the front focus effect, particularly when the cylinder is on the front surface of the lens. Therefore such a cylinder in a reading glass often may be satisfactorily worn even if it is slightly over power when measured for back focus.

Probably no other error in lens manufacture leads to more heated discussions than cylinder axis disparity. In the beginning of the correction of astigmatism, long, oval lenses were "fussed with" until the cylinder axis was correct to the last degree; then the lenses were adjusted as in Figure 246, and woe unto the optician who straightened them after the patient had become accustomed to them! Then followed the era of round lenses which became loose in the frames. Many patients learned how to turn their bifocal segments back into place after wiping the lenses.

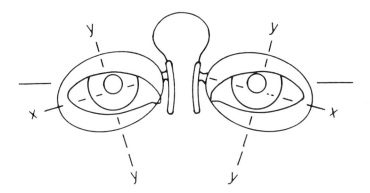

Figure 246. Common maladjustment of hoop spring eyeglasses.

When the lenses are inspected from the point of view of mechanical accuracy, 1 degree of error is 1/360th of a circle in any case. But when the error is viewed from the aspect of function, an altogether different conclusion is reached. The prescribed cylinder is a cylinder of the same power and *opposite* sign as the refractive error in the spectacle lens plane. The axes of the refractive error and that of the prescribed lens are identical. Therefore the prescibed lens neutralizes the refractive error. A cylinder of the proper power and sign rotated to such a position that the lens axis is not coincident with the axis of the refractive error is in reality an obliquely crossed-cylinder. In the hands of the laboratory technician it is "off axis"; in the hands of a refractionist, "crossed-cylinder."

Tolerance of the disparity is logically based upon its effect on vision. It is a function of the power of the lens and the amount of the disparity. Table XXXIX shows the power of the spherocylinder induced when a lens of the correct cylinder power is set obliquely to the axis of the refractive error. It clearly shows when the power of the lens and the amount of obliquity add a significant error to the correction.

TABLE XXXIX

Cylinder	5°	10°
0.12	—0.01 + 0.02	—0.02 + 0.04
0.25	—0.02 + 0.04	—0.04 + 0.09
0.37	—0.03 + 0.07	—0.07 + 0.13
0.50	—0.04 + 0.09	—0.09 + 0.17
0.62	—0.05 + 0.11	—0.11 + 0.22
0.75	—0.07 + 0.13	—0.13 + 0.26
0.87	—0.08 + 0.15	—0.15 + 0.31
1.00	—0.09 + 0.17	—0.17 + 0.35
1.25	—0.11 + 0.22	—0.22 + 0.43
1.50	—0.13 + 0.26	—0.26 + 0.52
1.75	—0.15 + 0.31	—0.31 + 0.62
2.00	—0.17 + 0.35	—0.35 + 0.69
	42½° off the prescribed axis	40° off the prescribed axis

The actual power induced by a very weak cylinder when the axis crosses the true position by as much as 5° to 10° is not measurable with regular lens-measuring equipment and probably would not be an optical problem for many patients. At 0.75D., an error of 5° given the effect of an .06 Jackson cross-cylinder diagonal to the prescribed axis characteristic of a crossed-cylinder held almost 45° from the prescribed power, and no new focal effect is induced in either of the principal meridians of the prescribed lens. The blur and inclination of the retinal image are almost identical with the effect of the routine cylinder axis check.

These data could supply background for the ANSI Z80.1 Committee in the establishment of cylinder axis tolerances. Since the sines and cosines of small angles are almost directly proportional, the induced errors increase regularly. A 1.50D. cylinder at 5° or a 0.75C. cylinder at 10° produce the effect of a 0.12 cross-cylinder, and a 2.00D. cylinder crossing the axis of the refractive error by 10° is the effect of a 0.37 Jackson cross-cylinder with the axis set diagonally.

The computations in Table XXXIX open the question of whether tolerances of axis errors should cover groups of lenses. Since the disparity adds a lens effect directly related to the dioptric power and axis, it seems that a simple rule might be developed to cover all lenses. For example, if it were decided that the induced cross-cylinder must not exceed one-half the weakest examining lens, then −0.05 +0.11 (which is the focal power induced on a 0.62D. cylinder 5° in error) is the limit of the conditions. Interpolating from this assumed permissible error, the chart (Fig. 247) shows the tolerance of cylinder axis disparity. It is not to be construed that these assumed limits are correct.

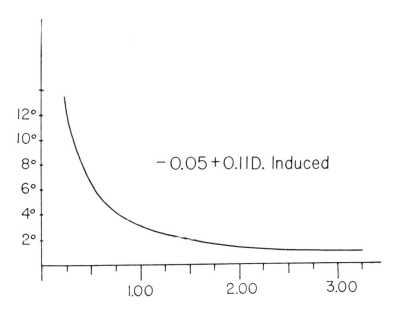

Figure 247. Tolerable cylinder axis error for various cylinder powers.

By the Bausch & Lomb limits, in Table XXXV,

$3°$ error at 0.50D. is $-0.026 + 0.053$
$2°$ error at 1.00D. is $-0.03 + 0.07$
$1°$ error at 2.00D. is $-0.03 + 0.07$

All of these crossed-cylinder effects are much smaller than the units of refracting equipment.

Shuron standard chart

$2°$ error at 2.00D. is $-0.07 + 0.13$
and the same rigid limit applied to
    0.25D. is $-0.01 + 0.02$

The Veterans Administration's requirements

$2.5°$ error at 0.75D. is $-0.03 + 0.07$
$1.0°$ for 1.00D. and up is not less than $-0.02 + 0.04$

In all instances the standards suggested as being within best laboratory procedure seem to fall well within the limits discussed above. In many instances the self-imposed tolerances are practically at the limit of accuracy of present-day laboratory equipment.

In Chapter 5 we are reminded by Maddox's table showing the torsion* of the eyes that all astigmatic patients must have a higher degree of adaptability if they are to comfortably sustain binocular vision. It is apparent that these individuals must not only make the revaluations of spatial projection in the corners of the visual field, they must also learn to tolerate the spherocylindrical power induced when the eyes turn on the z-axis and the lens axes do not follow.

After the power of the lenses has been measured and considered, the positioning of the lenses and the fitting of the frame are surveyed. This part of the inspection includes

1. Position of optical centers horizontally and vertically as related to interocular distance and pantoscopic angle
2. Position of x-axis
3. Position of multifocal segments
4. Vertex distances and their symmetry

---

*Van Wien, S.: Influence of torsional movements on axis of astigmatism. *Amer J Ophthal, 31:*1251-1260, October, 1948.

5. Fitting of frame pads on nose
6. Fitting of temples in front of ears
7. Fitting of temple ends (behind ears)
8. General tightness or security of glasses

The principles of proper fitting on which this appraisal is made are discussed in Chapter 7.

In conclusion, the inspection of a finished pair of glasses is somewhat in this order:

1. Final laboratory appraisal of the assembled glasses as a whole in which the quality of materials and workmanship is evaluated. A determination is made whether the product compares exactly with the specification of the order.

2. First inspection by the ophthalmic dispenser, who places the ink dots and lines on the lenses for the purpose of proper positioning of optical centers, multifocal segment dividing lines and centers.

3. Evaluation at the adjusting table at the time the lenses are positioned before the eyes.

4. Final verification of cylinder axes, prism bases, and optical centers when major adjustments have been necessary.

5. Inspection of the fitted glasses by the doctor or his assistant when the glasses are measured on the lensometer and the x-axes are marked on the lenses. The eyewear is then scrutinized on the patient's face to observe whether the placement of optical centers, x-axis, frame, bridge, pads, temples, and temple tips are as intended.

6. The graduation of the dispenser's handiwork comes with doctor's nod of approval after reviewing the performance of the new prescription. Regrettably, this last step is being overlooked in most cases in these days of rushing about. Many new practitioners have not been impressed by their teachers about this comforting gesture.

REVIEW

1. Fully discuss the two points of view to be kept in mind in setting and also observing tolerances when inspecting (or evaluating) lenses. When does the severity of a limit of tolerance exceed its utility?

2. Explain the reasonableness of including plus or minus almost half the unit of measurement with the measurement, e.g. 1.51 to 2.49 = 2. Explain how any closer approximation requires a unit smaller than 1.

3. With focal length of lenses the criterion, do the units used in a complete set of trial lenses seem correct? Are the units too small? Give your reasons.

4. Are the present-day limits of tolerances for lenses satisfactory, unrealistically narrow, or too generous? Cite the reasons for your opinion. Reference is made to ANSI-Z80, V.A., B & L, and other standards.

5. Why is it essential to measure the stronger lens first on a lensometer?

6. A prescription $+1.75 - 0.50 \times 90 \,\circlearrowright\, 6^\vartriangle$ Base Down deviates the Vertometer target too much to make a reading. How much prism, with the base in which direction should be placed in Vertometer?

7. Why is the target image not large for plus lenses and small for minus lenses?

8. For a lens $-0.50 + 4.25$, at what point would you set the lens power to start? At what point to find the optical center (axis) of the lens?

9. Why does a strong toric prism alter the optical effect of the curves ground on it? How is compensation made if necessary?

10. Why must the reading addition be measured from the front surface of the lens? Give all the steps to verify: In which direction should a compensation prism base be set to measure the lens?

$4.50 + 1.25 \times 180$
$+ 1.50$ add
segment down 5 mm

11. What will hand neutralization show that a lensometer may miss?

12. Why does so little of a pot of glass finish as an Ultex B?

13. What is an important side effect of moderate-sized reading segments set too wide or too narrow?

14. Could the ℞ +1.00 +1.00 × 60
+1.00 +1.00 × 120
+1.50 Addition
Univis D down 3 mm

be compensated? If yes, how?

15. Eyes with subnormal vision tend to "'ride" the focus depth nearest the eye. Why?

16. Old ℞ R +5.50
L +3.00

Lens centers 3 mm above pupils in primary position. How would you proceed?

17. Does a graph demonstrating the cross-cylinder generated by off axis cylinders suggest the best tolerance limit notion to you? Why?

Chapter 18

FITTING AND ADJUSTING

✦◆✦◆✦◇◆✦◆

The ophthalmic dispenser's final step in the filling of an ophthalmic prescription is in many ways the most important. The fitting and adjustment of the glasses to the patient's face is much more than the delivery of merchandise. The doctor's professional care, the dispenser's studied interpretation, and the laboratory's precision can be seriously impaired by a tactless, bungling adjustment and delivery of the glasses.

Two of the three qualities of a pair of glasses discussed in Chapter 9 may be in the patient's mind at once. He may wish to know immediately whether (a) they have the appearance that he had anticipated and/or (b) they give the visual results which he has expected. His first impulse is to get his hands on the glasses to look at them quickly, then put them on to "try out." Since he is not aware of the fact that oftentimes there is considerable work to be done in the fitting of the glasses after they leave the laboratory, it is natural that some explaining must be done. There is no reason why he should not have the privilege and pleasure of handling the glasses if he pleases, but every effort should be made to discretely prevent him from putting on the glasses until they have been adjusted. A first unfavorable impression, no matter how unfounded, can cause some difficulty. It is best to request a few moments to get the lenses set in the proper position before he attempts to test the new lenses.

The Dispensometer recently presented transcends all other instruments in placing the new lenses in the specified position. The slot in the datum line provides the opportunity for the location of the 180° (datum) line of the eyewear. The felt tip of the Pilot Razor Point® Pen fits nicely in the slot of the Dispensometer to make a perfectly placed and narrow indication of the datum line. A great assistant is the Dispensorule which holds any eyeframe so that its midline is always the midline (datum line, 180-line, pattern center line) of the B dimension of the lens. With it and a fine pointed felt tipped pen, all of the significant data can be put on the lenses: the y-axis, some dots on the top edge of multifocal segments, a line through the geometric center of the segment. With these data established you are ready to proceed with the fitting. The Dispensometer is now fitted on the eyewear, and the eyeframe with Dispensometer is placed in position on the nose. The position of the optical centers of multifocal segments can now be confirmed.

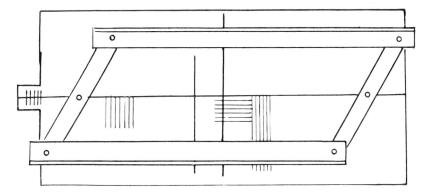

Figure 248. Willesden datum rule.

A thorough understanding of the mechanics of the fitting of glasses simplifies the undertaking immeasurably. The *fitting triangle,* discussed in Chapter 7, in which the fundamental statement "the vertical plane of a pair of lenses is established and supported by a horizontal triangle," is the foundation of spectacle fitting. Similar to the process of setting and leveling a photographer's tripod on an irregular surface is the compensating and contouring of a frame to fit the anatomical irregularities.

After the axis lines of the glasses have been marked and the general alignment of the frame has been checked, the spectacles are ready to be tried on the patient. The glasses should be held by

---

Martin Wells Head Caliper, Superior Dispensorule, Stimson Dispensometer all obtainable from Superior Optical Co., Post Office Box 15287, Santa Ana, CA. 92705.

the temples with the fingers in front of the tops of the ears. The bridge of the frame should be settled down onto the nose but the temples must not be released. By this approach the glasses are not actually placed on the patient's head. They are still in the dispenser's hands and can be quickly and easily removed. When the fitting is started in this manner, the patient is not free to "try out" the reading portions until the fitting is completed. Straight temple and heavyweight plastic frames cannot be held in quite the same way described above. These frames should be grasped at the end-pieces as they are placed on the face and the glasses should not be released.

At first the whole attention should be centered on the fitting of the bridge. The location and contour of the resting place for the pads is determined by the shape of the bone of the nose. Before the eyewear is placed in position, the nose should be palpated again with the fingertips. As previously discussed, the tissue of the nose can, on occasion, be quite deceptive. Until the inclination and slope of the nasal bone are known, even the shape and size of the pads are speculative.

The adjustability of the pads of metal frames and mountings permits some important variations in the placement of the lenses before the eyes. Within limits, the distance between lenses (DBL) can be changed independently of the separation between pads. The tops of the pads can be raised or lowered with reference to the geometric center of the lenses to control the position of the vertical centers and multifocal segments.

Plastic frames require an altogether different approach. Some small alterations can be made by filing and reshaping, but the pads and DBL vary together. A large part of the fitting of these frames is done at the time the glasses are designed—that is, when the choice of bridge design, DBL, and the shape of the nasal ends of the lenses is made. Oftentimes the most important decision on the part of the dispenser who is adapting the finished spectacles is made at this moment. If the weight and design of frame or any other detail causes the glasses to come to rest in an undesired position that can be corrected only by extreme or unusual adjustment, the best solution is often an exchange of frames at once. Before the frame is destroyed for other purposes and much time and patience are consumed, frequently the frame can be exchanged (or the lens shape altered) before the fitting actually begins. In this way, a satisfactory service is assured for everyone concerned. There is some virtue in knowing the right time to make a change. Expert fitting of plastic frames is not as simple as it looks, and even the most experienced dispensers design glasses that do not come up to their expectations in the finished product. The trained optician surveys the situation and makes his decision before circumstances and an obviously bad job force him to change his approach.

The apex of the *fitting triangle* supports 60 to 90 percent of the weight of the spectacles (see Chap. 7) and therefore the pads on the bridge assume an important responsibility both in the adjustment and comfort of the glasses. The contact surfaces should be contoured to the shape of the underlying structure of the nasal bone to distribute the weight as evenly as possible. The slope of the pad should be such that the upper edge bears ever so little more against the nose than the bottom edge. This compensation causes the spectacles to rather hang from the upper part of the pad and not allow the pad to create a furrow and cut into the tissue along the lower edge.

Metal frames and mountings are fitted with two types of pad surfaces (a) all metal, usually solid gold, or (b) plastic covered. The latter are molded over a metal base and can be shaped with pliers in much the same way that an all-metal pad is adjusted. Special contours or surfaces of the plastic pad can quickly be prepared with a sandpaper file (manicure emery board). A polisher such as the AO Pixie should be used to smooth the surface. Acetone often irritates the skin.

Adjustable pads are either of two kinds: (a) stationary or rigid or (b) movable or rocking. Most dispensers use either, but many spectacle fitters prefer one type to the exclusion of the other. Thus it would seem that each type must have advantages and probably some disadvantages. Those who choose the stationary pads maintain that because these pads can be precisely contoured a better and more stable adjustment is possible. They point out that normal wear in the pivots of rocking pads destroys both the accuracy and the intended comfort of the fitting. A large number of equally experienced and painstaking dispensers prefer a movable pad because they feel that the slight changes in slope and bevel that are assumed by the pad as it settles into place against the tissue of the nose provides a more delicate adjustment than can be done with pliers. They call attention to the fact that small pressures or jolts to the glasses do not cause the pads to dig into the flesh of the nose. At this point, it would be well to review the mechanics of pad fitting as developed by Fleck et. al. in Chapter 7. This research deserves more attention than it usually receives.

The designs of rocking pads have been modified by the frame manufacturers many times in an effort to perfect the performance of the bearing surface. In several designs the pad is attached to the arm on a kind of horizontal bearing that is intended to limit the movement to rotation on a horizontal axis. These pads continue to keep an equal pressure on the sides of the nose even if the frame is turned rather large amounts on its cyclopean z-axis. Other pads are supported on specially designed pins that serve as limited universal joints. It is with this type of pad to which advocates of rigid pads take exception. When the pins on the backs of some of these pads are badly worn, the pad may rotate on the pin. This can cause the spectacles to be askew or uncomfortable or both.

The size of the pads is not always easily determined in advance. Some manufacturers supply larger-sized pads on the larger-sized frames and mountings in order to be prepared for the additional weight of the heavier lenses. There are occasions, however, when fragile skin or extra strong and heavy lenses require extra large size pads on even small spectacle sizes. The major frame manufacturers offer at least three pad sizes which can easily be exchanged as required on rocking pad bridges.

As we have seen, the center of mass of a pair of metal framed or rimless spectacles is about 6 to 28 mm behind the plane of the lenses when the head is erect and Listing's plane is vertical. Therefore, the farther the position of the pads in front of this point, the smaller portion of the total weight of the glasses is borne by them. This also brings to our attention that pads on extended guard-arms to set the lenses away from proptosed eyes take almost all the weight of the glasses because of their proximity

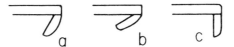

Figure 249. Various positions of zylo eyeframe pad.

to the center of gravity.

The fixed pads on plastic frames are capable of more adjustment than is commonly practiced. Again, the natural positions
of rest on the sides of the nasal bone are the starting points. They
are in the designer's thoughts when he orders the position of the
tops of the pads in relation to the geometric center of the lenses
as well as the contour (or soulé) of the nasal side of the lenses.
In much the same way that guard-arms can be raised or lowered
on a metal bridge, the pads can be removed and reset higher or
lower. When the nasal side of the bridge is to be filed to fit the
shape of the nose, the pads frequently must be removed so that
their thickness will not be reduced. The angle of the pads can be
changed quickly by removing them from the front, increasing or
reducing the bevel angle, and recementing them. The pads of
most plastic frames are more convex than the average contact area
on the nose and therefore fit rather well in most cases. Like most
compromises, however, the fitting can be improved for the individual case. The comfort of a large number of plastic frames can
be increased materially by the simple procedure of filing the pad
surface flat to match the inclination and bevel of the nasal bone.
A coarse bastard-cut file followed by sandpaper and machine
polishing or acetone accomplishes this fitting. A ten-inch coarse
rat-tail file is needed to undercut a bridge for a prominent nose.
Oversize pads are obtainable from the frame makers and can easily
be fitted to most plastic frames. In many cases they look best
when they are made of clear or pink plastic. If the surfaces to be
cemented are softened slightly with acetone before using plastic
cement, the cement sets very quickly; if the patient is instructed
to handle the glasses carefully for an hour or two, the pads will
be quite secure.

At this point the temples may be rested on the ear tops and the
spread of the temples at the endpieces surveyed. If the angles are

not wide enough the plane of the lenses will be bowed out at the endpieces. The temple angles and head width should have been on the laboratory order. The endpiece may be bent out slightly if the necessary adjustment is small. If filing is necessary, it should be confined to the temple, aside from a small touch on the front that may be required to perfect the mitered fit. English hinges require a slightly different approach. When the "temple-spread" is to be increased a small amount, hold the front plate of the hinge with parallel jaw snipe nose pliers and the temple with an end piece angling plier (like AO M168) and turn the hands to *force* the hinge. The temples can be opened several millimeters by this method. If a large adjustment is necessary a wedge of zylo at the end of the temple must be removed. A knife-edge file or jeweler's saw is required to do this properly. The angle should be increased cautiously. When it is overdone or for any reason an angle should be reduced, the tip of the hinge is bent away from the end of the temple and a small wedge of zylo is inserted. The metal fittings of an English hinge should not be filed.

Many heads are asymmetric. The temple-spread must account for this or the plane of the lenses will not be parallel with the base line (x-axis) of the eyes—that is, the pair of glasses will be rotated on its medial y-axis. The best observation for this phase of the fitting is made when the dispenser stands at the adjusting table and looks down at the patient's face plane.

The final spread of the temples should be just wide enough to put a small tension on the temples at the first point of contact which should be at the ear tops. To compensate for this, the plane of the lenses should be bowed back very slightly when they are off the face. The temples will then be held snugly against the head at the ear tops by the resiliency of the bridge of the glasses.

The temples must not take any of the weight or support of the glasses at any point in front of the ears if the *fitting triangle* is to be effective. The temples may touch against the face or hair dress but there must be no pressure if the glasses are to be worn with the greatest comfort and retain their desired position. Except in rare cases, the skull is widest at the ear tops. It follows that, if the temples exert pressure against the inclined surfaces, the force is forward. The greater the pressure and the greater the inclination, the greater the tendency for the spectacles to be forced off the wearer's face. As shown in Figure 113, only the support of the glasses from that portion of the temples behind the ears keeps the frame in place. Ideally, temples should be measured to the bend at the top of the ear (LTB) rather than the whole length (a manufacturer's identification). As paradoxical as it may seem, the patient's report on this maladjustment is that "my glasses slide down my nose and also hurt behind my ears." Even though the temples are properly fitted, the pull caused by the pressure in front of the ears causes pressure behind the ears.

A crease in the hair dress and sometimes in the flesh under the temples in front of the ears is the telltale sign. Even if the sides of the head are nearly parallel, there still is the possibility of discomfort from head pressure in front of the ears. When the pressure is greater on one side than the other, the line of force is directed to the contact point of the frame on the opposite side of the nose and thus the weight of the glasses is unbalanced. As soon as the temples are cleared and the points at the tops of the ears are in contact, attention should return to the position of the lenses.

It is seldom found that the crotches at the tops of the ears describe a line parallel with the x-axis of the eyes. The glasses will be elevated on the end corresponding to the higher crotch. It is immediately apparent that raising the end of the temple on that side or lowering the temple on the opposite side by the proper amount will adjust the x-axis of the glasses into proper alignment with the base line of the eyes. The choice of the temple will be indicated by the relationship of the lens centers and the inclination of the lenses to the face-plane. The vertical centers of the lenses are set to be compatible with the line parallel with the supraorbital prominence and the lower orbital rim as discussed in Chapter 10. The angle between the face-plane and rotation of the lenses on the x-axis is established. The angle required to accomplish this at the temple-joint is dependent upon the position of the temple-joint with reference to the geometric center of the lenses and the position of the crotches at the tops of the ears. Fry and Ellerbrock* have made some careful research on this subject

---

*Fry, G.A. and Ellerbrock, V.J.: Placement of optical centers in single vision lenses. *Optom. Weekly, 32*:933-936.

and their data show that even in a moderately small group the ears varied from 6.65 mm above to 15.60 mm below the base line of the eyes. Either or both of the temples are angled to adjust the inclination (pantoscopic angle) of the glasses. Finally the x-axes of the lenses are trued up to stand parallel with the Helmholtz Base Line.

Corneal reflections are used to verify the setting of the lenses with the base line. This adjustment can be very accurate because the distance from endpiece to ear top is about three times as far as from bridge to endpiece. Therefore a bend of about 3 mm at the ear is about 1 mm at the endpiece, and, as we have seen, 1° of cylinder axis.

The next step in the fitting of the glasses requires the dispenser to stand in such position that he can see how the temples fit against the head behind the ears. Medium and heavyweight plastic frames with short straight temples fitted to skulls with parallel sides in the area behind the ears are held in place by friction from direct pressure against the head (Fig. 117*a*). The security of these glasses is established by the slope and bevel of the nasal bone and the tolerance of pressure against the sides of the head. The permanence of the adjustment is dependent upon the weight and resiliency of the material (bridge and temples). These frames are especially desirable as "on and off" reading glasses. They serve handily as reading glasses to be worn in bed, where the head is tipped back and where the length of temple behind the ear may be uncomfortable against the pillow. These frames are difficult to adjust for all-time wear if the lenses are heavy, the nose has parallel sides or is unusually flat and/or if the frame is very lightweight and flimsy and will not continue to maintain sufficient head pressure.

When the temples are slightly longer or the head is shaped like Figure 113*b*, and the tips of the temples can be turned ever so slightly toward one another, the glasses become increasingly secure. The "fitting triangle" appears and the *lines of force* from the temple tips to the bridge pads are established. No head pressure is necessary and only enough pressure is needed at the tips (last 1 to 3 cm) of the temples to hold the full weight of the glasses when the plane of the face is turned parallel to the floor.

A temple that is turned down slightly at the tip is called the "club," "spoon," or "ambassador" temple design. It provides increased leverage. To the advantage of the *lock* in the vertical meridian by turning in the temple tips is added the contouring in the other planes over the mastoid processes which act to pull the temples down on to the ear tops. Since these temples are usually somewhat longer and/or larger at the tips than regular straight temples, the glasses are secured with fewer grams pressure per square centimeter.

Skull temples are lighter in weight and longer than straight or club temples. The frames on which they are regularly fitted are lighter in weight. These temples are fitted differently. There should be only enough head pressure to hold the temples snug against the head at the tops of the ears. The temple is abruptly bent just past the top of the ear and turned to contour with the skull but *not* snug in the crotch behind the ear until the point x in Figure 115a is reached. The *lock* of the temple is from that point to the tip. When the skull slopes rapidly toward the neck in this area, little pressure is required. If the shape of the head and ear is not favorable in this area, the temple can be adjusted like an extended club temple (Fig. 115b) in which the lock is accomplished over the mastoid process. There are occasions when the ear shape and/or head shape in combination with the point of rest on the nose do not provide contours that make it possible to lock the temples securely. These are the patients on whom riding-bow temples should be fitted when possible. Even with the best adjustment, skull-fitting temples will not hold the spectacles securely because the skin in the area of the ears moves, caused by the facial muscles in the acts of talking and laughing. The temples will gradually slip up at the ear tops and the wearer must frequently push his glasses into position on his nose and press the temples back into place.

A hot salt or glass bead pan is indispensable for plastic frame fitting. Hot water or other forms of heat can be used, but nothing else seems to supply concentrated heat at specific points of the frame quite as does hot salt. It is particularly handy for contouring temple-tips. A large unpainted wooden mixing spoon makes a good holder for a small quantity of the salt or beads to soften a nasal pad. A better means to apply hot salt to a small area, such as pads, is to fasten a small funnel on an arm about a foot above the salt pan. Use the wooden spoon to fill the funnel. The small stream of hot salt is enough to soften any small area of the frame.*

All temples for metal frames and mountings follow the same rules of fitting that have been outlined for the heavier plastic frames. Regular weight metal frames are too resilient to be regularly fitted with straight temples and held in place by direct head pressure. The additional *lock* of skull or riding-bow temples is almost a necessity for security and comfort. In no case are any of these temples adjusted to fit snugly in the upper part of the crotch behind the ear. The area in the center of the crotch at the back of the ear is very sensitive in most cases. When the external ear is pulled forward, a small cordlike structure appears under the skin surface. If the temple is tight enough to press against this point, some persons experience severe pain. As shown in Chapter 7, tightness in the area only confounds the intended *spring* or *lock* effect of the portion below the midpoint of the back of the ear.

With the temples fitted, the dispenser is now ready to check over the whole fitting. A routine procedure is now a time-saver and often prevents regrets. Begin at the bridge and give the setting of the nasal pads another inspection. The change in inclination of the lens planes may have affected the fitting. Check the alignment of the x-axis of the lenses with the eyes. A quick approximation can be made by having the patient raise his eyes to the point that the line of ink dots is tangent to the lower margin of the iris. This observation is most accurately made when corneal reflections are the points of reference as discussed in the measurement of interocular distance. The vertical height of centers and multifocal segments is checked with the Dispenso-meter for the last time. The patient turns his head or the dispenser approaches the patient from the side to confirm the angle of inclination from the profile position. The symmetry of the vertex distances of the lenses is compared from above. The lashes on the upper lids are usually very near the same length and can be used as indicators. The separation between lens and eye can be

---

*Archer, John: Personal communication, 1955.

accurately estimated by watching the sweep of the lashes when the eyes are opened and closed a few times. Very strong lenses and iseikonic spectacles must also be checked on the Essel Pupillometer from the profile position as described in Chapter 16. After the clearance of the temples on the sides of the head is checked, only the balancing of temple tightness remains. There seems to be no more delicate test for this adjustment than to rest the elbows on the adjusting table and carefully lift the glasses off the nose with the second fingers, then pull the glasses slightly forward. Uneven fitting is usually felt rather easily. When in doubt, the first *direct* remark with reference to the fitting may be made to patient. It should not be "Are the bows comfortable?" A frank answer to the first impression of a new pair of glasses may be difficult. It could be "No." A better question might be "Does the pressure feel equal on your ears?"

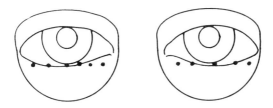

Figure 250. Properly set lenses.

After a pair of glasses has been most carefully balanced and the vertex distances precisely fixed, an occasional wearer will comment that one lens seems much closer than the other. Before he answers the remark, an optician should make sure of the cause, make his decision as to what should be done, and not alter his course. In the first place, the glasses may be out of adjustment in spite of careful work. Check the measurements with a Pupillometer or a millimeter rule from the side. If the glasses are true, the usual reason is a slightly fuller cheek or higher cheekbone on one side, or the brows may be asymmetric. Any of these anatomical vagaries will give a larger space or angle under one lens than the other. When the patient's head shape is the cause, either of two courses may be followed. If the lens power is very small and the asymmetry is not extreme, it is often easiest not to discuss the subject. Balance up the glasses for cosmetic effect. If the lenses are moderately strong or are multifocals, the lenses will be inaccurate and probably unsatisfactory if they are rotated on the y-axis and set out of the true frontal plane. In this case, it is best to refer tactfully to the necessity for accuracy of lens position, and so on, for the performance and comfort of the prescription. Sometimes an offer to favor that side as much as is safe for doctor's inspection is all that is necessary.

Another comment by the patient sometimes is that one segment seems higher than the other. A critical person can observe smaller differences than the optician can see, without assistance from equipment. Remove the judgment from personal opinion. Reset the Dispensometer.

Single vision lenses require no special technique at this point. Myopes all turn to look at distance and presbyopes are ready for a reading card. If the light level at the adjusting table is not high, a supplementary lamp should be turned on *before* the patient attempts to read. The doctor's findings were made under controlled conditions and a first effort with the lenses in a dim light can create a bad first impression with the new lenses. Unless the doctor has a habit of indicating visual acuity of his prescription or coding his prescriptions when acuity is subnormal, a dispenser must be cautious at this moment. A tactless remark like "Now you can read the small print" may cause no end of confusion. A much better comment is "Here's some work for your new glasses."

A *first* bifocal prescription or change in multifocal design gets off well to a first start by this method. Set the card on the adjusting table in natural reading position for the patient, turn on the reading light, put on the new glasses, but do not let go of the endpieces. With the fingertips hold the patient's head near primary position, then ask him to *look* at the reading chart. Now have him look over your shoulder at distance, then back at the reading card. Repeat this a few times while you are telling him the story of how to use his lenses. Finally release his head and let him practice a few times at developing the "marksmanship" that lets his eyes drop to the proper place to use the new near-point windows.

Once in a great while the patient may have some questions with reference to his glasses. Particularly is this true if vision is not as clear as expected at some point. There are four or five possible factors that singly or in combination may be the cause of the patient's perplexity. He may have eye disease. Although he may be aware of that, his hopes for radical improvement with lenses have not been realized and he is frustrated. Previous discussion of the accommodative-convergence relationship shows how some patients may have a temporary difficulty until the new conditions are accepted. In the case of multifocals, the patient may be confusedly trying to use his lenses at a distance different from the one that he and the doctor worked out so carefully. The glasses may not be correctly adjusted, but the routine should eliminate this possible cause. Finally, the doctor may also take exception to his prescription and alter it in the future after he has had an opportunity to judge the effect of the new lenses.

At the outset, it is obvious that an ophthalmic dispenser cannot make firm and authentic replies to all the questions that could be asked under these conditions. There is no set of answers that would be applicable in all cases. One's remarks should be tactfully based upon the fundamental situation and the inquiry or suggestions should be directed toward the obvious methods of relief. In the first place, make the comment that you have not yet given the glasses their final inspection (which, incidentally, you have not). Take the glasses to the lensometer, refer to the original copy of the prescription and check the lenses as if they were unknown glasses. Dot the centers and compare with the laboratory order. If there is a previous prescription, read it and note the differences. If there is a radical or suspicious change, ask the doctor to confirm the prescription. In this interval out of the patient's presence, the correct approach may be conceived. When the glasses are known to fill the prescription accurately, the patient is told to take them to the doctor for verification.

The patient should now be instructed in the handling of his glasses. These remarks should not be reserved for first-time wearers of glasses. Many individuals who have worn glasses for years know little about their glasses. Plastic frames are sufficiently heavy that they can be managed with one or both hands. Probably the best method is to grasp both endpieces with the fingertips and with the temples opened wide push the temple-tips back on the sides of the head to slip into position closely over the ear tops. A pair of skull-fitting temples may need another little tap on the temples near the tops of the ears to settle the tips of the temples into place. Demonstrate what a high temple does by lifting a temple off your own ear top. Remark what it does to all of the doctor's care in arriving at a precise prescription and also how it totally interferes with multifocal lenses.

Few persons handle a pair of riding-bow glasses correctly. A method about to be described is not the only way and many competent opticians may not consider it the best way. It has been used by a large number of fitters for many years. It can be taught quickly and will preserve the adjustment. If it is routinely used by a dispenser during his adjusting, he conditions the wearer to the "feel" or rhythm which assists him in the act of learning to handle the glasses.

To THE OPTICIAN: Open the temples for the glasses to be worn. Take the right endpiece between the thumb and forefinger of the left hand. Hold the left temple at the extreme tip between the right thumb and forefinger. If the wearer is a man, hook the right temple behind the ear and pull forward until it is about in the fitted position. Place the bridge on the nose in the proper position and let go of the endpiece with the left hand. The left temple will now be outside of the left ear. Raise it directly upward without straightening the bend at the top of the temple. When the temple has been raised slightly higher than the ear top, it will drop into place behind the top of the ear. A slight straightening of the temple concludes the fitting. A slight change in the technique is necessary for women and possibly to keep the plan simple it should be applied to all persons. Hold the glasses as before—endpiece with one hand and temple-tip with the other. First put the glasses on the nose, then raise the temple over one ear top without straightening the temple and let it fall in place. Take *both* hands off the glasses. Take the other temple-tip between thumb and fingertip. Raise this temple over the ear top and let it drop back into position without straightening the temple. It will be observed that when these instructions are followed, the points of contact with the glasses are widely separated. It is actually difficult to wrench or put much strain on the glasses as they are held. Since the glasses will not fall off when one temple is in position and the bridge is in place, the glasses are not held while the second temple is put in place.

To THE WEARER: Open your riding-bow rimless glasses for use. Take hold of the very tip of the right bow with your right thumb and forefinger in such a way you can easily see your thumbnail. Bring the glasses back toward your face and put the nosepiece in the proper position. Lift the right bow up high enough to put it over your ear top. Do not straighten out the hook at the end of the bow. Treat it as if it would break easily. When the bow is in place, let go of your glasses with *both hands*. Do not fear; they will not fall off. Now take hold of the tip of the left bow the same as you did on the right and lift the hook high enough to slip into place over the top of the ear.

This procedure works the same for zylo or rimless riding-bows. It is not varied for cable-comfort or xylo tip riding-bow. Children learn it as well as any method. If parents understand it thoroughly, it helps to keep children's glasses in better adjustment. Aged persons may have difficulty if their hands are not nimble. Probably zylo-covered skull temples should be used routinely for these patients.

Over a period of time the constant handling of the glasses by any method will loosen the temples slightly. If they are riding-bow and the wearer keeps them in a snug case part-time, the tension introduced by the case will almost compensate for the straightening of the temples while they are worn and handled. In most cases, the glasses will be slightly loose after a while. Reviewing the method of handling, one notes that the shaping and contouring of the end of the temple was carefully preserved when the temple was held at the very tip. Therefore, necessary tightening is merely a matter of reducing the angle at the top bend only. Many dexterous persons can be taught how to place the index finger inside the bend and bend down with the thumb from the outside for temporary relief. If the shape of no other part of the temple is molested, they cannot get into trouble. If the bend has been too abrupt, the bottom part of the ears will soon be uncomfortable and the pads will begin to bother. A slight reversal will cure the case temporarily. Interested parents should be shown these points because it is not always convenient to disrupt a school day to bring the child in for Aftercare Service and some children are at great disadvantage without their glasses in school.

At this point is a good time to give instructions in the use and care of glasses. It is sheer customer neglect if the story of the care of plastic lenses is not told now. This is a repetition of what has previously been read. *"Never wipe these lenses when they are dry. That is how they become scratched.* Hold the lenses under running water to flush off any hard particles on them. Moisten the fingertips and rub them on a bar of face soap (not Lava®) and rub the lenses lightly while the water is still running on them. Wipe the lenses with Kleenex®. Always rub up and down, never crosswise. Then you will know whether you ever scratch your lenses. With this care you will still have good lenses when they are replaced by your next prescription."

It seems human nature to be willing to make our greatest effort to take good care of something very new. Most people abuse glasses and in the end the abuse must contribute to eye fatigue. It is so easy to assume that a wearer knows how to handle a pair of glasses just because he has had glasses before. A glance at the old case or old lenses may contradict that idea at once. Tell each wearer how to handle his glasses, and how to avoid scratching his lenses. Tell him that scratched lenses are fatiguing and if bad enough actually reduce visual acuity. Tell why lenses can not be reground because accuracy is impaired, also that lenses are made as thin as permissible by FDA regulations in the first place and cannot be reground. Repeat why air-tempered lenses cannot be reground. Tell why some bifocal types cannot be reground because the size and shape of the reading portion will be tremendously reduced in size and the accurate fitting destroyed. Tell how carelessness may make it necessary to replace the lenses long before a prescription change.

Teach the patient how to wipe his lenses. Plastic frames, of course, do not require the care in handling that must be given to rimless glasses and metal frames, but a few moments should be spent with every patient on the handling and washing of spectacles. In times gone by some opticians said such extravagant things about spectacle lenses that patients handled their glasses in awe. Tell patients that glass lenses are polished with cloth in the lens factories and that any clean soft cloth will not injure an ophthalmic lens surface. Remark that lens cleaner is convenient for glass because it dissolves grease, and that oiliness from contact with the skin reduces lens efficiency. Tell patients they may wash their glasses with hand-soap and water from time to time. Tell patients to use a worn-out toothbrush to clean up the metal parts of the frame if they wish and that a brush with soap and water is good to clean up the edges of lenses in a plastic frame. Then tell them that you are not trying to push the job off on them, that you are equipped to do the job quickly and easily if they are afraid to do it. Reprove patients for the abuse of their old lenses and tell them to mend their ways with their new ones. Tell them that the glass in multifocals is not always the same hardness all over, that scratches cannot be removed.

After all proper instructions and recommendations are made to the patient, advise him, "with all the best care you can give these glasses, they are going to get out of alignment. Even an optician's glasses get bent. The important thing is that you come in from time to time to let us look them over and service them for you. Pay attention to the date on your Appointment Card and do not neglect to come in for service before the month expires. Even if they feel all right, come in as often as your Appointment Card requires and let us straighten and tighten them up. The Aftercare is a part of the service of making these glasses for you. Remember that the doctor's prescription and our work in interpreting it are no more accurate than the fitting of the glasses." It is not only necessary to tell patients that Aftercare is necessary, they must be told that you are prepared and willing to do it and that your interest in their eyes and glasses continues. Note the parting remark is *not*, "If you have trouble, come in," or "Come in when your glasses are out of adjustment." The first remark assumes a negative attitude. The second suggests that the wearer has the knowledge and means to find (like an optician) when his eyewear is out of alignment.

Tell your customer that with the best of care that in time his eyewear will be out of alignment and that you stand ready in your commitment to aftercare to give these lenses all the care they need until doctor decides they should be replaced.

When the customer returns take out his record and look at it a moment before you work on the eyewear. Make a record of the date of Aftercare Service and your initials on the Record Card. Chide your customers when they do not return before the expiration of their Appointment Cards.

Regularly using the record at alignment time will put an obstacle in the way of a competitor (without a record) seeing your customer.

The first Appointment Card notifies the patient he is neglectful if he does not have his glasses serviced from time to time and that you are cordially awaiting the opportunity to care for him. Some persons seem to respond when the thought is impressed that the price of the glasses includes the Aftercare and they should avail themselves of it for the health and hygiene of their eyes. When large numbers of spectacle wearers are observed in theaters, restaurants, church, or sports, it is quite evident that the care of glasses and the need of at least occasional reconditioning has not been sufficiently impressed. There is a possibility that some of the glasses never have been properly fitted and that the wearers are unaware of the degree of comfort attainable through the professional assistance of a competent optician. However, there are many other pairs of glasses that suggest that they must have been accurately fitted at one time and that their present condition is only a matter of abuse or neglect. Well-fitted, comfortably fitted glasses that are kept that way are good salesmen for both the doctor and the optician.

Records over many years show that more than 33 percent of the traffic in a prosperous ophthalmic dispenser's store is patients returning for Aftercare Services. If the percentage is lower than that amount, customers are going elsewhere for the services. This patient turnover impedes growth. Studies show that the reasons they do not return are (a) they were not impressed that the service could be done better by the original dispenser and that he still had an interest in the glasses, (b) delays or loss of time in connection with services, (c) attitude of indifference or at least lack of enthusiasm which caused him to feel unwelcome, and (d) technical inadequacy—that is, fitting difficulties or discomforts that were not relieved. All these situations are easily correctable. The proper parting remark disposes of the first impression. The others are a matter of relations and conduct after the patient has returned. When the "only an adjustment" attitude is changed to an "invited caller with whom relations are being renewed and improved," the second and third situations are relieved. There is no other continuing service through a lifetime that have such a long cycle as eye examination and glasses. Most persons see their dentist much oftener. The patient's call for a small service or adjustment to his glasses is an important opportunity to renew acquaintance with him. The enthusiasm with which he is received and the attitude of everyone who contacts him at the time of this service are important. Anything less than graciousness may suggest to the patient that an offer was made that was not seriously intended. Some persons are extremely sensitive about any kind of a gratuity, therefore extreme tact is necessary. When a patient has interrupted his own routine enough to come in for an eyewear Aftercare, as far as he is concerned something is sufficiently wrong to justify the effort. No adjustment should be blithely done and passed off lightly as being a matter of small importance, but it is not honest to exaggerate the act of reconditioning the glasses. The matter is important but usually not grave.

The widespread use of plastic frames has reduced the frequent returns of the days of rimless eyeglasses, but the servicing on these frames cannot be done as quickly or as simply. A few quick "passes" at an adjusting table are seldom sufficient or satisfactory. The preferred procedure is to take the patient's glasses from him and give them to a technician at the laboratory bench for the checkup. The receptionist or whoever greets the patient can easily say, "when our customers come in for their Aftercare Service, we like to do a thorough job because it usually requires some effort to get in for Service."

At the laboratory bench, the glasses can be thoroughly inspected and corrected. All the necessary tools and accessories are readily available to replace screws, tighten endpieces, and so forth. Careful cleaning and repolishing of the metal parts can be efficiently done. Even the person who feels that he is in a great hurry will spare the time when he realizes that a thorough job is being done. An ideal arrangement is to take the patient's prescription from the file and put it in the tray with the glasses to be tightened and straightened. Several advantages accrue. When the laboratory man has the prescription before him, he can align the lenses precisely. The dispenser has the advantage of the prescription and any special comments on it while he is delivering the reconditioned glasses. He can reply to the question about the date the glasses were made, which is usually at least 50 percent longer than the wearer realizes. Sometimes, too, there may have been some recent development that is particularly applicable for the patient plus the advantages previously mentioned.

When the serviced spectacles are brought from the laboratory, they should be lined up with the Dispensometer in the same way they were at the original fitting. The dispenser should always compare strong lens prescriptions with the record. After the fitting of the frame is completed, the lenses should be cleaned. If the lens surfaces are scratched, some comment should be made and a warning given about proper care. The patient is now given the opportunity to express his impression with reference to his vision. Among these patients are some who have had a rapid decline in vision from some pathological cause. If the glasses are known to be set precisely as they were before, it is a logical deduction for the patient that he should see the doctor about his eyes. The reading card should always be presented to presbyopes and as they move from *early* to *middle* and *advanced* presbyopia, the Hutchinson card is convenient to let the patient also evaluate his acuity at intermediate distance.

REVIEW

1. What is the geometric principle which causes a datum rule or Dispensometer to center a pair of glasses so that the midline of the lenses falls on the 180° line?

2. Why should the new eyewear be carefully controlled the first few times the lenses are placed in front of the wearer's eyes?

3. When should the temple spread and pantoscopic angle of

new eyewear be set to specifications?

4. What do temples that are tight in front of the ears do?

5. Do you think the time saved in not procuring sufficiently long temples is offset by repeated adjustments and realignments with the risk that a competitor may solve the misfit? Express your resolution.

6. Give the steps for the cleaning of CR39 lenses.

7. Discuss why reference to record and recording each transaction is advantageous.

8. Discuss the importance of an organized plan for Continuing Aftercare Service.

Chapter 19

ORTHOPTIC DEVICES

◆◆◆

A portion of the services of an ophthalmic dispenser is to act as a source of supply for the fusion training equipment that doctors may prescribe for patients to use at home. In the same vein of thought that a dispenser can well afford to have at least a superficial knowledge of refraction to serve the doctor and his patient best, it is equally important to have some idea of the uses of the implements for orthoptic training.

One of the simplest requests is an order for a single or group of square plano prisms. The doctor will have instructed his patient in the way the prism is to be used. There are at least two purposes for which it is found useful. In the same way that Positive and Negative Relative Convergence was measured, the function of fusion can be exercised. The doctor may have instructed his patient to put a lighted candle or an object on a sheet of white paper and move the prism in and out of the line of sight while the eyes hold fixation on the object. If the eyes continue to hold fixation, they would necessarily have to turn to compensate for the prism displacement. As shown in Figures 54 and 123, the direction is determined by the position of the base of the prism. When the object is seen singly, the eye behind the prism must look toward the image that is apparently displaced toward the apex of the prism. Thus a prism (or prisms) placed Base Out before the eyes causes the eyes to converge when single vision is maintained and, conversely, the eyes diverge when the prism is Base In. As variation to the procedure, the doctor may have instructed his patient to approach the object or candle closely holding the prism Base Out, then slowly back away from it with the prism held in position. The amount of the deviation of light caused by the prism is comparatively small at first, but as he backs away, the amount of deviation gradually increases. Further, when he is very close to the object, he accommodates and normally converges a rather large amount. As he increases his distance from the object, less accommodation is required, but the increasing displacement caused by the prism demands an increasing amount of convergence if he is to continue to see singly. This exercise is sometimes called a "backward marathon." The project, of course, is for the patient to attempt to increase the distance from the lightsource each time before he has double vision. The doctor may order one or more rather strong prisms or a series of weaker prisms for this exercise. In the second instance, the patient is told to stack up the weaker prisms as they can be overcome and thereby increase the prism effect. The doctor may also prescribe the use of a prism at home to awaken a sense of double vision which may have become dormant if one eye is turned out of line. A piece of red glass or cellophane is frequently placed over the prism in this procedure to emphasize further the presence of the second image.

Some children who have crossed-eyes finally have seriously impaired vision in the turned eye. This condition, called *amblyopia ex anopsia*,* can be improved by one means only—the eye must be made to do its work again. This is accomplished generally by covering the other eye or setting up conditions that demand the vision of the "turned" eye to accomplish the task. In the first instance, Bel-occluders, Pro-Optic and clip-on occluders are widely used. The clip-on occluders are safer out of doors because the wearer still has some indirect vision on that side. The Bel-occluders, which cover the eye completely, are preferred for indoor use when the child is reading or otherwise employed at the near point.

An optician must not presume to know when nor why the occluder or prism is to be used. When there seems to be some confusion about the wearing time or training procedure, it is best for the patient's parent or the optician to ask the doctor for a review of the instructions.

The Dobson Amblyopic Reader† is another approach in the

---

*Scobee, R.G.: *A Child's Eyes.* St. Louis, Mosby, 1949, pp. 59-69.
†Dobson, M.: *Amblyopia Reader.* London, Rembrandt Photogravure, 1940.

treatment of this condition. This book is printed in two colors of ink. The child wears a red filter lens over the better eye while the book is read. The filter causes all red objects and letters to disappear before the better eye and thereby the amblyopic eye is stimulated to see everything printed in red.

The same principle is applied in the New Era Duo-Chrome Drawing Set. A pair of red and green color filters are put on over the glasses and the child attempts to trace green lines that can be seen with one eye and a red colored pencil tip that is seen better with the other. The drawings are printed with pale green ink; when the green filter is placed before the better eye the picture disappears on that side, while through the red filter the picture is quite pronounced.

The Maddox Cheiroscope is also made as a home training device. In its simplest form, the frame is made of wood. As shown in Figure 251, one eye sees a reflection of the picture in the holder at the side and because of the angle of the mirror, the virtual image is projected straight forward. When the amblyopic eye attempts to guide a pencil to trace the image as it appears on the drawing paper, the eye is being trained to see again. This instrument is a kind of stereoscope.* When the drawing on the paper is a duplicate of the picture in the holder, the eyes receive the separate images and interpret them as a single picture in the same way that identical images are received by the two eyes in normal binocular vision and are superimposed (fused) into a single impression. All instruments for the training of binocular vision are based upon the principle of a stereoscope or (when mirrors are

*Cantonnet, A. and Filliozat, J.: *Strabismus.* London, M. Wiseman, 1939, pp. 33-76.

Wells, D.W.: *The Stereoscope in Ophthalmology.* Boston, Mahady Company, 1926, pp. 15-17.

Gibson, H.W.: *Clinical Orthoptics.* London, Hatton Press, 1947, pp. 58-69.

Giles, G.H: *The Practice of Orthoptics* London, Hammond, 1947, pp 230-231.

Krimsky, E.: *Binocular Imbalance.* Philadelphia, Lea & Febiger, 1948, pp. 365-416.

Lyle, T.K. and Jackson, S.: *Practical Orthoptics.* Philadelphia, Blakiston, 1949, pp. 21-29.

Smith, W.: *Clinical Orthoptic Procedure.* St. Louis, Mosby, 1950, pp. 79-92.

Velasek, J.: *Theoretical and Experimental Optics.* New York, Wiley, 1949, pp. 101-105.

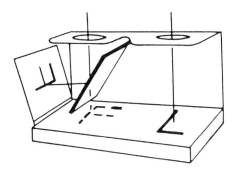

Figure 251. Scheme of Maddox cheiroscope.

used) haploscope. A large number of the prescriptions are for the various charts and cards to be used with the different forms of stereoscopes. An understanding of the purposes of the cards requires some knowledge of the stereoscope as an optical device.

The photographs taken for regular stereoscopic viewing are made from the negatives of a camera with two lenses. The axes of the lenses are 3 inches apart. One could say that the camera has an interocular distance of 76 mm. The stereoscope made to view the pictures has +5.00D. spherical lenses in it, the centers of which are separated by 76 mm, the same as the camera. As can be seen in Figure 252, a pair of luminous points at the centers of the cards are projected as parallel rays. Therefore, if a pair of "ideal" eyes are placed in any position in front of the lenses, the two points in the objects will be superimposed without any accommodative or convergence effort and the illusion is a single star or light-source at great distance. It is immediately apparent that a stereoscope has no "pupillary distance" and performs the same for child or adult. It is also evident that if the eyes need correction lenses, the picture would be out of focus in precisely the same way it would be with uncorrected distance vision. Also, if the eyes have a tendency to turn or actually do turn away from parallel when fixation is at infinity, the images of the luminous points would not be superimposed. They would be separated, and so long as the eyes functioned simultaneously, the luminous points of light would be double.

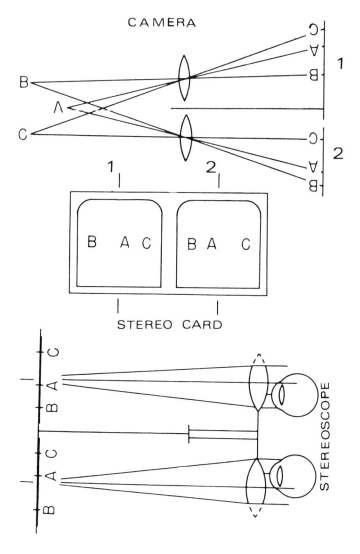

Figure 252. Analysis of stereoscopic photography and stereoscopic cards.

As a stereoscope is designed, the slide bar supporting the card holder is somewhat longer than the focal length of the lenses in the hood. The blurred picture for a slightly hypermetropic patient without glasses is cleared if the card is moved away from the

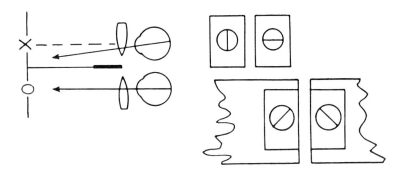

Figure 253. Analysis of fusion training with stereoscopic cards.

hood. A nearsighted patient sees the picture clearly if the card is pulled toward his face.

The double vision to which we have just referred can be corrected by only one method. The luminous points must be set at the points where the projection of the patient's visual axes intersect the card. Figure 253 shows how the centers of the cards must be closer together than 76 mm for eyes that converge, and, conversely, must be wider apart for eyes that diverge. The ordinary stereoscopic photograph is not adjustable, so this compensation must be accomplished otherwise.

If the card cannot be adjusted to the eyes, it becomes necessary to adjust the eyes to the card. Referring again to the discussion of Relative Convergence, it was noted that a stimulation to either accommodation or convergence caused a reflex stimulation to the other. The adjustment of the steroscope is accomplished by this interrelationship. It will be noted in Figure 254 that when the card is brought inside of the focal distance of the +5.00D. lenses, accommodation is stimulated, but the centers of the pictures subtend increasing *divergent* angles when the card is drawn closer to the eyes. Beyond the focal point an uncorrected hypermetrope relaxes accommodation, but convergence must be stimulated to account for the diminishing angle between the card centers. Thus it is seen that when the card is moved either direction from the focal point of the lenses the functions of accommodation and con-

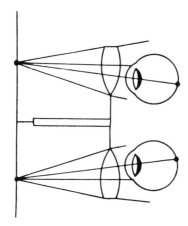

Figure 254. Fusion training with ordinary stereoscope.

vergence are inversely stimulated and inhibited. When the card is drawn toward the eyes, accommodation is stimulated and convergence is inhibited (in fact, the eyes must diverge) ; when the card is moved past the focal distance of the lenses, accommodation is relaxed and convergence is stimulated. Therefore, any person who has no or at most a small refractive error can use a stereoscope without glasses after some slight adjusting of the slide, if his eyes are not too badly out of alignment horizontally.

When proper glasses are worn, the user of the stereoscope whose eyes are parallel or slightly divergent can still use the instrument. If the eyes turn out (exophoria), the card is slowly drawn toward the eyes to stimulate accommodation and likewise inhibit convergence the proper amounts to turn the fixation lines to corresponding points on the stereoscopic photographs. It is now apparent that, if the patient's eyes are convergent (esophoria or esotropia) and he is emmetropic or wears his regular correction, he cannot use the stereoscope for pictures with centers 76 mm apart. At the focal distance of the lenses, his projected visual axes intersect the card at a distance less than 76 mm. If the card is moved farther away, the picture blurs from overcorrection. If the picture is brought closer to his eyes, accommodation and convergence are stimulated. The maladjustment between fixation lines and the centers of the pictures is further aggravated as the eyes continue to converge at a greater angle.

A large number of the patients for whom fusion training is prescribed are children with convergent strabismus. It has been shown that cards with standard separation of centers would be useless for them, and that the greater the degree of squint, the closer the centers of the cards would have to approach one another. Provision has been made for these very conditions in the series of training cards designed by Javal, Sattler, Guibor, and Berens. The pictures in these groups are not mounted as stereoscopic photographs. The two halves of each picture are on separate cards. A special holder is provided so that the distance between centers can be shortened materially. The Keystone View Company accomplishes the same result when the pictures are affixed to separate stereoscopic mounts. These training cards are called Split-Slides.

It might be interesting to consider the limit of convergence error for which compensation could be made with sliding adjustable cards. The focal distance of the lenses in the stereoscope (+5.00D.) is 0.2 meter, therefore each 2 mm of displacement of similar objects on the stereoscopic card causes a deviation of $1^\triangle$. If the individual cards are 30 mm in diameter and the normal distance of separation is 76 mm, the cards can be moved toward one another until they touch. In this position the visual lines must converge $23^\triangle$ to see the pictures singly ($76 - 30 = 46$ mm $\div 2 = 23^\triangle$ or about 12 arc degrees).

But again, the stereoscope is adaptable (Fig. 255). A model is available with clips to hold auxiliary prisms in front of the lens cells. Except for very large objects, however, it is recommended that not more than $15^\triangle$ be added to each side because of the blur

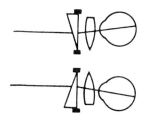

Figure 255. Supplementary prisms on stereoscope.

caused by the introduction of excessive chromatic aberration and distortion which interfere with fusion.

Worth* described fusion as having three degrees. Although orthoptists have made some further subdivisions in recent years, his classical definitions are still popularly used. Degree I is defined as simultaneous macular perception. This degree has been reached when the bad habit of monocular vision of the squinting patient has been broken up to the point where the central portions of the two retinas are mentally perceiving the images which fall upon them at the same time. The card in the training set typical of Degree I is the bird and cage. One eye sees the cage and the other sees the bird (Fig. 256). When the bird appears to be in the cage, both eyes are seeing, and more important, perceiving at the same time. When the centers of the pictures can be adjusted to the point where they favorably agree with the angle of the patient's squint, and thus permit the objects to be viewed with central (macular) vision, then it can be said that the patient has Degree I fusion. The definition of the training cards for Degree I is a pair of pictures in which no part of one picture is in the field of the other eye, but the two objects depicted have some kind of mental association: bird and cage, ball and basket, lion and cage, etcetera. These are the "A" series in the AO Wells Series of Training Cards.

The next development is to superimpose similar images and demonstrate some ability to hold them together against convergence stress. The typical card of Degree II is the letter "F" on one card and the letter "L" on the other, which, when they are superimposed or "fused," give the impression of the letter "E." The vertical line of the letter "F" is common with the line of the letter "L." The two legs at the top of the "E" are supplied by the "F"

*Worth, C.: *Squint.* London, 1929.

Chavasse, F.B.: *Worth's Squint,* 7th ed. Philadelphia, Blakiston, 1939.

Giles, G.H.: *The Practice of Orthoptics.* London, Hammond, 1947.

Lyle, T.K. and Jackson, S.: *Practical Orthoptics.* Philadelphia, Blakiston, 1949.

Krimsky, E.: *Binocular Imbalance.* Philadelphia, Lea & Febiger, 1948.

Lyle, T.K.: *Worth and Chavasse's Squint.* London, Balliere, Tyndall & Cox, 1950.

Ogle, K.N.: *Binocular Vision.* Philadelphia, Saunders, 1950.

Scobee, R.G.: *Oculorotary Muscles.* St. Louis, Mosby, 1947.

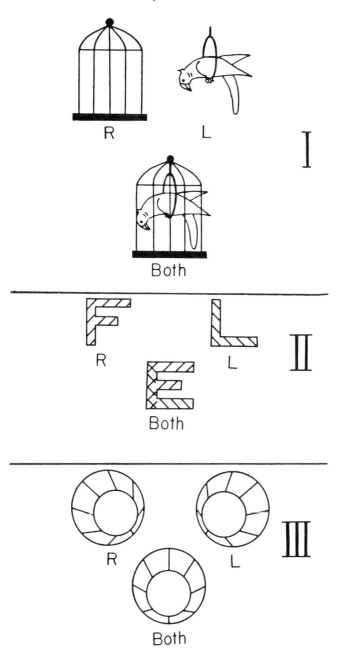

Figure 256. Analysis of three grades of fusion training cards.

and the leg at the bottom is supplied by the "L." In the parlance of orthoptists, the vertical line is called the *lock* and the legs are termed the *controls*. The lock is the part of the picture appearing on both sides. The controls appear on one side and not on the other. They are the proof that both eyes are perceiving the picture simultaneously and that fusion is actually taking place. Examples of the cards for Degree II are the jack o'lantern with one eye missing in each picture. When both eyes are seen simultaneously the viewer is seeing with both eyes. In another set, the letters "on" appears in one picture and "ne" in the other. When the "n" superimposes, the letters spell the word "one." These are the "C" series in the Wells set.

The third and final accomplishment is depth perception or stereopsis and is termed Degree III. When a three-dimensional object, such as a cube, is placed a short distance from the eyes, one sees the shape from different angles of parallax with the two eyes. Figure 256 shows two views of a basket as seen by the right and left eyes when both eyes see the basket, the slightly dissimilar images are fused and the sensation of depth or volume is created. It is suggested that some cubical object, such as shoe box or large book, be set about three or four feet away and the object be surveyed with one eye, then the other, and finally with both eyes open. Let this be repeated from several different angles. It is important to gain an appreciation of the noticeably different retinal images formed by the right and left eyes. Note how the nearest point of the object always seems to point toward the nose as first one eye and then the other is covered. Thus we find that the images seem to rotate in such a way that the images of the objects closest to the eyes require greater convergence.

Place a regular stereoscopic photograph in a stereoscope and study it carefully. Choose the item that seems to be the closest and the one that seems to be the farthest away. Remove the photograph from the stereoscope and note whether there are any apparent differences to be found in the right and left pictures. Are there any lines or shapes in the pictures that suggest the perspective lines of the cube in Figure 256? Take a millimeter rule or a pair of dividers and measure the distance in the two pictures between corresponding parts of the object that appears to be farthest away. Now compare the measurement of the object that seems closest. It will be noted that the corresponding parts of the nearest object are much nearer together. This is what is to be expected when the picture is compared with the visual experiment above. The nearest object requires more convergence than an object at greater distance.

Stereoscopic pictures designed to test and train Degree III fusion are usually specially prepared with *controls* much like the two-dimensional Degree II cards. It is necessary to make sure that neither eye suppresses vision while these similar pictures are viewed. Oftentimes the card has many numerals distributed over the picture or lines or other geometric designs in the foreground at different distances while the two stereoscopic photographs in the background become the *lock*.

This type of card is used not only to develop and train the binocular vision of squinting children but also to develop the visual skills and build fusion reserves for adults The Keystone View Company makes a number of different series of cards for special purposes. By way of example, the Alpha set is termed a Base Out or convergence stimulating set. If this set is opened and the distance between the objects at the apparent greatest distance is measured, it will be found that the object will be 76 to 78 mm apart. The closest object will be found to be several millimeters narrower. If the same scene is measured on the succeeding cards, it will be found that while the distances in the background do not vary, the same objects in the foreground are closer together in each succeeding picture. Each new card requires a greater convergence effort to fuse the pictures. If the latter cards are viewed in a stereoscope, it will be found that the effect of depth has been exaggerated and that all objects in the picture are grotesquely elongated toward the viewer. It has now been shown that one can identify the intended use of a series of cards with a millimeter rule. The Beta set for Base In effect or divergence stimulation shows the greatest variation in the background at the points where convergence is inhibited.

Recently Bausch & Lomb has developed some sets of cards to do the same type of training described above without the use of a conventional stereoscope. The unique application of polarized light is named Orthofuser.® A pair of Polaroid® spectacles is supplied in which the axis of polarization is axis 45 for one eye and axis 135 for the other. Several special pictures are supplied on which two polarized films are mounted. The right eye sees one film and the other is polarized out. The left eye sees the other picture but not the one seen by the right eye. The pictures are covered with a series of controls set for highly exaggerated stereoscopic effects. This training routine is essentially a near-point exercise because the device has no lenses to inhibit accommodation. It is desirable to have such a routine available for doctors because the greater part of the symptoms reported by patients come from difficulties in the use of the eyes at near-point.

The Keystone View Company also provides some special sets of charts for squinting children, but as has been shown, a standard stereoscope is limited for higher angles of squint. A Home-Trainer is available with a sort of desk top for a card-holder. The slide-bar of the stereoscope fits into a slot in the top. This device is excellent for stereoscopic cards in which the halves of the pictures are separately mounted to permit slidable adjustment. These "split slides" are available to train all three degrees of squint. The table also makes a convenient surface for the drawing routine when the doctor has prescribed it. This enterprising firm makes frequent changes and improvements in the training series. Their catalogues and manuals are highly informative and instructive.

Make the acquaintance of and visit the office of an orthoptist. Inquire if there is anything that you can do or materials you should have available. Take a demonstration of the synoptiscope, synoptiphore, or troposcope if possible. The average orthoptist will respond to your interest in the work.

A dispenser must be just as careful in the discussion of this very profound subject as he would be in a discussion of pathology or refraction. It is important that an ophthalmic dispenser know what these instruments and products are used for and be able to assist the doctor in any way that he may request in the explanation of his order for the use of the apparatus—but at that point he should abruptly stop! Strabismus, its diagnosis, surgery, and treatment have had the attention of the keenest minds in the professions for centuries and still is far from a finished subject.

No dispenser can afford to venture any opinions about any part of this work.

The publication, *Your Child's Eyes,* written by R.G. Scobee, M.D., is invaluable. It is written in layman's language and simply but accurately tells the story of binocular vision. Parents of cross-eyed children or others who wish to understand the purpose of orthoptic training will be authoritatively informed by this small book published by C.V. Mosby, St. Louis, Mo.

REVIEW

1. Describe the optics of a Maddox Cheiroscope.

2. Discuss a stereo-camera and the stereoscope that views the pictures.

3. What is the special usefulness of split slides?

4. Describe the three degrees of fusion as projected by Worth. Give the typical card used to identify each category.

5. Explain how Polaroid is used in the viewing of stereoscopic pictures. What are the advantages?

Chapter 20

REFLECTIONS AT SPECTACLE
LENS SURFACES

◆◆◆◆◆◇◆◆◆◆◆◆◆◆◆◆◆◆◆◆◆◆◆◆◆ ◆◆◆◆◆◆◆◆◆◆◆◆◆◆◆◆◆◆◆◆◆◆◆◆◆◆◆

A small part of the light that strikes a lens surface is reflected. This part of the incident light is focussed as if the lens surface were a curved mirror. Under some conditions, usually indoors, this reflected light forms visible images that are occasionally troublesome to spectacle wearers. These images can be formed by a large number of combinations of reflection and refraction at the surfaces of a lens but only a few of them are significant. This subject was so thoroughly discussed by W.B. Rayton of Bausch & Lomb in 1917* that little has been added to date.

The problems of surface reflections are like the location of this chapter. They are near the end. Surface coating in its diverse forms has almost obliterated a troublesome complaint of years gone by. Probably it was at first a frustration because information was sparce.

Recently the Hoya Optical Company of Japan has established a stock depot and laboratory in Torrance, California, under the name of Hoya Lens of America. One of their first innovations was the presentation of lenses with multiple surface coatings which almost completely transmit all the light incident upon them. Thus the lenses are nearly invisible and produce practically no reflections. This is a great advance over lenses with a single coating of a single chemical. These new lenses obliterate the difficulties discussed in this chapter.

---

*Rayton, W.B.: Reflections in spectacle lenses. *J Opt Soc Am,* 7:1917. Reprinted in *Ophthalmic Reference Book.* Bausch & Lomb, 1941.

von Rohr: *Ueber Spiegelbilder und Brillen glaeser.* Zeitschrift fuer Opthalmoligische Optik, Dec. 5, 1913.

Morgan, M. and Peters, H.B.: *The Optics of Ophthalmic Lenses.* Berkeley, U of Cal Pr, 1948, pp. 92-96.

The following are the conditions under which specular images cause a spectacle wearer some difficulties: (a) The image formed by the lens surfaces must be close enough to the fixation line to be superimposed upon the object fixed or near enough to it to cause a distraction. In other words, direction of the reflected and refracted rays must be nearly coaxial. (b) The image must be bright enough to stand out against its background, Reflections are seldom noticed out of doors because of the high level of illumination. (c) This reflected light proceeds from a bright object in space which is determined only by the position of the light source and the spectacle lens curves. This wave front enters the eye as if no correction were being worn. It is sharply in focus if the image plane is within the range between the far-point of the uncorrected eye and the near-point of accommodation. In practice, the patients who are troubled most are myopes up to —6.00D. to —8.00D. and young hyperopic persons who have weak lens prescriptions and large accommodative amplitudes. In both instances the image planes are distances that range from 15 to 70 cm. As we give brief attention to the literature the reasons are apparent.

The amount of light reflected from a source normal to a lens surface as found by Fresnel is

$$I_R = \left(\frac{n-1}{n+1}\right)^2 I$$

where I_R = intensity reflected
I = original intensity
n = index of refraction.

When we take $I = 1$ and $n = 1.523$, the index of regular ophthalmic crown glass,

$$I_R = \left(\frac{1.523-1}{1.523+1}\right)^2 = 0.0428$$

Therefore, slightly more than 4 percent of the light is reflected, and, of course, 95.72 percent is transmitted by the front surface. When this same formula is applied to the second surface

$$0.0428 \times 0.9572 = 0.0410$$

another 4.1 percent is returned in the direction of the object

$$0.9572 - 0.0410 = 0.9162$$

and slightly less than 92 percent of the original intensity is transmitted at the second surface.

Rayton showed that three types of reflections account for 99.99 percent of the light incident upon the lens from the front side. When the reflections of luminous objects situated behind the lens are added, practically all the "ghosts" and "bright spots" have been accounted for. His identifications of the five most significant cases are

I. The image of an object behind the lens imaged by reflection from the back surface of the lens.

II. The image of an object back of the head imaged by reflections from the front surface of the lens together with two refractions through the back surface.

III. The image of an object in front of the lens imaged by reflection from the cornea and the front surface of the lens and refraction at both surfaces.

IV. The image of an object in front of the lens imaged by reflection of the cornea and the back surface of the lens after refraction at both surfaces.

V. The image of an object in front of the lens imaged by double reflection within the lens and one refraction at each surface.

The formulas for the location of the image distances are prepared from an assumed vertex distance of 12 mm. The lens is assumed to be infinitely thin for convenience. An assumption of thickness would make the calculations unduly tedious and add nothing significant to the conclusions. The effect of refraction at the lens surfaces is not considered. It, too, is insignificant in weak lenses and accumulates a dioptric value of only 1.5D. at the limit of +20.00D. with the incidental lens thickness. To put the formulas in convenient form for immediate investigation of a specific problem, each reflection type is equated to the dioptric curve of the front surface of a lens that would place the image at the far point of the uncorrected eye. In other words, the solution to the formula is the worst form of that lens power. Each of the formulas will be applied to a —3.00D. lens which corrects a myopic eye with a far point of 33 cm.

(I) $D_1 = \dfrac{(1+n)}{2} D$

$= \dfrac{2.523}{2} \times -3$

$= -3.78D$

(II) $D_1 = -\dfrac{(1-n)}{(2)} D$

$= -\dfrac{1-1.523}{2} \times (-3)$

$= -0.78D.$

(III) $D_1 = -\dfrac{(n-1)}{(2)} D + \dfrac{(n-1)}{(2)} 62.5$

$= -\dfrac{.523}{2} \times (-3) + \dfrac{.523}{2} \times 62.5$

$= 0.78 + 16.34$

$= +17.12D$

(IV) $D_1 = \dfrac{(n+1)}{(2)} D + \dfrac{(n-1)}{(2)} 62.5$

$= \dfrac{2.523}{2} \times (-3) + \dfrac{.523}{2} \times 62.5$

$= -3.78 + 16.34$

$= +12.56D.$

The formula for the case of interreflection becomes

$$D = \dfrac{(3n-1)}{(n-1)} D$$

which is satisfied when $D = 0$ regardless of the shape of the lens. This reflection is the bothersome one in very weak power lenses when the lens curves are nearly concentric. It is a function of lens power and cannot be removed by any change in lens profile. On occasion the patient can be pacified by increasing the dioptric power of the base curve. The "bright spots" are not removed, but they are sometimes ignored if the position in space is changed.

When reflections I, II, III, and IV are reviewed as applied to —3.00D. it is seen that the front curves calculated have no relationship to standard ophthalmic lens curves.

I $= -3.78D.$

II $= -0.78D.$

III $= +17.12D.$

IV $= +12.56D.$

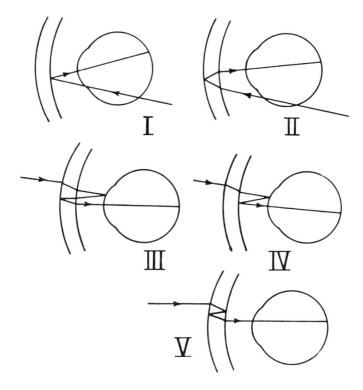

Figure 257.   Illustration of different surface reflections.

For example, an Orthogon —3.00D. sphere uses +5.35D. front curve.   In all instances, the incident light from the object is assumed to come from infinity.   In practice, a proper combination of luminous objects at some finite distance and change in vertex distance of lens could still provide an annoying reflection.

When all the factors are considered, it can be shown that to find a reflection-free form for all prescriptions approaches an impossibility.   The change in refractive power of the eye in the act of accommodation alters the requirements.   All astigmatic eyes with two focal planes corrected with lenses having two focal planes also complicates the project.   Reflections III and IV in which the surface of the cornea is involved produce very small images which frequently can be obliterated by a small change in the vertex distance. Reflection III is potentially the problem in the correction after cataract surgery when the front surface of the correcting lens is about 12 mm in front of the cornea.

SURFACE COATING

Some time elapsed between the discovery that some optical instruments with oxidized lens surfaces transmitted more light than those with new fresh lenses. Finally physicists solved the problem by vacuum coating new lenses with a very thin (0.000147 mm) low refractive index metal deposit and thereby quickly obtained a predictable "bloom" on lens surfaces that vastly surpassed the effect obtained by the lengthy ordeal of "weathering." Now instead of glass lenses transmitting about 92 percent and reflecting about 8 percent of light, the new coated lenses sometimes transmitted almost 98 percent.

The attention of ophthalmic optics concentrated *not upon transmission* but upon the new means to reduce reflected light. Concave lenses would now not appear so glassy. All lenses would be less conspicuous. The problem of bothersome surface reflections would be solved.

The phenomenon is accomplished by what physicists call destructive light interference. Returning to waves on a placid body of water, interference is the effect of the meeting of waves of equal strength. At this point the radiating rings of waves lose their identity and shortly the water is surprisingly placid again. The interference of the waves annulled the wave action of one another. The thin coating on the lens surface interferes with the returning (reflected) waves from the back surface of the metallic coating and destroys the reflection.

Figure 258 is an attempt to represent the reflection of a single undulation of a light wave after passing into a coating one quarter of a wavelength thick. When the undulation strikes the metal-glass interface it is returned 180° out of phase (mirror reversal) with the oncoming waves. By the time the undulation has returned to the metal-air surface it is a half wavelength out of phase with the oncoming waves and is destroyed. Let it be understood that the drawing is only a schematic presentation attempting to show why practically all of the light waves that fall upon an antireflection coating are transmitted and do not return as reflected light.

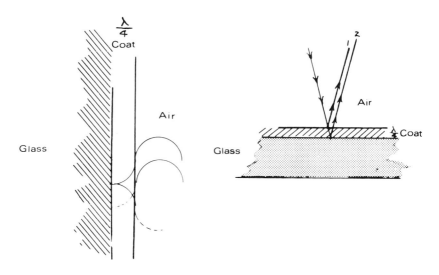

Figure 258. Analysis of surface reflection interference.

Another way of stating the case is that the wave which has gone through and returned through a coating which is one quarter of a wavelength thick has travelled one half of a wavelength. Therefore the crest of the reflected wave meets the crest of the oncoming wave and is neutralized.

Since each color has an individual wavelength, the thickness of a coating could be perfect for only one color. The color yellow was chosen because it is at the point in the spectrum where visibility is the keenest. This selection causes the coating to be somewhat too thick for the shorter wavelengths at the blue end of the spectrum and also a little too thin for the longer wavelengths at the red end. In the proper lighting a coated lens reflects a magenta or purplish cast.

The first public participation in the benefits of the new development was motivated by producer David Selznick when he stipulated that all of the lenses in the motion picture projectors be antireflection-coated to show his new picture, *Gone with the Wind.*

A gain in light transmission is effected when light strikes the coating material which has a very low refractive index (magnesium fluoride n $=$ 1.38). Instead of a transmission loss (by reflection) at the first glass surface of 4.3 percent, the reflection from magnesium fluoride is only 2.55 percent. This gain of almost 2 percent at each front surface of a lens results in the transmission of more than twice the usual light at the tenth lens. Aside from this remarkable increase in transmitted light from this factor, Robertson* states that the annulled reflected light is also added to the beam. He remarks that this phenomenon occurs in any system of interference fringes and that can be proved mathematically, but he asks his reader to accept it as a fact without proof.

After seeming to be striving to avoid any reference to mathematics, Ralph Drew* capitulated on page 311 of his *Professional Ophthalmic Dispensing* to give ten pages to a particularly lucid exposition of lens surface coating thoroughly documented by formulas.

A cosmetic effect which is imperceptible to the spectacle wearer is the elimination of light reflections on the front side of his lenses. Frequently lighting conditions are such that a public speaker's facial expression is erased when spectacle lens reflections hide his eyes. Surface coating removes this problem. Surface reflection III discussed in this chapter which may be bothersome to cataract lens wearers can be obliterated.

A process of hardening the metallic surface coating has been developed which is very effective. With reasonable caution, lenses which are treated with Permacote, Duracote, or similar process are not delicate. Nevertheless the lens washing procedure for hard-resin lenses is an extra insurance.

Like the heat-treating of lenses, antireflection coating of spectacle lenses is a lens improvement that is gaining in popularity

*Robertson, John K.: *Introduction to Optics Geometrical and Physical.* New York, Van Nostrand, 1961, p. 168.

*Drew, R.: *Professional Ophthalmic Dispensing.* Chicago, Prof Press, 1970.

and is seldom forsaken after a wearer has enjoyed the benefits of the process.

REVIEW

1. Using the reflection numbers, why is reflection V so bothersome?

2. Surface reflections suggest coating on (a) one surface, why? (b) both surfaces, why?

3. Show the wave front path through the antireflection coating.

Appendix A

OPERATIONS PROGRAM

◆◆

There is a basic procedure for ophthalmic dispensing which, although varied by the personalities of individual dispensing firms, cannot be materially reduced without some loss of acceptance by prescribers or of business success by the dispenser.

An ophthalmic dispensing business can survive from now into the future only on the *basis of service,* and this service cannot be a "service" in name only. The drug chains and discount houses are better capitalized, buy lenses and frames cheaper, use cheaper help, and have minimum rent and "four walls" expense. Further, they usually do not base their operations upon high quality opticians. They are not necessarily operating to improve dispensing quality. Their corporations have only one objective: profit.

They can not compete with you in service because they do not have the personnel or the budget for service. The elements to compete are (a) a good basic optical education and understanding of the fitting of eyeframes and lenses, (b) presenting a hospitable appearance and courteous conduct of all personnel, (c) keeping good records and delivering the highest grade workmanship, and (d) obviously and persistently doing everything possible to assure the customer will return with his next prescription, irrespective of who may write it. Accomplishment of this program assures a rapidly increasing professional success.

What follows is a complete description of Operations Procedure that has had the contributions of many men within and outside my firm for many years.

There is only one opening remark, "How may I (or we) serve you?" Never say, "May I serve you?" because an occasional customer will give you the correct answer, "Yes".

Greet the Customer

There are a few remarks that must invariably be expressed in greeting the customer whether the greeter is a receptionist or the proprietor. For the prospective customer with a new prescription ask, "Have we made glasses for you before?" For the apparent shopper, suggest "Lets move over here and look at some of these new frame designs." For the person who wishes his eyewear serviced, ask specifically, "When did we make these glasses?" You are not as much concerned about *when* but *whether*. You need to know because you can immediately go to the record file and take out his record. Date stamp the record jacket to record the visit and prepare the record for the dispenser to put the service and his initials beside it. At the fitting table the dispenser takes the record from the envelope and looks at it for a moment to note if there are any special remarks, such as "Temples should be snug." "Avocations are sailing and tennis." This routine of looking at records is also done by your dentist. It subtly reminds the patient that the dentist knows more about his dental history than anyone. This aspect of the routine, like returning to the same dispenser, helps build the association that causes him to return with his next prescription.

In the same way people return to the same hair stylist, it is logical that customers continue with the same optician. The initials on the record jacket indicate who should care for the customer next time. The exception is when something discordant occurs. The optician should then *sign off*. Any number of code signals can be used. A simple one is to draw a red ink line under the date of last service.

The routine of withdrawing the record from the file *every time* a customer visits the store develops a record that is necessary for a routine described later.

Receptionist's Memo

The receptionist's memo (see Fig. 259) is filled out for each customer. The daily accumulation of them sets up a journal of the day's transactions.

A one-man store proprietor may think, "Why should I do this? I am the only dispenser in the store." A file of these is a store-

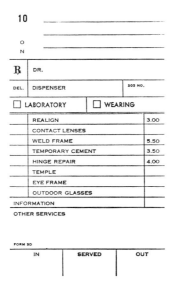

Figure 259. The receptionist's memo.

O and N indicate relationship with customer. Encircled N indicates new prescription from a new customer. Encircled O is for customer with record in file who has come in for any service, including ACS (Aftercare Service).

Encircled N/C indicates new prescription brought in by previous customer whose old record has been cancelled (removed from file). Encircled N/C2 means new prescription from customer who has had two previous prescriptions filled.

At the time of the receptionist's first contact, one of the remaining activities will be checked if the service is not a new prescription or delivery.

℞ is encircled when the visitor has a new prescription to be filled. The doctor's name with initials follows.

DEL is encircled if the customer has come in for his eyewear.

DISPENSER, the dispenser who serves the customer places his initials in this box.

The receptionist enters in the next box the serial number of the order form (which she has put with the memo) when a patient has brought a prescription to be filled. This small act is valuable assistance in the event of future identification for the IRS or auditors.

The next line is helpful when a customer has brought in eyewear to be serviced. It prevents a dispenser asking for eyewear which is in the Laboratory or hunting in the laboratory for eyewear which the customer is still house of information of how many new prescriptions one man can handle in a day, how long it takes on the average for every service, how many *Aftercare Services* (formerly called adjustments) are made, length of time customers wait to be served.

When the store has grown to need more than one optician, an authentic schedule is available to measure the efficiency of the new firm member.

The serial numbers assure that customers are served in order. When, at the end of the day, yesterday's last number is subtracted from this day's last number, the number served is indicated.

These memos are filed in a dated glove envelope. They provide perfect information for traffic studies, whether the store is too busy or not busy enough for the number of personnel, and much other sales research information.

Contact Lenses Memo

A separate memo is used for contact lens customers (Fig. 260). Aside from name, address, doctor's name, and order number, all of the detail is filled in by the contact lens fitters. These memos are filed back of the receptionist's memos in the envelope for each day.

Order Form—Envelope

Paraphrasing the theme of an ophthalmologists educational course I would say that prescription record keeping is the "heart"

---

wearing (aphakic).

Aftercare service describes the work we formerly named adjustment or re-alignment. Note that it is priced. Later in this appendix, the whole routine will be described.

The next two items relieve the dispenser of the embarrassment of asking the customer *how* he can serve him when the customer has just told the receptionist what he wishes.

The bottom line is used to show the exact clock time when the customer came *in*. The dispenser records the time when the customer is *served* and again records the time when the customer goes *out*. More details may be added; that is, how long the customer waited before being served, the length of time the dispenser spent with the customer, and the time of day when the customer was served.

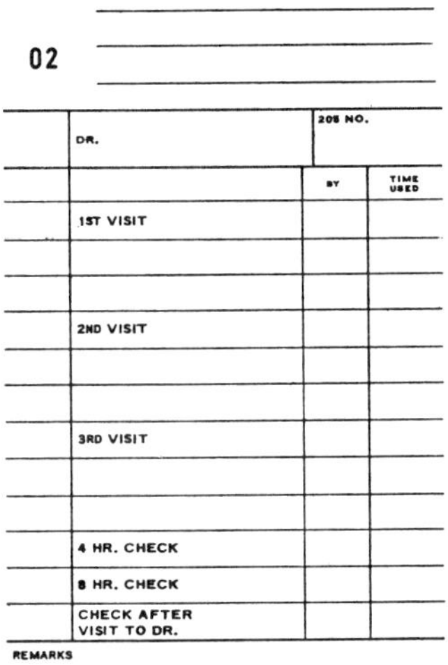

02

		208 NO.	
DR.			
		BY	TIME USED
1ST VISIT			
2ND VISIT			
3RD VISIT			
4 HR. CHECK			
8 HR. CHECK			
CHECK AFTER VISIT TO DR.			

REMARKS

Figure 260. The contact lenses memo.

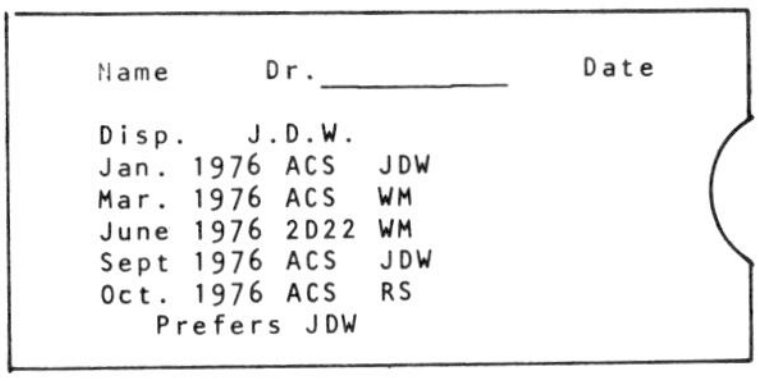

```
Name        Dr._____       Date

Disp.    J.D.W.
Jan.  1976 ACS   JDW
Mar.  1976 ACS   WM
June  1976 2D22  WM
Sept  1976 ACS   JDW
Oct.  1976 ACS   RS
       Prefers JDW
```

Figure 261. The order form envelope.

of the operation. On these, the minute details of the eyewear provided for the customer and further significant information about
the customer are indicated. Five by seven inch file cards, are
needed to have enough space on them for all of the specifications
for laboratory orders; there is not space for the customers service
records.

After years of many changes, we have settled on order forms (see
Fig. 262) which have as many as four carbon copies. This procedure makes copying unnecessary—even laboratory orders and
surfacing orders. Do not hesitate to change, if necessary. The
order form is used at the fitting table by the dispenser.

The original is folded into an open-end envelope. These plain
envelopes are made of five colors of paper. At the start of each

year, there is a color change and when (the sixth year) a color is to be repeated, all of the five-year-old records are taken out of the file and stored in a "transfer file." This file is largely for a psychological reason: Many dispensers have believed that "Old records are necessary and valuable." Thirty years experience in many stores refutes that statement. Most doctors would question the refilling of a six-year-old prescription. With the kaleidoscopic changes of eyeframe designs, there is faint hope of duplicating or getting parts for a six-year-old eyeframe. However, a record can be retrieved in the rare instance if it is needed. The tinted envelopes are advantageous in filing and in recognizing the age of the records.

As shown in Figure 261, the customer's name, the doctor's name, the date of the prescription, and the first dispenser's initials are typed on the top edge of the envelope. At each visit of the customer a date stamp, the purchase or service, and the dispenser's initials complete each entry. These data prove to be valuable records for surveys of customers' returns.

The folded prescription copy placed in the open-end envelope is easy to handle and the plain envelope provides space to record all return visits of our customers.

Our procedure requires that the prescription record be furnished the dispenser at every contact with a customer. When he reviews the record, he is completely informed about the eyewear. Even a one-man operation has time to say, "Pardon me for a moment while I get your record." It is expected that this routine will finally teach your customers that the record is needed for Aftercare Service, realignment, or adjustment. When this is accomplished, your customer will routinely return to you.

Order Form and Prescription Record

The order form (see Fig. 262) has a small perforated tab at the top to provide a customer receipt. The third tab (not shown) is an accounting record for a deposit on the order; the fourth tab (not shown) can be used as a "sale completed" tab to accompany the balance of the money received.

The original is kept for the firm's records as already described.

This form can be made with as many as four carbons:

(1) Goldenrod is the laboratory order.
(2) Pale Yellow is the accounting control copy.
(3) Pink is used at store as memo for replacement of store inventory (sunglasses, eyeframes, magnifiers).
(4) White, Heavy paper, is used as the surface grinding order. This copy accompanies the goldenrod to the laboratory.

Use of carbon copies reduced our laboratory payroll by one person, a savings of $8000 per year. She wrote surface-grinding orders.

Summary

A complete cycle of the store's activities has been studied. Based upon the uniqueness of the activity of ophthalmic dispensing in which the original product is serviced and cared for as long as the buyer has use for it, no other service is similar. No other provider, whether of clothes, homes, automobiles, or shoes, shows such interest in his product after it has been delivered. In fact, many large separate businesses are founded upon the servicing of previously sold products.

SUPERIOR OPTICAL CO.

DEPOSIT IS NON-REFUNDABLE

A MONTHLY SERVICE CHARGE WILL BE MADE ON ALL PAST DUE ACCOUNTS.

℞ № __ 4801

O				
N		90	TAX	
NAME			AMOUNT	
			TOTAL	
	M.D.	REC'D BY	DEPOSIT	
DATE	OPTICIAN	THANK YOU	BALANCE	

O S P C A		℞ № 4801	
N			
NAME		90	TAX
STREET			AMOUNT
CITY	ZIP	PHONE	TOTAL
NO. PRS / SV		M.D./DATE / /	DEPOSIT
M.	FITTED BY / CHECKED BY / FINAL INSPEC. / DELIVERED BY /		BALANCE

LABORATORY	SPECIAL LENS INSTRUCTIONS	VOCATION

	SPHERE	CYLINDER	AXIS	PRISM	△ BASE	THICK	LENS CAT. NO.
R.							
L							
R				NOS. /		△	
L				S.O.			

A D D	SEGMENT +	INTEROCULAR DIST. NEAR R R L L	CENTER +	BASE	STOCK USE

LENGTH	+ TOT. DEC.	+ EDX	− SEG	= MBS	METAL / RIMLESS	EYEFRAME S L

SHAPE	ABC	LENGTH	DBL	TOTAL	ZYLO	FABRICATED BY: S L

| HIDEABEVEL | STOCK USE |

SPECIAL EDGING INSTRUCTIONS

EYEFRAME CAT. NO.	COLOR NO.	EYE	BRIDGE	LENGTH	TYPE	SPREAD	ANGLE

CUSTOMER'S MATERIAL	EYEFRAME INSTRUCTIONS	ENGRAVE FRAME ☐	R
DESCRIPTION			L
CONDITION	REMARKS:		
ENCLOSED AT STORE TO COME			
			FRM
			TOT

Figure 262. The prescription order form.

Care is exercised in recording the name. Names of doctors are not recorded as Dr. John Doe but as John Doe, M.D., John Doe, D.D.S., John Doe, D.V.M., or Mary Worth, R.N.; a professional price is granted to Doctors of Medicine and Registered Nurses. The spouse of a doctor is also entitled to a professional price; the doctors' name is added in parentheses following the customer's name. Children are identified with the name of the father or responsible elder above the name of the child, simplifying credit responsibility. The telephone number is the one where the customer can be reached in the daytime.

Definite effort is made to accept full payment, or at least a substantial deposit at the time of the order, with the balance upon delivery. Credit cards are accepted in lieu of credit. Small dispensing firms seldom have enough working capital to afford many Accounts Receivable. A question asked at the conclusion of the order should automatically be repeated with scant pause: "Your eyewear will be $64.75 including tax. Do you wish to take care of it now or leave a deposit?" Practice those words many times until they become automatic.

At the right, the boxes *No Prs SV and M* are to prevent the calling of a customer when one pair of a multiple order is completed. It is also a reminder to check up on the balance of the order when the first pair has been checked in.

Fitted By is obvious. Each order is read and verified by another dispenser (a pharmacy also does this) before it is sent to be fabricated. *Final Inspection* is when the order is completed after receipt from the laboratory. *Delivered By* with space for the *Date* shows the initials of the dispenser who delivers the order.

The square marked *LABORATORY* is seldom used. It is best to make no definite or even approximate statement about completion time. The word "Rush" is completely avoided, because it is ambiguous. "Rush" may mean either to do the work in a hurry, thus increasing the risk of mistakes in detail or of spoilage and lost time, or "Rush" may mean to unfairly do this work before other work that is already in the laboratory. When the occasion arises that a dispenser makes a specific promise (for a patient who is leaving town or has an emergency) the whole responsibility is in the hands of the dispenser. The dispenser must discuss the order with the laboratory superintendent over the phone, so the dispenser can find whether the required lenses and/or frame are in stock. When the laboratory superintendent says the work can be done, the dispenser returns to his customer and reports that the superintendent believes the order can be completed in time. The dispenser writes "confirmation" across the order and sends it directly to the superintendent. Now the dispenser starts his vigil. The morning of the day BEFORE the order is to be delivered, the dispenser calls to find whether the order is completed or its point of progress. If there has been spoilage or other delay which may mean the order will not be ready to ship at the end of the day, the dispenser telephones his customer AT ONCE and tells him what has happened. In this case, the dispenser telephones the laboratory again in the middle of the afternoon to get the final word. If the order has been completed or is very near completion, the message should be relayed to the customer. Less attention to such a special order can be disastrous. Every dispensing firm which has haphazardly handled a special order knows the devastating poor public relations that can ensue.

The next section below is headed "*Special Lens Instructions.*" In this space special comments with reference to the lenses are written. To the right is *Vocation.* The importance of this and proper presentation of this information is discussed in Chapter 9.

The space to copy the prescription (Sphere, Cylinder, Axis, Prism, Base) concludes with Thickness. By FDA regulations, the minimum center thickness has been established but the space is still justified to record the center thickness of plus lenses. Center thickness is an essential specification when replacing one lens of a pair. This detail may be ordered on a new pair of lenses when the new lenses are being made to duplicate the appearance of an old pair. The space to the right justifies the effort required to establish catalogue numbers for lenses. Any lens style and its tint or surface coating can be shown in the space. Since the size of multifocal segments is a part of the number, no additional space is needed to show the segment width.

Under the heavy line, the first three squares are the place to put the optical difference of the right and left lenses, as was discussed in Chapters 10 and 12 on Prescription Analysis. The next square identifies the Univis® segment numbers used to balance the anisometropia, if the prism effect is large, the next square is used to record the amount of prism of the Slab-off (S.O.).

Below this line are the boxes for the reading addition. The following divided box is for the position of the top edge of the segment. The "O" is the datum line (180° line or the line through the center of the pattern). Segments for trifocals frequently are above (+) this line. Most bifocal segments are somewhat below (−) this line. No other reference to segment position is necessary or desirable. The next pair of boxes are for the *Interocular Distances* (P.D.). Each side (Dist. and Near) has spaces for monocular measurements. Learn to itemize them for symmetric measurements; such as 31/31 not 62.

The next box is for the position of the optical centers as determined by the Dispensometer® for the pantoscopic angle of the eyeframe. This information is an absolute necessity when making one lens. Vertical prism is the calamitous result of neglect of this lensometer finding. The next box (Base) is used when the lenses must be made on a base other than the one established by the lens designer of the particular lens ordered.

The next line of boxes could be considered the most important information on the order. They establish the minimum size of the lens blanks to make the specified lenses. This information must be found by the dispenser; it is necessary to establish the lens price. If the lens is oversize it may require a call to the stock department to find availability and to warn the customer about a delay in obtaining materials. The detail for these boxes is simple: *Length* is the *A* dimension of the lenses. To this is added the *Tot. Dec.* (total decentration). This is found by subtracting the total Distance Interocular from *Total* on the next lower row of boxes. For example: $A = 54 + DBL18 = 72$; Distance Interocular $= 63$. Therefore *Tot. Dec.* $= 72 - 63 = 9$. The difference between the equivalent diameter (as shown on the manufacturer's specification sheet) and the "A" length is the equivalent diameter extra *(EDX)*. This is on the short tag on the left temple of the eyeframe selected. The next box is not needed since all Flat Top bifocal manufacturers are decentering their segments for the right and left. The sum of the three boxes described $(54 + 9 + 3 = 66)$ is the MBS: thus 68 or 71 mm blanks are required. Now the stock clerk, surface grinders, and edgers are all informed.

The next row of boxes begins with *shape*. In Chapter 9 our lens pattern rack was described and illustrated. It showed that each shape was identified by two letters and a number from 1 to 24. This information is also on the short tag on the left temple. By this simple means each one of the 7,000 different patterns in the rack is individually identified. In this instance the *SHAPE* box would be filled like this:

SHAPE	
BK7	
Eapirit	

Now any person in the whole laboratory can immediately put the proper pattern in the job tray. Production is accelerated. No lengthy conferences about "What is this bleep shape?" The next box has lost some of its usefulness since our pattern rack has been in use. The *ABC* identifies the category of the shape by the convention of my *Lens Pattern Book* (1957). At that time there were as many as six patterns with the same name and many of them had two or more differences in shape. Hence in those times this was indispensable. *Length* still refers to the "A" length and *DBL* is the measured lens separation. The specification on an imported eyeframe may vary either way. *TOTAL* is the sum of the "A" length and DBL. It is necessary in finding Tot. Dec. for Minimum Blank Size. The four words arranged vertically are concerned with the edge of the lenses. The group of boxes with S or L in them are to show whether the materials or laboratory work are done in the store (S) or laboratory (L). This is for accounting and inventory purposes and to locate an unfinished order. When the store has an eyeframe which is not the precise specifications but can be used, the dispenser puts a box around the S to avoid the delay if the stock department does not have the item on hand. The next line *Special Edging Instructions* is used for such purposes as Mayo Rim, etc.

The entire next line describes the eyeframe to be used: the *Catalogue Number, Color Number, Eye,* Size, DBL *(Bridge),* Temple *Length, Type, Spread* (caliper measurement minus 5), *Angle* (temple angle of eyeframe as constructed), *Eyeframe Instructions* such as "Reduce wrap around." When an X is put in the *Engrave Frame* square, the desired engraving is printed in the *Remarks* space below.

Under *Customer's Material,* indicating the customer is using old frame, *Description* has space for the Catalogue Number or name followed by *condition* — this usually refers to the age of zylo frames and is judged as good, fair, or poor. *Enclosed, At Store,* and *To Come* are circled as appropriate.

In the lower right corner of the form, the prices of the right and left lenses are written separately, followed by spaces to enter prices for oversize lenses, tint, dye, frame, etc.

CAPITALIZE ON AFTERCARE SERVICES*

◆◆◆

After many years of comparatively quiet operations of the optical business or profession with trained opticians (for the most part) guiding the destiny of the business, there has come an abrupt change with expert merchandisers (not opticians) proliferating at an unusual pace.

Some changes include (1) consumer's advocates who scream through the media that the public is being "ripped off" by opticians; (2) bureaucrats in Washington who chime in loudly that glasses are unfairly high; (3) drug chains that make a travesty of dispensing; (4) optical manufacturers who cut across regular channels to make eyewear for HEW, union, and HMO plans.

When we stop to think of it, all of these groups are directed at taking ophthalmic dispensing away from opticians. For our survival we are forced to reduce this erosion of our business.

These changes will not pass away but are expanding regularly, created and multiplied in the atmosphere of our present haphazard methods. No opticians organization has done more than beat their chests and say, "We dispensing opticians are better" Such pronouncements fall on deaf ears. To the promotors of the drug chains it may sound like the whimpering of the defeated.

Dispensers who attempt to compete with "discount houses" on *their* terms are doomed. Even if the "price cutters" use good lenses, they buy them for at least one third less than small operators. For those with few scruples, there is hardly a bottom cost for lenses, and their labor cost is less: Untrained help is the rule. Their "four walls" expense is less than we could imagine.

Even to continue as most of us now operate will only prolong our ultimate decline. Our salvation is to set up customer care

---

*From a seminar lecture for the Southwest Optical Dispensers Association delivered in Dallas, Texas, October, 1977.

with which they can not compete. Let us capitalize our unique-ness. My firm has weekly executive meetings; one of the most important subjects ever discussed was on impressing the signifi-cance of visual care to our customers. These discussions set the stage for a merchandising analysis group. The analysts began at our receptionist's memos which record the customer's name and purpose of his visit.

After all of our many previous surveys and investigations based on the memos, we were surprised at what the analysts emphasized. Like Edgar Allen Poe's story of "The Purloined Letter," the letter was so obvious (fastened on the wall) that it was not noticed. The analysts centered on this simple fact: one-third of our customer traffic was service on eyewear. The adjusting of glasses has been the "ugly duckling" of our profession. The attitude toward adjusting has varied from firm to firm. Some operators almost displayed their aversion to and displeasure at the perform-ing of this detail because it took time and did not reach the cash register. A few tried to charge for it and came to the conclusion that it "chased away customers." It appalled us when our analysts recommended that we explore a means to *capitalize* on this monster.

Analysis showed that a large percentage of non-customer services were being rendered for those who had had their eyewear supplied by discount houses, optometrists, and dispensing oph-thalmologists. Our service was more satisfactory to the wearers than that of the suppliers of the eyewear. In substance, we were supplementing the service of our competitors.

We took this information seriously, but it took many executive meetings for us to first visualize, then prepare a program by which we could use the eyeglass wearer contact as the means by which we could reinforce our relationship with our own customers and otherwise increase our business. At that point, like most other dispensers, this part of our daily service was handled haphazardly and, consequently, with no consistent advantage to our firm.

Finally we came to the conclusion that by an organized pre-sentation, we could use this part of our firm's activity to accom-plish two purposes. It could be used to impress upon our cus-tomers the importance of the care of their eyes and eyewear by participating in a scheduled Aftercare Service. To discontinue the gratuitous care of eyewear supplied by our competitors, *we would do an about-face.* No longer would we release our customers to make a dispenser's analysis as to when his eyewear needed realignment and service. *We would take control* of the situation as would be becoming for conscientious dispensers and set a schedule for the return for service for each customer for his best interests.

After some trial and error, which could be expected, we have perfected a relatively simple and effective method to accomplish our whole purpose. It brings our customers closer to us than we or other opticians have ever experienced.

The details of the procedure are simple, but we have found they must be routinely and enthusiastically pursued or the whole notion could collapse. Two obvious changes are made: (1) At the conclusion of the delivery of eyewear, each customer receives a generously illustrated booklet (Fig. 263) which describes our firm and its services; (2) in a slot in its back page is placed an Appointment Card (Fig. 264); (3) it is impressed upon the customer to return any time the eyewear feels uncomfortable, but to not defer returning beyond the last day of the month on the Appointment Card.

Analysis of our records showed that a few customers had been

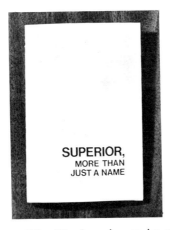

Figure 263. The Superior service story.

APPOINTMENT CARD

This card is to remind you to come in for aftercare service for your eyewear at any time should they become uncomfortable. In any event, be sure to return for realignment of your eyewear before the end of:

JULY

Remember, doctor's carefully written prescription cannot perform as intended unless your lenses are perfectly positioned before your eyes. This is a part of Superior's Aftercare Service provided to its valued customers at no additional charge.

SUPERIOR OPTICAL CO.

Figure 264. The appointment card.

returning with reasonable regularity, but the vast majority were irregular and many seldom returned. This Appointment Card organizes their attention on the care of their eyes and eyewear. We have found that regular renewal of our acquaintance with customers develops a friendship and appreciation of our Continuous Aftercare Service.

The date of the Appointment Card (the period between return visits) to some extent becomes a matter of judgment of the dispenser, but the original schedule should be made with these considerations.

(1) Children should not stay away for more than two months. Eyewear delivered in June should be seen by the end of August. The Appointment Card is given to the mother with some remarks about the importance of the lenses being properly placed before the eyes to perform as doctor intends. Experience has shown that even with the best of intended care, most children's eyewear needs service in sixty days. Of course, there are exceptions. In such cases, extend the Appointment Card to ninety days.

(2) Customers wearing lenses for aphakia should be regularly seen within ninety days, so lenses delivered in June would require a September Appointment Card. Remember, this does not imply the customer must not return before that date. It goes without saying they should come in at any time the eyewear is uncomfortable. The card means: Do not wait *longer* than the end of the

month to come in.

(3) Multifocal wearers should be given three or four month Appointment Cards, depending upon the complexity of the prescription.

(4) Single vision lenses, either distance or reading, should start with four month cards. The length of time should be adjusted to meet the customer's best interests.

The dispenser places the three letter abbreviation of the month on the Appointment Card in the left hand margin of the prescription record envelope in ink, colored ink preferably. This serves as the key for the date of the next card.

For the customer who returns in the interval before the date on the card, remark, "Don't forget to come in again before the end of _____." If he comes back after the expiration of the card, make something of it. Talk about "neglect of your eyes." Present a new card for the customary interval from the date of this visit. Defend regular appointments as important to sustain the purpose of Continuous Aftercare Service.

While we are all busily engaged in making changes from our old individual routines, we must not forget that we are also in the process of changing haphazard habits of our customers in the care of their prescription eyewear. If we are negligent in converting them into some regularity with reference to their returns for Aftercare Service, this whole effort could deteriorate. For the growth, not decline, of our business, it must succeed and grow.

When you give your customer his first Appointment Card at delivery, you should talk about the return for Aftercare Service. Even if his eyewear is comfortable, he should return before the end of the month on the card.

Before your receptionist files the records, she should put a colored filing flag on the upper edge of the prescription record envelope to identify the month on the next appointment card. Four colors for the quarters of the year are excellent.

If perchance the customer forgets his return date, your receptionist will use the flag to send the customer a reminder postcard around the middle of the following month. In this way, the customer will realize that you are serious about your service. In the rare instance that the customer does not return after the postcard, he should be sent another card thirty days later. We must do all that we can to convert all of our customers to let us use our professional judgment about the constant perfection of the fitting of their eyewear. When this is accomplished, we have divorced our customer from the "merchandised" spectacles of the "discount houses" and drug chains.

The Aftercare Service must not be, or look to be, perfunctory. In many instances your customer has had to make considerable effort to come. Make his trip worthwhile. It is essential to take the eyewear into the laboratory to polish and clean it. If the improved lustre of the frame is noticeable, comment on it, even use a mirror if possible.

For eyewear that is out of line, a comment such as, "It is a good thing you didn't stay away any longer." At the other extreme, for eyewear that is shipshape, say in effect, "For your extreme good care of your eyewear, I am going to increase the length to your next appointment, but don't let that encourage neglect."

A card on our reception desk announces that we have a minimum charge of three dollars for service on eyewear that we have not made. Analysis has shown that those who were not our previous customers were the patients of optometrists, dispensing

A $3.00 MINIMUM CHARGE WILL BE MADE ON ALL SER- VICES TO EYEWEAR *NOT MADE BY SUPERIOR OPTICAL.*

This minimum charge may be applied as credit towards the future purchase of prescription eyewear.

Figure 265. The minimum service card from the receptionist's desk.

ophthalmologists, or discount houses.

At first we were unsure of the effect of regularly charging those who were not our customers for service. We were pleased to hear many of these people say, "I have wondered why you haven't charged for this before." Our customers appreciate Aftercare Service even more when they note that other people pay for each visit.

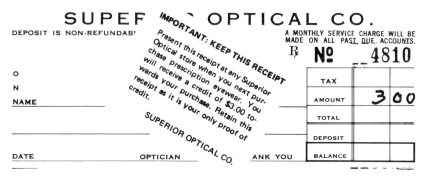

Figure 266. Credit sticker on a receipt.

We have introduced an important innovation with this charge. We have a small sticker that we put on the receipt which gives credit to the customer on a future purchase. We have found that the supermarket coupon notion has carried over. The receipts are brought in. There is also the non-customer's thought, "This wasn't a payment, it is a deposit on my next pair of glasses."

We enthusiastically redeem these receipts, because they mean that we are developing new customers who have come to us because of the quality of our service, and the advertising expense has been small.

This new service income (and with us it is more than $2,000 per month) could be thought of as "bottom line" income because it is labor and "four walls" expense for which we previously had no return. Actually, it pays for the additional time spent on more appointments with our own customers.

Like many other merchandising "breakthroughs," the "bare bones" of this procedure is not remarkable. Think of other successful projects that are also essentially simple. All that Colonel

Sanders has is an organized franchisable program to sell good fried chicken. All that Avon did was to renew the house-to-house sale of fragrances and soap. Think about their impressive success. The secret in these instances, and at McDonalds, is an enthusiastic and unvarying presentation.

Had all dispensers adopted a Continuing Aftercare Service some years ago, many people would now be aware of such service. How much better the profession could have presented its case before the Federal Trade Commission and other consumer groups when we explained that eyewear is only a portion of dispensing service. As an aside, it is easily assumed that the leaders in dispensing had not evaluated the importance of Aftercare. All men and organizations stopped their descriptions of ophthalmic dispensing at the delivery . . . quite the same as the discount operators. Otherwise, the first reply to a question about price might have been like this: "Records show that the average pair of glasses is worn at least three years. By our appointment card system our customers see us a minimum of three times a year. For this service we charge Three Dollars to those who are not our customers. Hence 3 years $\times$ 3 visits $\times$ \$3.00 is \$27.00 for service. For example: Lenses at \$35.00 plus Frame at \$25.00 = \$60.00 less \$27.00 Service equals \$33.00 for the spectacles."

Price cutting drug chains would have to recast their entire programs to include Continuous Aftercare Service. "Wholesale plus a dispensing fee" would have to be recalculated if it were to compete with Continuous Aftercare Service. Acceptance of the full responsibility of ophthalmic dispensing might not be so attractive to optometrists and ophthalmologists if their patients expected to return three or more times a year.

Equipment required at the time of designing the eyewear and used again at each Aftercare Service sets us apart from haphazard or even routine dispensing. It emphasizes the uniqueness of a full service. We use a (1) Head caliper (Fig. 267); (2) Essel Pupillometer P.D. and Vertex Distance (Fig. 268); (3) Dispensometer (Fig. 269); and (4) Datum Rule (Fig. 270).

1. The width of the skull in millimeters at the ear tops should be placed on the record and laboratory order. Time spent in widening or narrowing the temple spread of laboratory work

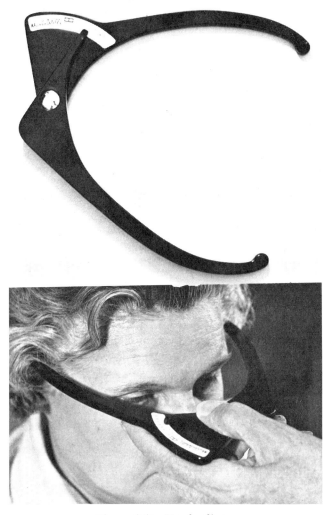

Figure 267. Head caliper.

is wasteful of fitting table time.

2. The monocular visual axis distance, vertex distance, obtained with the Essel Pupillometer is, of course, placed on the record and laboratory order.

3. The Dispensometer locates the pupil center position, eyeframe inclination from which the pantoscopic angle and vertical

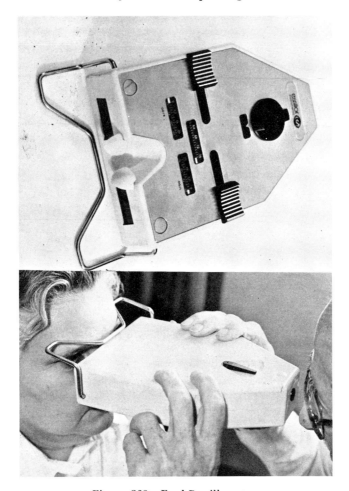

Figure 268. Essel Pupillometer.

optical center are determined, and the top of multifocal segment.
4. The Datum Rule locates the datum line and provides for precise specifications.

Use of a Dispensometer for a New Eyeframe

1. Open the Dispensometer and place it on the selected frame.
2. Place eyeframe on the face.

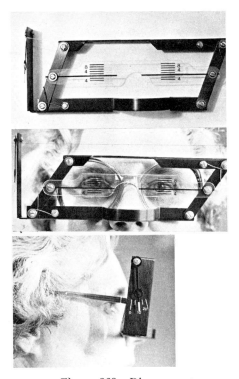

Figure 269. Dispensometer.

3. Have the patient hold his head with his face-plane vertical.

4. Read the angle of the front of the eyeframe on the inclinometer.

5. Observe the height of the pupil centers above the 180° (Datum) line. This indicates the normal placement of the "center" of the Ultravue, Varilux II, or Younger 10/30.

6. Divide the inclinometer reading by two. Specify the optical centers of the lenses to be that amount below the pupil centers. It will frequently be above the 180° (Datum) line.

7. Note the location of the cilia line of the lower lid. This is the average position of the top edge of a bifocal segment.

Caution: Remember to use the distance from the calculated optical center position to the top edge of the segment to specify the segment position below the center.

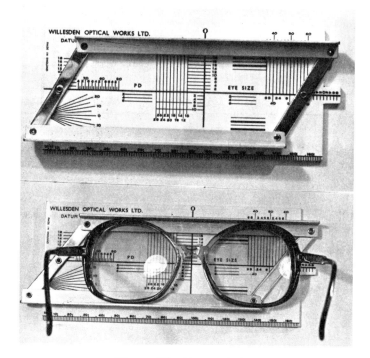

Figure 270. Datum Rule.

EXAMPLE:

>Optical center 3 mm above 180° (Datum) line.
>Segment edge 2 mm below 180° (Datum) line.
>Specify 5 mm below optical center.

Use of a Dispensometer for Customer's Old Frame

1. Spot old lenses in your lensometer. Put some dots on the top edge of segments.
2. Discuss whether the reading portions in the old lenses were conveniently placed.
3. Place Dispensometer on old eyewear and put the old eyewear on the face.
4. Determine the new segment position, if a change is to be made.
5. Read the inclinometer and determine the vertical position of the optical centers for the new lenses. Remember to divide pantoscopic angle by two.

6. Note pupil position if progressive power lenses are to be supplied.
7. The Datum Rule confirms the Datum line and lens detail accuracy.

We are insistent that all of this equipment be routinely used. *We know that "discount house" opticians do not have and perhaps would not know how to use this apparatus.* We must do a better job and we must be different.

When a customer returns for Aftercare Service, the eyewear is immediately taken to the laboratory where the frame is buffed to freshen up its appearance. The lenses and frames are washed with soap and water. The screws are tightened and swaged if necessary. The lenses are centered and dotted on the Vertometer. The equipment needed in the fitting area are (1) Vertometer; (2) Dispensometer; (3) Essel Pupillometer; and (4) Datum Rule.

The Dispensometer is fitted on the eyewear before it is placed on the face. The position of the optical center is compared with the prescription record and the eyeframe adjusted if necessary. The Essel Pupillometer vertex measurement confirms the symmetry of the vertex distances of the lenses.

This procedure requires your enthusiasm and, equal enthusiasm of your dispensers. It is important, too, that customers absorb some of this enthusiasm. It means more store traffic, but it does insure the return of your present customers with their new prescriptions and also increased "word of mouth" references. It removes the haphazard conduct of the past and replaces it with an environment of organized "customer service."

GLOSSARY

◆◆

A., A.U. Abbreviation for Ångstrom Unit, 10^{-10} meter $= 10^{-7}$ mm.

Abbe, E.K. (1840-1905). German physicist at Carl Zeiss, Jena.

> **A. focimeter.** Instrument for measuring the vertex focal length of ophthalmic lenses or lens systems.

> **A. number.** See *constringence*, *v*-number.

abducens. The external rectus muscle.

abduction. Divergence. The outward rotation of a pair of eyes in the attempt to maintain single binocular vision when stimulated by a Base In prism or Base In prisms.

aberration. An imperfection in a lens or optical system which prevents a point focus.

Abney, Sir W. (1844-1920). English physicist.

> **A. formula.** Describing the ideal pinhole camera $y = k \sqrt{x}$, where $y =$ pinhole diameter, $k =$ a constant (0.20312 mm); $x =$ distance of aperature to plate.

abnormal retinal correspondence. A condition in which areas of the retinae of a pair of eyes normally having no common visual stimulation adapt to macular stimulation in one eye and an extramacular point in the other eye. This extramacular point is referred to as false-macula.

absorption. The interception of radiant energy as it passes through a medium in which the energy is converted into heat, chemical energy, or photoelectric energy. For example, ultraviolet light is converted into fluorescence or phosphorescence. most optical media have selective absorption—that is, absorb certain radiations (colors) differently.

> **a. lenses.** Colored or neutral lenses used to reduce visible and/or dangerous invisible radiations or to reduce glare.

accommodation. The act of altering the dioptric power of the crystalline lens to permit objects at different distances to be clearly seen.

accommodative amplitude. The total amount of dioptric power by which the eyes are increased by maximum effort of the ciliary muscle. The dioptric power increase of the near-point over the dioptric power of the far-point.

achromatic. Without color.

> **a. lens.** A lens corrected for axial chromatic aberration by uniting a convex crown glass lens and concave flint glass lens.

acuity. Sharpness of vision.

> **letter a.** The conventional measurement used in clinical refraction. Designated fraction d/s in which d is the distance between observer and the letter (Snellen) chart and s is the size of the smallest letter recognized. For example, 20/60 is letters which subtend a normal 5 minute angle at 60 feet seen at 20 feet.

> **vernier a.** The ability of an eye or the eyes to discern an offset in a line, such as micrometer gradations. This acuity is much more sharp than letter acuity. Average eyes detect a break in a line at about 12 seconds and trained observers can observe an offset of as little as 2 seconds.

addition (add.). Dioptric power added to distance prescription to supplement accommodation for some finite distance, such as reading. The dioptric power of a bifocal segment.

additive. A series of lenses designed so that their individual dioptric powers can be added by arithmetic, such as the lens systems of refracting instruments and corrected trial lens sets.

adnexa. Term used to describe adjacent anatomic structures or accessories, such as lids, extraocular muscles, or lachrimal apparatus.

afocal. Without a focus, particularly a plano lens. A thick plano-meniscus but producing magnification used to correct aniseikonia. An iseikonic lens.

after-cataract. An intraocular disease caused by remnants of the lens remaining in the eye after cataract surgery by the extracapsular method in which the contents of the lens capsule are removed and allowing the capsule to remain in the eye.

after-image. The persistence of a visual image after the stimulus, usually intense light, has been discontinued. The image changes in color from the color of the stimulus to the complement of the color.

after-image test. A subjective test in which one eye is stimulated by a bright horizontal light and the other eye stimulated with the light rotated to a vertical position.

Airy, Sir G.B. (1801-1892). British astronomer. Designed cylindrical lenses (1827) for correction of *astigmatism* discovered by Sir Thomas Young (1800).

> **A. disc.** The central disc of light in the diffraction pattern of the image of a point source of light. This spot is surrounded by alternate annular dark and bright areas. The radius of the bright central disc $= \dfrac{0.16\,\lambda}{y}\,f$ where $y =$ radius of the entrance pupil of the lens or optical system of focal length f. The wavelength of the luminous object is identified by λ.

amblyopia ex anopsia. Dimness of vision resulting from non-use, as, the nonfixing eye in strabismus.

amblyoscope. A haploscope modified by Claude Worth (1904) used for the training of the amblyopic eye or fusion. Enlarged modern models are synoptiphore, synoptiscope, and troposcope.

ametropia. The refractive state of a static eye in which the secondary focus does not fall upon the retina.

angle. The geometric figure produced by the intersection or meeting of two straight lines. Measured in degrees, radians, prism diopters, or meter angles.

> **a. alpha (α).** Angle between anterior-posterior or optic axis of the eye and the visual axis at the first nodal point.

> **a. gamma (γ).** Angle between the optic axis and the visual axis at the center of rotation.

Angstrom, A.J. (1814-1874) Swedish physicist.

> **A. unit (A.U.).** Unit of length used to specify wavelength of

light. One Å.U. $= 10^{-10}$ meters.

aniseikonia. Lack of congruence of the ocular images projected in the central field. The difference may be symmetric inequality or meridional differences. Special magnifying lenses which produce equality of projected image size are called iseikonic lenses.

anisometropia. The refractive error in which there is a decided difference in the prescriptions for the two eyes. The condition often leads to discomfort because the optical correction may cause dissimilar image sizes or unequal prism differences in extra-axial areas of the lenses.

anneal. The act of removing internal strain by heating metal or glass and slowly cooling it. This procedure softens metals.

antimetropia. Refractive error of the eyes in which one eye is hyperopic and the other myopic.

antireflection coating. A thin film of magnesium flouride deposited upon a glass surface by vaporization of the metal in vacuum. The optimum performance for one color (wavelength) of light is when $n_F = \sqrt{n_G}$ where $n_F =$ index of refraction of film material and $n_G =$ index of refraction of the glass. The thickness of the film to accomplish interference of the light rays striking the glass surface must be $t = \lambda/4$ is the reduced thickness of the film t/n and $\lambda =$ wavelength of the incident light rays.

aperture. The opening which permits light to pass through an element or the elements of an optical system.

aphakia. The condition of an eye without the crystalline lens in the path of incident light. Usually lens removal in cataract surgery, but also can be caused by luxation of the lens. Loss of lens adds more than $+ 10.00D.$ hyperopia to the eye.

aspherical. Not spherical. Such conic sections as parabolic or hyperbolic, also ellipsoidal. Used to reduce marginal aberrations in lenses for aphakia or field lenses in the eyepieces of some optical instruments.

asthenopia. Distressed vision. Literally weak vision. Commonly called eyestrain. It causes headache, photophobia, irritated or burning eyes, and dimness of vision.

astigmatism. The condition in which the focal lengths of opposite meridians of an eye or optical system are not equal, thus producing two separate line images of a point source.

atrophy. A wasting or diminution of a body structure due to failure of nutrition.

  optic a. May be congenital or due to some affection of the optic nerve or retina. A symptom is subnormal vision which can often be improved by magnification and liberal illumination.

atropine. A powerful mydriatic and cycloplegic made from belladonna.

axis. An imaginary line with which an object's functions or parts are symmetric.

  cylinder a. The meridian of a cylinder lens in which there is least or no curvature. One of the principal medians of a spherocylindrical lens or surface.

  optical a. An imaginary line joining the centers of curvature of a lens or symmetrical optical system.

  visual a. The line joining the fixation point through the nodal points with the fovea centralis.

B segment. One-piece bifocal segment 19 to 22 mm in diameter.

back focal length. Distance from back vertex (pole) to the secondary focus (F′).

back vertex power. The reciprocal of the back focal length in meters. The vertex power of the lens or optical system in diopters.

Badal, A.J. (1840-1929). French ophthalmologist.

  B. optometer. A visual acuity measuring device consisting of a plus lens (usually + 10.00D.) and test letters. The secondary focal point of the lens is placed at the anterior focal point of the eye, thus permitting the test object to approach or recede from the lens without change in the size of the retinal image. The essential sight-testing instrument for itinerant opticians in the late nineteenth century.

base-apex line. The line at a right angle to the refracting edge of a prism. The line on which an object appears to be displaced by refraction.

base curve. The meridian of least curvature on a cylindrical surface. It may be found on either the convex or concave side of a meniscus lens.

base line. The lens connecting the centers of rotation of the two eyes. First described by Helmholtz. The actual interocular separation (or distance). The measurement sought when finding "pupillary distance."

bent lens. A term used to distinguish the form of curved lenses, such as periscopic, meniscus, or toric lenses, from a flat lens of the same power.

best form lens. A term used by Whitwell, a British lens designer, to describe "bent" lenses which reduce marginal aberrations to minimum.

bevel edge. The V-shaped edge ground on the periphery of a lens (about 135° angle) to hold the lens in a spectacle frame.

biconcave. A lens with both surfaces concave, usually identical curves.

biconvex. A lens with both surfaces convex, usually identical curves.

bifocal. A spectacle lens with two areas, one of which has more dioptric power than the other.

    cement b. A lens on which extra lens power in the form of a wafer segment is attached with balsam cement to the major portion of the lens.

    Franklin b. A split bifocal made of sections of two lenses held together in a frame. It is the first bifocal, invented by Benjamin Franklin.

    fused b. A bifocal made by fusing a lens of stronger power into a depression in the major lens.

    one-piece b. A solid bifocal ground with two curves on one of the lens surfaces.

    perfection b. A split bifocal with a curved dividing line.

binocular. The term used to describe simultaneous use of the two eyes in the act of vision.

blind spot of Mariotte. Projection in the visual field of the head of the optic nerve. This scotoma is not noticed (negative) in binocular vision since it is 15° temporal in each eye.

blindness. Inability to perceive light, absence of the visual sense.
   b. legal. 20/200 visual acuity or less.

blur circle. A patch of light which is the faulty image of a point of light. It is caused by the diffraction of a small aperture, inaccurate placement of the projection screen, or the abberations of the lens or system. See *circle of least confusion.*

Boeder, Paul, Ph.D., Goettingen (1902–. . . .). Mathematician, author, teacher. Made important contributions Dartmouth research in aniseikonia.
   B. isobars. Isobars used in charts to indicate amounts of Prism Diopters.

Brewster, Sir D. (1781-1868) Scottish physicist.
   B. stereoscope. A stereoscope with two mirrors inclined 45° to the lines of sight of the eyes, which receive reflections of objects on the right and left sides. These reflections are fused to form an image in relief (depth perception). Cf. haploscope.

bridge. The central part of a frame or mounting which joins the two lenses. Types (metal): W, C (crank), A (arch), K, X, Chinese (reversible), Pad, Saddle. Types (plastic): Saddle, English, French, Keyhole, Pad, Inset, and Unifit. Styles (metal): cylinder, swelled, and wire.

broken circle, Landolt. A test object for the measurement of visual acuity consisting of a circle subtending a 5-minute angle for normal acuity. The thickness of the ring and the gap each subtend a 1-minute angle. The test is sometimes called the letter "C" test.

C-Line. Fraunhofer line (red), (Greek lambda) = 6563 A.U. Used in measuring dispersion of media and calculating achromatic lenses.

calipers. A tong like instrument with a scale at the wide end to make internal or external measurements.
   optical c. Used to measure lens thickness, usually in units of 0.1 mm.

camera. A light-tight box with a convex lens or system of lenses by which objects in space are imaged upon a photographic film or plate on the inside of the opposite side of the box. This is the form of a schematic eye.

carborundum. Silicon dioxide used as an abrasive.

cardinal points. Six points on the axis of a lens or lens system defined by Gauss and used for ray tracing and the preliminary design of an optical instrument. The three pairs of points are focal, principal, and nodal points. Perpendicular to the axis through these points are planes which facilitate the diagramming of ray paths.

cataract. Opacification in various degrees of the crystalline lens. substance or capsule which can diminish visual acuity from normal to bare light perception. It may be congenital or caused by metabolic derangement or by trauma. Vision is reestablished by the surgical removal of the lens and capsule.

   c. lens. A strong (usually + 10.00D. to + 16.00D.) lens to correct aphakia.

cellulose acetate. A thermoplastic which is not easily flammable. It is used as the material for spectacle frames. Safety plastic.

cellulose nitrate. A highly flammable thermoplastic which was formerly used as the material for spectacle frames. Also known as celluloid, xylonite, zylonite, zyl.

center. A point on the axis of a lens between the nodal points through which extra-axial rays pass undeviated.

   c. of curvature. The geometrical center of a spherical surface.

   c. of rotation. An imaginary point which has been proved to move or vary as the direction of the versions of the eye change. It is a necessary assumption in spectacle lens design. It is assumed to be located 13.25 to 14.6 mm behind the anterior pole of the cornea.

centrad. (∇) A unit of circular measurement (0.01 radian). Suggested by Dennett as a unit to measure ophthalmic prisms. Prentice's Prism Diopter has superceded it.

cerium oxide. A medium used to polish glass.

chamfer. A slight safety bevel on the edge of a lens to prevent chipping.

Chevasse lens. A clear plano meniscus lens with a pebbled back surface used to produce lowered visual acuity; such as, 20/20, 20/400.

cheiroscope. An orthoptic instrument invented by Maddox with the effect of a haploscope on one side to train hand and eye coordination.

choroid. Inside the sclera at the back of the eye and under the retina is a layer of blood vessels that nourish the interior of the eye. It is also named the uvea.

chromatic aberration. Due to the fact that all colors have different indices of refraction in all media, blue rays come to a focus first, which are followed by the colors in spectral order to red, which has the longest focal length. Hence the best focus is surrounded by a halo of blue and red.

ciliary body. An extension of the uvea which is comprised of the ciliary muscle and ciliary processes. Its function is to assist in changing the shape of the crystalline lens in the act of accommodation.

circle of least confusion. The minimum spot of light in the interval of Sturm lying between the two line images of a spherocylinder. The distance of the spot from the lens, $D_c = \dfrac{D_1 + D_2}{2}$ where D_1 and D_2 are the dioptral distances of the line images of the lens. The size of the spot $= 2\, y\dfrac{D_1 - D_2}{D_1 + D_2}$ where y equals the diameter of the lens aperture.

claw. That portion of a rimless strap which contacts the edge of the lens.

Colmascope®. A polariscope used to test strain in glass lenses, as the stress in air-tempered (case-hardened) glass lenses.

coma. A lens aberration so named because it changes the focus of a point object not on the lens axis into a pear shape somewhat like a comet. The length of the tail of the comet varies directly with the angle of the point source with the lens axis and with the square of the aperture. Increasing the depth of a meniscus lens reduces the aberration.

compound lens. A generic spherocylinder lens (+ on + or = on −) as distinct from a crossed-cylinder, contrageneric (− on + or + on −).

cone. One of the two types of nerve endings of the retina. In the macular area they are tightly bunched to produce maximum visual acuity. They are sensitive to color, much less sensitive to motion.

conjugate foci. A pair of object and image points which are interchangeable. Light diverging from either point focusses at the other.

conjugate movement. Movement of the two eyes in which the angle between the visual axes remains constant during fixation upon different points at the same distance in the field of vision.

constringence. Abbe number, ν value. The reciprocal of the dispersive power of an optical medium, $\nu = \dfrac{n_D - 1}{n_F - n_C}$ in which the indices of refraction refer to the C, D, and F Fraunhofer lines: C (orange), D (yellow), and F (dark blue). Originally this relationship was stated $\dfrac{n_F - n_C}{n_D - 1}$ which regularly produces a fraction ranging from approximately $1/33$ to $1/60$ for optical glasses. These were difficult to use in calculations and Abbe proposed the reciprocals be used, such as 33 to 60 as developed from the first formula above.

contact lens. A thin plastic shell, shaped like the front of the eyeball, which is held in position by the suction of a thin layer of tears. This lens is used to correct refractive errors including irregularly shaped cornea, as a cosmetic lens to change iris color, or to cover unsightly scars.

    corneal c. 1. A contact lens 7 to 10 mm in diameter that rests on the cornea only, not on the sclera as previously constructed.

control. An object in an orthoptic training target that is seen by only one eye. It is used as a perception test.

convergence. The movement of the eyes in which the internal recti turn the visual axes to intersect at some finite point.

    accommodative c. That portion of convergence reflexly stimulated by the act of accommodation.

    fusional c. That portion of convergence either positive (increasing the angle) or negative (decreasing the angle) to supplement accommodative convergence turning the visual axes precisely to the fixation point.

coquille. Blown glass plano lenses usually used for goggles, approximately 12.00D. curve; mi-coquille lenses have a curve of about 6.00D. Nowadays, lenses of this class are made by "dropping" (sagging) a flat lens with heat.

cornea. The transparent anterior portion of the scleral coat of the eye. The radius of curvature, about 8.00 mm, is less than the sclera. The power of the cornea is about 43.00D. (about 75% of the dioptric power of the eye).

corresponding points. Pairs of points on the two retinal surfaces which when stimulated give the percept of a binocularly seen object. These receptors have identical lines of direction; for this reason images stimulating either of them are interpreted as arising from the same point in space.

cross-cylinder. Spherocylinder lenses with sphere and cylinder of opposite signs and the cylinder twice the power of the sphere, thus producing a lens with a spherical equivalent of 0.00. Used in the subjective measurement of cylinder power and the location of the cylinder axis. Called Jackson cross-cylinder.

Crookes, Sir William (1832-1919). English physicist and chemist.

C. glass. An absorptive glass designed for ophthalmic use which absorbs ultraviolet and infrared radiation and in its lightest shade has slight effect upon visible light. The darkest shade absorbs more than 50 percent of visible light.

crystalline lens. The biconvex lens situated behind the iris of the eye. It is suspended from the ciliary body by a yoke of zonular fibers. By the force of the muscle fibers surrounding the lens its center thickness increases, its diameter decreases, and the anterior portion bulges forward. This increases its dioptric power to focus the eye upon objects near to the eye. This act is known as accommodation.

cullet. Waste glass remelted in a subsequent pot to promote fusion of the constituents and form a lining for the new pot.

cyclopean eye. An imaginary eye lying midway between the eyes which performs as the reference point for estimates of direction for binocular vision.

cyclophoria. A tendency for the eyes to rotate on the z-axis. When the top of the eye moves toward the nose it is called incyclophoria. When the rotation of the top is out toward the temple, the condition is named excyclophoria. Horizontal Maddox rods separated by about $6^{\triangle}$ to produce parallel lines is the means of testing.

cycloplegia. The ciliary muscle paralyzed by drug action. The function of accommodation halted by the paralysis. Drug: atropine and homatropine are the commonest cycloplegics.

cylinder bridge. A metal bridge for a spectacle mounting or frame. Cross section of the portion which rests upon the nose is the side of a cylinder; the bearing surface is convex. The width is usually 3 or 5 mm.

cylindrical lens. An ophthalmic lens having at least one of its surfaces cylindrical or toroidal. A lens used for the correction of astigmatism.

> **axis, c.** The only meridian of a cylindrical lens without focal power.

D-line. Fraunhofer line D (yellow); $\lambda = 5896$ Å.U.; D_2 line, $\lambda = 5890$. Syn. sodium lines.

datum line. A line at the midpoint and parallel to the horizontal tangents to the top and bottom of a lens. The 180-line. The x-axis of a lens through the geometric center of the lens.

decentration. The act of placing the optical axis of a lens in a different position than the geometric center of a spectacle lens. The unit of measurement of the displacement is Prism Diopters. Lens power in diopters times decentration in centimeters equals Prism Diopters.

density. The term applied to light absorbing ability of a filter. The formula is $D = \log (I_0/I)$ where I_0 is the intensity of the light in the object space and I is the transmitted light. D is always a whole number. It is the characteristic of the logarithm of the reciprocal of the fractional transmission of light. $1.00 = 0.10$ transmission, $2.00 = 0.01$ transmission, $3.00 = 0.001$ transmission.

depth of field. Distance that an object may be moved (along the axis of a lens or optical system) without creating blur circles larger than a tolerated amount.

depth of focus. The sum of the distances on either side of perfect focus that an object can be moved (along the axis of a lens or lens system) without creating blur circles larger than a tolerated amount.

depth perception. An experience in visual perception in which the comparative distances of objects are recognized. This synthesis of the slightly different images caused by the slightly different images from the parallactic angles are the foundation of the phenomenon. Geometrical perspective, overlapping contours, image size differences, and light and shade also contribute. Third-degree fusion.

deviation. Bending or turning in another direction. The deviation of visual axes in strabismus (squint), the deviation of a ray which is refracted at an interface.

dexter. Right side, e.g. oculus dexter (O.D.), right eye.

dextroversion. Version or turning to the right side.

didymium glass. An absorption glass containing the element didymium, which strongly absorbs light in the yellow portion of the visible spectrum.

diffraction. The small amount of light spreading into the umbra at an aperture. An occasion when light does not move in a straight line as postulated in geometrical optics.

diopter, dioptre, dioptry. Unit of focal power in ophthalmic optics. The reciprocal of the focal length of a lens or optical system expressed in meters. 1 meter focal length $= 1/1 = 1.00$D.; 0.50 meter focal length $= 1/0.2 = 2.00$ D.; 0.20 meter focal length $1/0.2 = 5.00$D.

diplopia. The condition in which images of a single object fall upon noncorresponding points of the two retinas and cause the perception of double vision.

Dispensometer®. An instrument to measure the pantoscopic angle of an eyeframe as worn and to determine the location of the upper end of the corridor of a progressive multifocal, the optical center and/or the top line of a bifocal or trifocal segment.

dispersion. The separation of light into its spectral constituents, such as white light separated by a prism into a continuous spectrum. All optical media have different indices of refraction for different spectral colors, hence dispersion of colors. The dispersion of optical media is measured by the differences of index for a portion of the whole spectrum usually N_f (blue) — N_c (red).

dispersive efficiency. See *constringence*.

dispersive power. The ratio of the difference of the dispersion of two colors (usually N_f and N_c) to the mean dispersion N_a: $= \dfrac{N_f - N_c}{N_d - 1}$ This is the reciprocal of the constringence.

distometer. A device to measure the distance from the corneal apex to the pole (vertex) of a lens, the vertex distance.

Donders, F.C. (1818-1889). Dutch ophthalmologist who stimulated the interest of medical doctors in the practice of refraction with his classical textbook.

Duane's table. An amplification of Donder's table in which the maximum, minimum, and average accommodative amplitudes for the life span are recorded.

ductions. Disjunctive movement of the eyes in the effort to sustain binocular vision when prism is introduced before either or both eyes. The breadth of fusion is measured by the amount of prism which can be overcome while binocular vision is sustained.

effective focus. The focus of a lens measured from the back vertex (vertex focus).

Eikonometer®. An eyepiece micrometer.

　ophthalmo-e. An instrument for the measurement of the difference in size and/or shape of ocular images. Used in the study of aniseikonia.

emmetropia. The state of an eye without refractive error in which visual acuity is at maximum for distant vision without accommodative effort.

endpiece. The extension attached to rimless lenses, metal frame eyewires, or plastic frame rims which contains the joint or hinge to which the temples are attached.

entrance-pupil. The opening (real or virtual) in an optical instrument through which all of the light rays of the object space pass.

Eonite®. A unique glass made by Schott Optical Glass Co. which, by the use of additional nitrates and other chemicals, gives ultra-strength when chemically tempered.

equivalent focal length. The focal length of a lens or system measured from the principal point of the related area.

equivalent lens. A geometrical optics concept of an infinitely thin lens having a focal length equal to the equivalent focal length of the lens or system. It is the core of thin-lens optics.

esophoria. Heterophoria in the horizontal meridian, latent over-acting convergence.

esotropia. Convergent strabismus. Crossed-eyes. Convergent squint.

exit pupil. The image of the aperture stop formed by the ocular lenses of the system. The image of a brilliant object in front of an optical system projected on a white surface. If its minimum diameter is larger than the pupil of the eye, all of the rays from the object do not reach the retina.

exophoria. Heterophoria in the horizontal meridian, latent underacting convergence, or divergence.

    physiological e. The insufficient amount of convergence concurrent with accommodation for near-point. It is obscured by fusion convergence.

exotropia. Divergent strabismus. Wall-eye.

extraocular muscles. The six muscles which cause movement of the eye: internal and external recti, superior and inferior recti, and the superior and inferior obliques.

eye. (1) the sense organ which contributes to the sense of vision. (2) Abbreviation for length of eyewire of metal or rim of a nonmetallic frame.

eyeframe. Generic for all prescription lens holders, that is frames, mountings, or eyeglasses. First used by Perc Westmore, motion picture make-up artist.

eyeglasses. Framed or rimless glasses held on the nose by spring pressure, pince-nez.

eyewear. Generic for all prescription spectacles or eyeglasses.

F-line. Fraunhofer line, $\lambda = 4861$ A.U. (blue). The short wavelength (N_f) used in measuring mean dispersion and also in calculating achromatic lenses.

f-number. Designation of photographic lens, relating the effective diameter of the aperture to the focal length of the lens. Example: f/4 means effective diameter of the lens is $\frac{1}{4}$ the focal length.

false-macula. The extramacular area of a squinting eye which is stimulated with the macula of the fixing eye and finally acquires some functional correspondence with it.

far-point. A point which is conjugate with the macula when accommodation is relaxed. In myopia it is less than infinity (6 meters). In hyperopia it is a virtual point behind the retina. Also P.R. *(punctum remotum).*

> **f. p. sphere.** The curved surface described by the far-point of an eye as it rotates.

field of vision. That portion of space before the eye in which objects are visible. These angular limits are conceded to average 60°, up 75° down, 60° in, and 100° out. The vertices of these angles are at the center of rotation of the eye.

Fieuzel glass. A yellowish green absorption lens which because of its iron content absorbs ultraviolet light.

fitting triangle. The imaginary triangle which has its apices at the tops of the ears and the point of contact on the bridge of the nose.

fixation axis. The line joining the point of fixation with the center of rotation of the eye.

Fizeau, Armand. (1819-1890) French physicist.

> **F. experiment.** Means of measuring (1849) the speed of light by the use of rapidly revolving mirrors.

flat-top. A type of multifocal in which the segment is flattened at the top.

flint glass. A glass with high refractive index containing lead.

fluorescein. A dye used in solution to inspect the fitting of contact lenses.

focus. A point through which rays of light converge or from which rays of light appear to diverge when entering or emerging from an optical system.

equivalent f. The point measured from the nearer principal plane toward which or from which rays of light really or virtually move.

Foucalt, J.B. (1819-1868). French physicist.

F. knife edge test. Test for measuring the focal length and precision of curvature of concave parabolic mirrors.

fovea. A small pit or fossa.

f. centralis. The depression in the macular area where visual acuity is the keenest. Syn. yellow spot.

Franklin, Benjamin (1706-1790). American scientist.

F. bifocal. The earliest form (1784) of a two-focus lens consisting of equal halves of distance and reading focus.

Fraunhofer, J. (1787-1826). German physicist.

F. lines. Dark absorption lines seen in a spectroscopic image of the solar spectrum, which are characteristic of chemical elements.

Fresnel, R.J. (1788-1827). French physicist and engineer.

F. formula. The criterion by which the amount of normal (perpendicularly incident) light is reflected at the interface of two different media $\dfrac{(N_2 - N_1)^2}{(N_2 + N_1)^2}$ where $N_1 =$ first medium and $N_2 =$ second medium. For air to crown glass $=$ about 4% per surface.

F. lens. A lens surface with concentric zones of small prisms which deviate parallel rays to a point focus like a convex lens.

F. prism. A surface composed of narrow prisms of identical deviation which give the effect of a single larger prism. When constructed of plastic, provides a tremendous weight advantage.

Ful-Vue® Trade name of a spectacle frame or mounting in which the temples are attached $15°$ to $30°$ above the datum line. Also a flat-top multifocal.

fusion. The function of merging simultaneous retinal images into a single perception.

breadth of f. The term applied to the limit of the amounts that convergence or divergence can be altered with Base In or Base Out prisms while single binocular vision is sustained.

Gallelei, Galleleo (1564-1642). Italian astronomer and physicist.

    G. telescope. A telescope with a convex objective lens and short focus concave eyelens. It produces an erect image with a small field of view, for example, opera glass, field glass.

gamma rays (γ rays). Rays emitted by radium, 6 ten-billionths to 30 billionths mm in wavelength.

Gauss, J.K.F. (1777-1855). German mathematician and physicist.

    G. theory. A method of tracing paraxial light rays through a series of centered optical surfaces in which the lens, mirror, and refracting surfaces are replaced by focal, principal, and nodal points and their corresponding planes. This system of "ray optics" made Gauss the "father of geometrical optics."

geometrical center. The point in a regular geometrical figure (circle) which is equidistant from all points on the circumference. In other than a round spectacle lens, the point is the intersection of the diagonals of the "box" tangent to the horizontal and vertical dimensions.

glass. The material used for most optical lenses and devices. It is an amorphous substance composed of fused silica (sand), lime, soda, and/or other elements to produce desired characteristics for special refractive purposes.

    tempered. Finished glass lenses or products which have been heated to almost the melting point, then quickly cooled by compressed air to form surfaces of strained glass surrounding the central portion. This procedure greatly increases the impact resistance of the glass. A similar and even more effective procedure of heating the glass in molten salts (potassium nitrate for crown glass), in which ion transfer accomplishes case-hardening.

glasses. Colloquial name for eyewear.

glaucoma. An eye disease caused by impaired drainage of aqueous humor which results in increased intraocular pressure.

Finally, the peripheral nerve fibers of the retina are atrophied, ending with blindness of central vision for total blindness. A treatment is a drug to reduce the pupil size and thus clear the chamber angle in the area of the canal of Schlemm.

gold. A precious metal used in the manufacture of spectacle frames. Fine gold is referred to as 24 carat. Lesser carat ratings denote the number of 1/24ths of fine gold and the remainder of alloys such as silver, copper, and nickel. Hence 12 parts fine gold, 12 parts alloy = 12 carat. In the U.S.A. the letter K. (karat) is used for metal. Standard gold-filled quality is 1/10 12K = 1/20 or 5 percent fine gold. Without plier marks which break through, it is remarkable how long this thin skin of gold will last in direct contact with the skin.

von Graefe, A. (1828-1879). German ophthalmologist.

> **G. test.** A method of detecting and measuring heterophoria by disassociating binocular vision with a vertical prism before one eye.

Gullstrand, A. (1862-1930). Swedish ophthalmologist.

> **G. schematic eye.** See *reduced eye*.

haploscope. A mirror-type stereoscope. The object carrying tubes are rotatable on the vertical axis to measure the direction of the z-axes of the eyes or depending upon fusion to train positive and/or negative fusional amplitude.

Helmholtz, H. von (1821-1894). German physiologist. Widely acknowledged as the inventor of the ophthalmoscope. Author of the classic *Physiological Optics*.

> **H. Base Line.** The line connecting the centers of rotation of the eyes. The length of the line is the visual axis separation or pupillary distance, and the x-axis of the prescription lenses is congruent with this line.

heterophoria. The tendency for one eye to turn from the fixation point.

heterotropia. The actual turning of one eye from the fixation point.

Hi-lite. A low density, high index glass made by Schott Optical Glass Co. which, unlike previous flint, contains titanium instead of lead.

Holmes, Oliver W. American poet, philosopher.

    H. stereoscope. A stereoscope in which the stereogram is placed at the focal distance of two convex lenses which have their centers separated by the distance of the centers of the pictures of the stereogram. See Figure 252.

horopter. The sum of the points seen singly while fixation remains at a single point.

Huygens, C. (1629-1695). Dutch physicist.

    H. construction. The graphical method of depicting the deviation of a ray of light at the interface of two dissimilar media.

hyperopia. An error of refraction in which the image conjugate with an object at infinity would not have focussed when it strikes the retina of an eye with relaxed accommodation. Additional plus dioptric power is needed to bring the image plane to the retina.

hyperphoria. Heterophoria in the vertical meridian in which there is a tendency for one eye to deviate upwards relative to the other.

hypertropia. An actual deviation of the z-axes in the vertical meridian.

hypophoria. Vertical heterophoria in which one eye tends to deviate downwards relative to the other. This can be differentiated from hyperphoria in the other eye only by evidence of paresis or paralysis of elevating muscles.

illiterate E. A letter or symbol repeated on a test chart in all four positions. The test is to indicate in which direction the legs of the letter are pointed.

image. A semblance of an object produced by refraction or reflection by a lens or mirror system. It is a real image if it is inverted and can be projected on a screen such as a camera ground glass. A virtual focus is erect and cannot be projected on a screen. It is viewed by looking toward the last lens surface of the system.

index of refraction. The ratio of the velocity of light in one medium to the velocity of light in the next medium. Also the ratio of the sines of the refracted and incident angles.

$$\text{index} = \frac{\text{V first medium}}{\text{V second medium}}$$

infinity (optical). A distance which is great as compared with the aperture or focal length of an optical system. Six meters (20 feet), the distance used for refraction, is over 1000 times the width of the pupil and about 400 times the focal length of the eye. At 6 meters the size of the pupil subtends an angle of less than 4 seconds at the first nodal point.

interocular distance. The distance between the centers of rotation. Helmholtz Base Line.

inverse square law. The means by which light intensity at two points from the source is measured.

iris. (1) A stop or aperture in an optical system whch limits the size of the beam of light passing through it; (2) the colored element of the uveal tract which lies in front of the crystalline lens. It regulates the quantity of light entering the globe of the eye. It has sphincter muscles which control the size of the aperture (pupil).

isobar. A line drawn on a diagram or plan which shows equal quantities or units. Used by Boeder to demonstrate prism power at extra-axial points in lenses.

isosceles. Having two equal sides, as an isosceles triangle.

Jackson, Edward (1856-1942). American ophthalmologist. Founder, *American Journal of Ophthalmology.*

    J. crossed-cylinder. Plus on minus lens with a spherical equivalent of zero used to refine cylinder power and/or axis.

Jaeger, E. (1818-1884). Austrian ophthalmologist.

    J. types. Ordinary type in graduated sizes from 6 to 36 point size used to test near vision.

keratitis. Inflammation of the cornea.

    herpetic k. Accompanying an attack of herpes zoster.

    interstitial k. An effect of congenital syphilis. It is recognized by the deposits in the interstices of the substantia propria of the cornea causing a diffused image which is not correctable with lenses.

keratoconus. Anomalous development of the cornea in which the cornea assumes a conoidal shape. Also known as conical cornea.

keratograph. A corneal reflection camera which uses an illuminated Placido Disc as an object, thereby measuring the corneal curvature and imperfections.

keratometer. An instrument used to measure the curvature of small areas of the cornea by reflected light.

keratoplasty. Plastic surgery of the cornea in which a section of a donor's clear cornea is grafted into an opaque cornea.

Kryptok bifocal. The first fused bifocal, patented by Borsch in 1904.

Kurova®. Trade name of a series of marginally corrected lenses.

laevo-version. Turning of the eyes to the left.

laminated glass. A safety glass like automobile windshields made with a layer of transparent cellulose nitrate or cellulose acetate between two sheets of glass. The plastic holds the fragments of glass in place in the event of breakage.

Landolt, E. (1846-1926). French ophthalmologist.

> **L. broken ring.** A test letter which for normal vision is a circle 5 minutes in diameter with a 1 minute wide ring at the periphery in which a 1 minute by 1 minute square is removed, creating a capital C. The position of the opening is in one of four directions.

lap. A metal tool used in the grinding and polishing of lens surfaces. Regular laps are cut for n = 1.530.

L.E. Abbreviation for left eye.

lead glass. Optical glass containing lead oxide. High-refraction index promotes its use for fused bifocal segments. Its high chromatic aberration (low ν-value) makes it objectionable. Syn. flint glass.

lens. A transparent medium bounded by two geometrically describable surfaces one of which shall be curved = this is, spherical, cylindrical, toroidal, or aspheric.

> **l. blank.** A slab of optical glass which has been molded or cut to a size and shape which is suitable for grinding and polishing into a lens.

l. cutter. A machine provided with a diamond or steel wheel to cut uncut lenses to the proper shape for edge-grinding.

l. measure. A two-legged spherometer with a dial that reads in diopters. It reads lens meridians. Therefore a cylinder is the difference in the reading of the minimum and maximum curvatures. These instruments have historically been made for $n = 1.530$.

lenscorometer. A micrometer to measure the lens-cornea (vertex) distance. Syn. *distometer.*

lensmeter. An electronic instrument composed of a laser and computer to give a digital reading and print-out of ophthalmic lens powers to 0.01D.

lensometer. An instrument conceived by Abbe to measure the dioptric power of a lens or system at the back vertex; American. Optical Co. trade name. Syn. focimeter, dioptrometer, vertometer®, vertex refractionometer.

lenticular. A strong lens which has a central area (usually 30 to 40 mm) ground to the prescription. The margin has a shallow curve to reduce weight and/or thickness.

Listing, J.B. (1808-1882). German physiologist.
L. plane. The plane through the center of rotation of the eye parallel to the focal plane. This plane is used for reference. It does not move.

loupe. A binocular magnifier in which the lens axes are inclined on the fixation axes or a magnifier which uses Base In prisms to relieve convergence along with the accommodation relieved by plus lenses.

lorgnette. A spectacle which is attached to a folding case that also serves as a handle to hold the lenses before the eyes.

macula. The point of clearest vision at the center of the retina.

Maddox, E.E. (1860-1933). English ophthalmologist, an authority on heterophoria and extraocular muscle function.
M. rod. A cylindrical glass rod (or series of them) approximately 20 mm long and 3 mm in diameter which images a spot of light as a streak at a right angle to the rod. This

is used to dissociate fusion and permit the measurement of heterophoria.

magnesium fluoride. Transparent mineral $n = 1.36$ which is sufficiently less than glass to serve as a film for the diminution of reflected rays.

magnification. The property of some optical lenses or systems of projecting a real inverted image of larger area than the object.

   virtual m. An object at the anterior focal plane of a convex lens is magnified to an amount $M = pD$, where $p =$ original position of object; $D =$ dioptric power of lens. Object set at 40 cm is viewed through a $+ 10.00D$. lens $M = .4 \times 10 = 4X$.

major reference point. That point on an uncut lens which satisfies all of the specified distance prescription requirements and is marked MRP.

medium. A substance that transmits light.

meniscus lens. A lens with a profile similar to a crescent, one surface convex, the other concave.

meridian. A lens plane perpendicular to the optical axis of a lens or optical system. A diameter of a round or oval lens.

meter angle. Angle at the center of rotation of a visual axis with fixation on the median line at one meter. The value varies directly with the interocular distance. Rule: M.A. = D. of accommodation $\times \dfrac{\text{I.O.D. in cm}}{2}$

mi-coquille. A blown plano lens. A section of a globe approximately 7 inches in diameter.

Micron. See *mu*.

minify. To reduce the apparent dimensions. The opposite of magnify.

minimum deviation. The deviation of a ray of light that passes through a prism perpendicular to the base-apex line, thus having identical angles of incidence and emergence.

miotic. A drug that constricts the pupil, such as eserine or pilocarpine.

monocular. Refers to only one eye. One side of a prism binocular.

mu: μ. Abbreviation for micron, .001 mm, meter^{-6}. Sometimes used to signify index of refraction: $\mu = 1.523$.

multifocal. A lens having more than one focal power in the United States. A lens having more than two focal powers in the United Kingdom.

mydriasis. Dilation of the pupil.

myopia. A refractive error in which the far point of the unaccommodated eye is at a finite distance before the eye. Short-sightedness, near-sightedness.

n. Usually the symbol for index of refraction, $n = 1.523$.

near-point. The closest point at which accommodation can be momentarily maintained. *Punctum Proximum.* (p.p)

near-vision point (N.V.P.). Term originated by Bugbee describing the point in a lens intersected by the z-axis in the act of reading. Usually about 8 mm down and 2 mm nasalward from the distance optical center of a lens.

Negative Relative Accommodation (N.R.A.). Term describing number of diopters accommodation can be relaxed with plus lenses without interrupting near-point fixation.

Negative Relative Convergence (N.R.C.). Term describing number of Prism Diopters Base In that can be tolerated while maintaining binocular single vision.

neutral filter. A light filter which dampens illumination by reducing the visible spectrum about equally, thereby causing no visible color changes.

Newton, Sir Isaac (1642-1727). English scientist.

N. rings. Interference rings which surround the point of contact of a convex surface with a flat surface or in the contact of two curved surfaces. Most easily seen in monochromatic light.

N. telescope. A reflection telescope used by astronometers.

nodal points. Two of the cardinal points of Gaussian geometric optics which coincide with the principal points when the first and last medium have the same refractive index. When an object ray is directed toward the first nodal point, it emerges without deviation into the image space from the second nodal point.

normal. The perpendicular to a surface at the point of incidence of a ray. It is the extension of a radius of a spherical surface at the point of incidence.

object. In optics, the identification of a point or area from which radiation (light) is emitted or reflected. This radiation can be formed into an image by an optical lens or system.

occluder. A device that excludes light from one or both eyes.

O.D. Abbreviation for *oculus dexter,* right eye.

one-piece bifocal. A bifocal invented by Connor which has two spherical surfaces on one side. Called solid bifocal in Europe.

ophthalmic. With reference to the eye and its functions.

ophthalmo-eikonometer. An instrument designed to measure the size and shape of ocular images in the diagnosis of aniseikonia.

ophthalmologist. A medical doctor who has had three or more years of graduate education in eye care. He diagnoses and treats eye diseases, does eye surgery, and prescribes lenses. Eye physician, oculist, ophthalmic surgeon.

ophthalmoscope. An instrument invented by Babbage and/or Helmholtz to illuminate and permit the viewing of the interior of the eye.

optic. Pertaining to light or the sense of sight.

optical axis. The line connecting the centers of curvature of a lens or system of lenses. The cardinal points lie on this line or its extensions. The anterior-posterior axis of the eye.

optical bench. A bar upon which are mounted slidably adjustable holders for lights, lenses, mirrors, and/or screens. It is used to make demonstrations and/or measurements of the optical functions of these parts.

optical center. A point on the lens axis midway between the nodal points.

optician. One skilled in the application of the science of optics, including optical lens and/or instrument designing or manufacturing.

    certified o. An optician certified by examination by the American Board of Opticianry.

    dispensing o. One who limits his activity to the filling of doctors' prescriptions including the manufacturing of eyewear and the fitting of it to doctors' patients.

Guild o. A dispensing optician who has no financial connection with doctors and who limits his activities to dispensing under the Code of Ethics of the Guild of Prescription Opticians.

Master o. An optician certified by a senior examination by the American Board of Opticianry.

optics. The portion of the science of physics which deals with light and the function of vision.

geometrical o. Deals with the tracing of rays of light through a lens or optical system.

physical o. Deals with the nature of light and its manifestation in diffraction, interference, polarization, reflection, and refraction.

physiological o. Deals with the investigation of the human eye as an optical device.

visual o. Deals with the image-forming system of the eye.

optometer. An instrument for the measurement of the refractive state of the eye.

objective o. One provided with an optical system which measures the vergence of light leaving the patient's eye. Examples: Gullstrand's refractionometer, Rodenstock refractionometer.

subjective o. One which is based upon an artificial far point created by a convex lens. One based upon the coalescence of two luminous spots.

Orthogon®. The trade name of a series of marginaly corrected ophthalmic lenses after the formulas of von Rohr modified by Rayton.

orthoptic training. A method of correcting defective vision such as strabismus or accommodative-convergence imbalance by stereoscopic and other ocular exercises.

O.S. *oculus sinister,* left eye.

O.U. *oculi uterque,* both eyes.

Panoptik®. The trade name of a series of fused flat-top multifocal lenses invented by Hammond and made by Bausch & Lomb.

pantoscopic angle. The angle of spectacle lenses when rotated on the Helmholtz base line to bring the lenses parallel to the inclination of the upper and lower rims of the orbit.

papilla. Head of the optic nerve.

parallax. The apparent displacement or change of position of an object when viewed from different places, such as the alternate use of the right and left eye.

paraxial. Close to the axis of an optical lens or system. Rays of the Gaussian system of geometrical optics. Close enough to the axis that the trigonometric functions of ray slopes are equal. Within 1° is usually considered a satisfactory approximation.

P.D. Abbreviation for interpupillary distance which has been confused by frame manufacturers referring to the total of the distance between lenses plus the "A" measurement of a "boxed" lens as the P.D. of a frame.

perimeter. An instrument used to measure the limits of the indirect field of vision.

phorometer. Trial frame equipped with Risley prisms, Maddox rods, and Stevens phorometer attached to a floor stand or wall bracket.

Phoroptor®. An instrument for determining the refractive errors and muscular balance of a pair of eyes.

Placido disc. A disc upon which equidistant concentric circles of black on white are presented. The center of the circle has an aperture bearing a convex lens. Light reflected from the disc upon the cornea makes a corneal reflection which indicates curvature irregularities such as irregular astigmatism, keratoconus, and/or corneal scars.

Polaroid®. A sheet of cellulose acetate containing crystals of an iodine compound which are all oriented in one direction. The plastic is sometimes laminated in glass. Light polarized by this material is used for stereoscopes, 3-D pictures and movies, glare-protecting lenses, and a test for strained glass including case-hardened glass.

pole. Either extremity of the lens axis at the point it intersects the lens surfaces, vertex.

Positive Relative Accommodation. The amount of accommodation measured in Diopters that can be stimulated while convergence remains fixed. The measurement is made by adding minus spheres binocularly to the point that vision begins to blur.

Positive Relative Convergence. The amount of convergence measured in Prism Diopters that can be stimulated while accommodation remains fixed. The measurement is made by adding Prism Base Out to the point that vision begins to blur.

presbyopia. Literally, the sight of old age. The condition of vision due to diminished accommodative amplitude which removes the near-point farther from the eye than is convenient for reading.

prism. An optical element bounded by two flat surfaces inclined toward one another. The edge at which they intersect is called the apex. The angle between the surfaces is termed apical angle.

  dissociating p. A prism with sufficient deviation to cause diplopia placed before an eye to provide the conditions to measure ocular imbalances.

pupil. An aperture or its image of a lens or an optical instrument. The aperture of an eye created by the opening of the iris of the eye.

radian. The unit of angular measurement generated at the center of a circle by an arc which is the length of the radius of the circle. $360° = 2\pi$ radians. 1 radian $= 57.29577°$.

ray. A straight line representing the direction of a ray or bundle of rays of light. An element of geometrical optics.

reduced distance. The actual distance divided by the index of refraction in which the distance is measured. In air, actual and reduced distances are equal, since n $= 1.00$.

reduced eye. The human eye simplified by Gullstrand by reducing the optical effects of the media to one lens with n $= 1.333$, radius of curvature 5.55 mm, focal length 60.00D., f $= 16.67$ mm, f′ $= 22.22$ mm. Also known as schematic eye.

refraction. The bending of a ray of light at the interface of two optical media of differing indices of refraction. The term used to describe the act of measuring an error of refraction of the eye.

refractive index. See index of refraction.

Refractor®. An instrument similar to Phoropter® invented by Doctors Aaron and Louis Green.

resolving power. The capability of an optical system to separate the images of two closely situated points in the object space.

retina. The innermost coat of the eyeball. It is composed of nerve endings which convert optical images into nerve impulses.

retinoscope. An instrument to objectively measure refractive error invented by Cuignet (1873), consisting of a mirror with an aperture through which the refractionist observes the reflection of light in the patient's pupil. The direction of the apparent movement of the illumination across the pupil indicates the refractive error.

>   **streak r.** A luminous retinoscope invented by Jack Copeland (1919) which projects a streak rather than a spot of light and, since the streak can be rotated, the astigmatic axis is located.

riding-bow. A spectacle bow or temple that extends to the lobe of the ear and is shaped to the crotch behind the ear.

Risley, S.D. (1845-1920). A Philadelphia ophthalmologist.

>   **R. prism.** A rotary prism which provides variable degrees of prism power by counter-rotating two plano prisms of equal power.

rods. One of the two principal nerve endings of the retina which are highly sensitive to low variations in illumination but relatively insensitive to color differences.

Scheiner, Christopher (1575-1650). Invented the optical means for the first optometer (1619).

schematic eye. See *reduced eye.*

sclera. The outer coat of the eyeball, a tough fibrous membrane.

scotoma. An impairment to vision caused by diminished or total lack of function of the retina in a limited area. It may be unnoticed (Mariotte's blind spot) or be seen as a black area in the visual field.

segment. That part of a multifocal which is used for finite distances, as reading.

Sheard, Charles, Ph.D. Physiologist. Designed and instituted the optometry course at Ohio State University. Edited the *American Journal of Physiological Optics*. Founded the American Board of Opticianry.

skull. A spectacle bow or temple that bends at the ear top and fits over the mastoid process.

slab-off. A method of creating a bicentric lens by grinding a prism-shaped slab from one surface of the lens, usually the convex surface.

Snellen, H. (1834-1908). Dutch ophthalmologist.

> **S. fraction.** A simple fraction used to record visual acuity. The numerator is the distance at which the test is given, the denominator is the smallest size of Snellen type seen at that distance. Although it is seldom so recorded, Snellen suggested that the type size be recorded in Roman numerals — 6/VI, 6/IX, 6/XII, 6/LX.

soulé. To cut off a portion of a lens, usually the lower nasal quadrant to give clearance for the side of the nose.

specified major reference point. The point on an edged prescription lens which meets all of the specification of the lens.

spectacle magnification. Increase in retinal image size induced by the placement, curvature, thickness, and dioptric power of prescription lenses. This magnification was reduced to simple formulas by E.D. Tillyer in research in aniseikonia at Dartmouth University.

spectacles. A pair of prescription lenses fitted to a frame or mounting to rest upon the nose and ear tops to correct a refractive error. Not a pair of eyeglasses which are supported by the nose only.

specular reflection. A reflection from a mirror surface.

sphere. A surface on which every point is equidistant from the center of curvature; a surface of revolution.

> **fixation s.** The spherical surface with its center at the center

of rotation and radius at the fixation point in primary position.

vertex s. The spherical surface with its center at the center of rotation and its radius of curvature the distance from the center of rotation to the posterovertex of the lens.

spherical aberration. Breach of a point image of a point object by rays refracted from the periphery of a surface to a shorter focal distance than paraxial rays.

spherical equivalent. The dioptric power of a cylindrical or spherocylindrical lens from the vertex to the plane of the circle of least confusion (the midpoint of the interval of Sturm). It is the spherical power of the lens plus half the cylindrical power.

spherocylinder. A lens with one spherical surface and one cylindrical (or toroidal surface).

standard notation. The method of denoting cylinder axis or prism base-apex axis, established in 1917 by the Technischer Ausschuss für Brillenoptik (T.A.B.O.) in which (from the patient's side) the horizontal axis 0–180° is the origin for angles measured clockwise beginning from the left side.

stereopsis. Third-degree fusion (Worth), in which objects in projected space are perceived at definite distances (relief).

strabismus. Anomalous fixation in which the nonfixing eye is turned in another direction, thus retinal images fall upon noncorresponding points. Heterotropia, squint, crossed-eyes, wall eyes.

temple. The shaft or bow of a pair of spectacles which gives support to the lenses.

Tillyer, Edgar D., D.Sc. (1881-1969). Physicist, lens designer, U. S. Bureau of Standards (1906-1914), charter member of Optical Society of America, director of Lens Research American Optical Co. Designed Tillyer marginally corrected lens series Nokrome bifocal, Ful-Vue multifocals, Giant ophthalmoscope, monocentric Ultex bifocal, Executive multifocals.

T. lenses. The first American-designed series of marginally corrected lenses. In their first form, special laps, templates, and master lenses were required. When Rayton presented a compromised series to use standard laps, Till-yer recalculated his series to be competitive.

torsion. Rotation of the eye on the fixation axis (z-axis).

trial frame. A spectacle frame into which trial lenses are placed during the refraction procedure.

trifocal. A lens with three focussing points, as distance, intermediate, and reading.

Tscherning, M. (1854-1939). Danish ophthalmologist.

T. ellipse. Graphs which determine the optimal F_2 curves of thin lens dioptric powers to produce the best form (marginally corrected) lenses.

u. Symbol commonly used in geometrical optics to denote the distance of the object from the vertex or first principle point (object distance).

ultex. A form of multifocal made by grinding two or more different spherical curves on one side of the lens. See *one-piece bifocal.*

ultraviolet radiation. Invisible radiation below visible violet from 4000 Å.U. to the beginning of x-rays at about 150 Å.U.

Ultravue®. American Optical's design of a progressive addition multifocal which has great promise. It has a wider reading area, thus moving the astigmatic zone farther from the center of the lens.

Univis®. Trade name of the first flat-top multifocal presented in the United States. The whole series comprises many designs.

uvea. The middle coat of the eye which consists of the choroid and extends to the ciliary body and iris.

v. Symbol commonly used in geometrical optics to denote the distance of the image from the back vertex or the second principal point (image distance).

Varilux II®. The most recent model of the Maintenez progressive addition multifocal is a vast improvement over previous models as is demonstrated by its acceptance. The makers have conducted lens fitting courses which assure better handling of the lenses.

vertex. The point on a lens or mirror surface intersected by the lens or mirror axis. In ophthalmic lenses, originally related by von Rohr to the back surface.

front v. The point from which the neutralizing or front focus of a lens is measured.

v. distance. The distance from the back vertex of a lens to the apex of the cornea.

v. power. The dioptric power of a lens measured from the back vertex. Reciprocal of v. focal length in meters.

v. sphere. The spherical surface with its center at the center of rotation and radius of curvature the distance from the center of rotation to the posterior vertex of the lens.

Vertometer.® Abbe focimeter, trade name of Bausch & Lomb, Inc., for same.

visible spectrum. That portion of the radiant energy spectrum extending from 3800 to 7000 Å.U. producing the sensation of colors from violet to red.

vista. The field of view of a spectacle lens.

visual. Pertaining to the eye and ocular perception.

v. acuity. Resolving power of the eye compared with a standard.

v. axis. The imaginary line joining the fovea centralis through the nodal points with the point of fixation in the object space.

v. field. The area in space in which radiant objects stimulate the retina. The boundaries of this area of a normal eye are the brow line, the nose, the cheeks, and (on the temporal side) the limit of retinal sensitivity of the nasal portion of the retina.

vitreous humor. The transparent gel filling the space between the crystalline lens and the retina. It is contained in a hyaloid membrane which is attached to the retina in the area of papilla.

von Graefe. See *Graefe.*

von Rohr. See *Rohr.*

Widesite®. Trade name of a series of marginally corrected lenses.

Worth, Claude (1869-1936). English ophthalmologist who concentrated upon heterophoria and strabismus.

W. ambyloscope. A hand-held haploscope with convex lenses on the ocular end to view translucent slides on the distant ends of the tubes. Convergence or divergence is stimulated by the angle at which the tubes are placed.

x-axis. For a prescription lens, (it is the horizontal, datum, or 180° line of the lens. For a pair of spectacle lenses, it is the line connecting the centers of rotation of the eyes, the Helmholtz base line.

xylonite. See *zylonite*.

y-axis. For a prescription lens, it is the vertical line perpendicular to the x-axis through the optical center of the lens. For a pair of spectacle lenses, it is the line perpendicular to the x-axis at the midpoint of the line connecting the optical centers of the lenses of the spectacles.

Young, Thomas (1773-1829). English scientist, called "father of physiological optics." Discoverer of astigmatism.

    Y. construction. A method of ray tracing through refracting surfaces using arcs scaled to the refractive indices.

z-axis. It is the optical axis of a lens and is perpendicular to the x-axis and y-axis. For a pair of lenses, it is an imaginary line midway between the z-axes of the lenses. It is directed toward the mean cyclopean center.

zonule of Zinn. Suspensory ligament of fibers extending from the ciliary body to the equator of the crystalline lens.

zylonite. Nitrocellulose, celluloid, the thermoplastic material formerly used for eyeframes which has been replaced by cellulose acetate. This is also referred to as zyl or zylo.

INDEX